THE HORMONE SOLUTION

THE HORMONE SOLUTION

STAY YOUNGER LONGER

WITH NATURAL HORMONE
AND NUTRITION THERAPIES

THIERRY HERTOGHE, M.D.

with JULES-JACQUES NABET, M.D.

FOREWORD BY DR. BARRY SEARS

THREE RIVERS PRESS • NEW YORK

Published in the United States by Three Rivers Press, an imprint of the
Crown Publishing Group, a division of Random House, Inc., New York.
www.crownpublishing.com

THREE RIVERS PRESS and the Tugboat design are registered
trademarks of Random House, Inc.

Originally published in hardcover by Harmony Books, an imprint of the
Crown Publishing Group, a division of Random House, Inc., New York,
in 2002.

Printed in the United States of America

Design by Barbara Balch

Library of Congress Cataloging-in-Publication Data
Hertoghe, Thierry.
   The hormone solution : stay younger longer with natural hormone
and nutrition therapies / Thierry Hertoghe ; with Jules-Jacques
Nabet ; foreword by Barry Sears.—1st ed.
      p.   cm.
Includes bibliographical references and index.
   1. Hormone therapy—Popular works.
      [DNLM: 1. Hormones—therapeutic use—Popular Works.
2. Aging—physiology—Popular Works. 3. Diet Therapy—Popular
Works. 4. Nutrition—Popular Works. WK 190 H574h 2002]
I. Nabet, Jules-Jacques. II. Title.
   RM286 .H47 2002
   615'.36—dc21   2002003147

ISBN 1-4000-8085-1

10 9 8 7 6 5

First Paperback Edition

To Drs. Eugene, Luc, and Jacques Hertoghe,
my predecessors who so brilliantly illuminated my way to the
world of hormone therapies—since the very beginning,
110 years ago.
To my family, so sweet to my heart:
to Claude, my love; to India and Jalla, our daughters; to my
mother, Marie; to my brother Eugene; and to my sisters,
Christine and Thérèse.
To all the pioneers and scientific researchers who have opened
up this modern medicine for the patients.

THIERRY HERTOGHE

To Helen, Paola, and David.

JULES-JACQUES NABET

AUTHOR'S NOTE

ACKNOWLEDGMENTS

We are indebted to the work of so many courageous pioneers and masters of medicine, especially Drs. Eugene, Luc, and Jacques Hertoghe, Walter Pierpaoli, William Regelson, Etienne-Emile Baulieu, Jonathan Wright, Bill Rea, Jens Möller, Georges Debled, Paul Ide, Barry Sears, Jacques Fradin, and William Crook, who have made this book possible through their wisdom and influence.

We want to acknowledge Jacques Hertoghe, Thierry's father, in particular, for his vast experience and competence in the field—and for sharing it so fully with Thierry.

We thank Drs. Ron Klatz, Bob Goldman, and Vincent Giampapa, pioneers in anti-aging medicine, for successfully opening up this field in modern society.

Also the contributions of close collaborators Drs. Thérèse Hertoghe, Walter Baisier, and Brigitte Riedelsheimer have been precious, as were and are those of Claudine, Helen De Winter, Dr. Edmond Devroey, and especially Marie Hertoghe, Thierry's mother, who provided tremendous assistance whenever needed.

CONTENTS

PART IV: THE HORMONE SOLUTION

Medicine is entering into a new era. In the coming century, health care will be increasingly based upon hormonal control. This is because hormones are orders of magnitude more powerful than drugs. More important, they can alter the expression of our genes. In essence, improved hormonal control brings us to the very core of human health.

I have had the pleasure of personally knowing Thierry for the past several years, which makes me even more in awe of his ability to diagnose hormonal disturbances in a wide variety of patients. As powerful as hormones are, it still requires the practiced eye to look for key signs that blood tests often fail to reveal. Thierry removes much of the mystery of hormonal interactions using very clear and concise language that is based on an unbroken lineage of four generations of endocrinologists in his family. Just as the great skills of craftsmen are often passed from one generation to the next, the intricate skills of astute observation of hormonal problems is likewise transmitted.

This is why this book is so valuable to both the physician and the layperson, since the skills of diagnosis are now accessible to all. For the physician, this means he will be better able to understand the complexities of chronic disease from a new hormonal perspective. For the layperson, they will understand the beginning signs that their hormonal communication patterns are becoming less efficient years before this inefficiency manifests into various chronic disease conditions. And for those with existing disease of unknown origin, this book may provide the insights as to the real basis of their condition.

To control your hormones is to control your life. This book will give you the tools to achieve that often elusive goal.

—Barry Sears, Ph.D.

PART I

HORMONES

CHAPTER ONE

WHAT HORMONES
MEAN TO YOU

Your body contains more than one hundred different types of hormones, and they pour into your bloodstream at the rate of thousands of billions of units per day. Hormones regulate your heartbeat and your breathing. Hormones make men men and women women. Hormones put you to sleep at night and wake you up in the morning. They control your blood pressure. They build bone, maintain muscle tone, and lubricate joints. Hormones govern growth. They make the body produce energy and heat. Hormones burn fat. Hormones govern the menstrual cycle and allow pregnancy (and birth) to occur. They fight stress, prevent fatigue, calm anxiety, and relieve depression. Hormones make and keep memories. Hormones maintain the correct level of sugar in the blood and tissues. They resist allergic reactions and infections. They soothe pain. Hormones control your sex drive, virility, and fertility. They stimulate your brain and your immune system.

It is by no means an exaggeration to say that hormones are crucial to every single function of the human body. You can't live without them.

But in the environment we live in at the opening of this new millennium—and particularly as we ourselves age—rarely do our bodies have the optimum levels of hormones. So we don't enjoy optimum health, whether that means arthritis or heart disease or flagging sex drive or gray hair and wrinkles or out-of-control weight gain. The program in this book, a combination of nutrition and hormone balance, can bring anyone into optimal health. The Hormone Solution is not a miracle cure or an empty promise. It is a reality. It is for anyone who feels tired all the time. Or forgets things. Or isn't sleeping well. Or feels more

MOST HORMONE LEVELS DECLINE WITH AGE

Nighttime Level of Melatonin in Blood

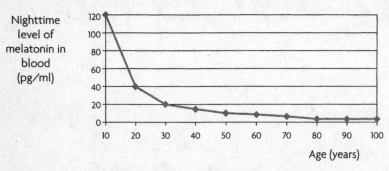

The level of melatonin at night declines with age.

Nighttime Level of Growth Hormone in Blood

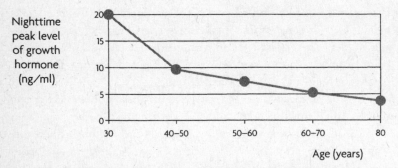

The nighttime growth hormone peak declines with age in men. At ages
70–80, about 50 percent of subjects have no significant serum GH
around the clock.

MOST HORMONE LEVELS DECLINE WITH AGE
(continued)

Level of TSH in Blood

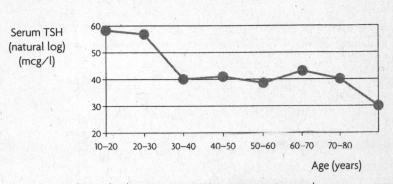

Relationship between serum TSH concentrations and age in 202 patients with hypothyroidism (thyroid gland deficiency).

Level of Thyroid Hormones in Blood

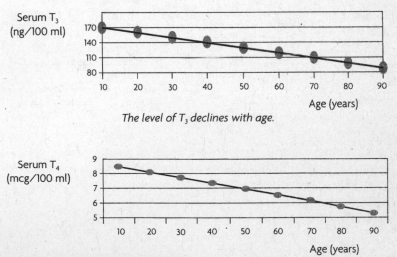

The level of T_3 declines with age.

The level of T_4 declines with age.

MOST HORMONE LEVELS DECLINE WITH AGE
(continued)

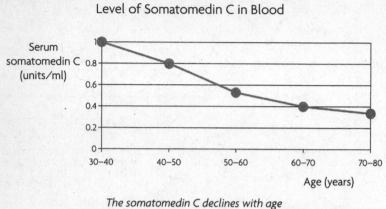

The somatomedin C declines with age
in blood of adults.

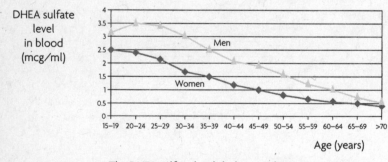

The DHEA sulfate level declines with age
in men and women.

MOST HORMONE LEVELS DECLINE WITH AGE
(continued)

Excretion of the Metabolites of Cortisol in Urine

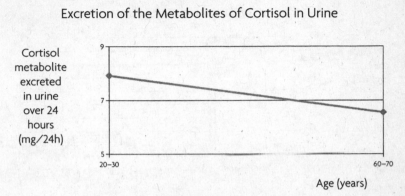

The level of the metabolites of cortisol excreted in the urine in 24 hours declines with age.

Level of Aldosterone in Urine

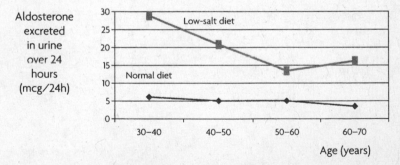

The excretion of aldosterone in the urine declines with age. This decline is amplified in low-salt diets.

MOST HORMONE LEVELS DECLINE WITH AGE
(continued)

Level of Estradiol in Blood of Women

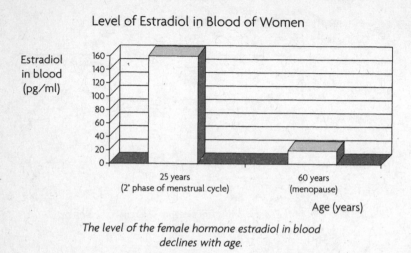

The level of the female hormone estradiol in blood
declines with age.

Testosterone Level in Women

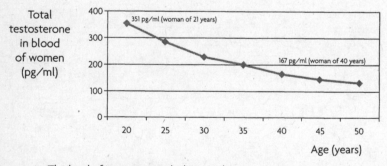

The level of testosterone declines with age in women. At 40 years
it is already less than half the level at 21 years.

MOST HORMONE LEVELS DECLINE WITH AGE
(continued)

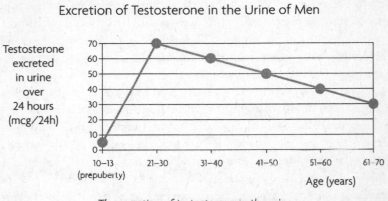

Excretion of Testosterone in the Urine of Men

Testosterone excreted in urine over 24 hours (mcg/24h)

Age (years)

The secretion of testosterone in the urine declines with age in men from 30 years on.

depressed and anxious than he used to. Or who is at risk for osteoporosis or cancer—among many, many other things. We've accepted these things as inevitable, especially as we age. We didn't like it, but we thought we had to live with it. *But we've been wrong.*

You probably know that some hormone levels decline with age. What's less well known is that almost *all* hormone levels drop, across the board, in men as well as women. Your endocrine glands cannot maintain the same production of hormones they did in your younger days. And that loss is the most crucial—and eminently correctable—underlying process that causes the signs and symptoms of aging as well as a host of other health concerns. With the proper physiological doses of natural hormones in combination with a hormonally supportive diet and vitamin and mineral supplements, you can retain your health—and your youth—more fully and for a longer time. I am *not* recommending the massive pharmaceutical quantities of the standard hormone prescriptions, like menopausal hormone replacement therapy (HRT), but rather the finely tuned individualized substances that are identical in structure and quantity to what young, healthy bodies produce.

When all our hormones are at optimal levels, our bodies are healthy, efficient, resilient, flexible, and strong. Through our twenties, that's what most of us experience. But even a small drop-off or slight imbalance, as happens to most of us by our thirties and forties, can create havoc. And not just for women! I was hit with the effects in my mid-thirties. I was gaining weight and overeating, and I often felt sleepy during the day. I had trouble concentrating, little energy, and stiffness in my joints. I was often cranky and supersensitive to stress. It got to the point where it was interfering with my work and my relationships and family life. And even though I was experienced in nutrition, hormones, and longevity, I felt indignant: I was much too young to be old!

Fortunately for me, with my medical training—and the wisdom passed down to me through three previous generations of hormone specialists in my family—I knew what to do. I understood that my hormones were shifting, and while growing older might be unavoidable, the negative consequences were strictly optional. With this book I intend to share with you the holistic health program I developed for myself and my patients of natural hormone therapy combined with specific diet and supplement regimens.

WHAT TO EXPECT

*T*his chapter gives an overview of how hormones work in the body and when and why they don't do their jobs. I'll tell you a little about how I came to practice in this field and how my philosophy of practice developed. We'll look at a few examples of how my patients have benefited from a program like the one in this book—and how I myself have responded to it. We'll talk about how hormone levels inevitably decrease with age, how that affects us, and what can be done about it. Finally, I'll discuss (and debunk) the fears a lot of people have about using hormones, before going on to give you a road map to the rest of the book.

TUNING UP YOUR HORMONES

*E*ach of the many hormones in the human body has its own job to do, but they all work together in an elaborately interwoven system. You can liken this exquisite synergy to an orchestra: Each instrument has its own melody or rhythm, but all are necessary to play a symphony.

Similarly, without balanced nutrition the body cannot make all the hormones it needs in the proportions it needs them. The first thing you need to do is to provide your body with the nutrients it needs to take

THE MAJOR HORMONE GLANDS AND HORMONES

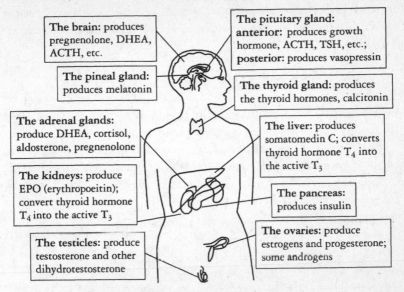

The brain: produces pregnenolone, DHEA, ACTH, etc.

The pineal gland: produces melatonin

The pituitary gland: anterior: produces growth hormone, ACTH, TSH, etc.; **posterior:** produces vasopressin

The thyroid gland: produces the thyroid hormones, calcitonin

The adrenal glands: produce DHEA, cortisol, aldosterone, pregnenolone

The liver: produces somatomedin C; converts thyroid hormone T_4 into the active T_3

The kidneys: produce EPO (erythropoeitin); convert thyroid hormone T_4 into the active T_3

The pancreas: produces insulin

The testicles: produce testosterone and other dihydrotestosterone

The ovaries: produce estrogens and progesterone; some androgens

care of itself. Much of our food is so refined and processed, we can run into problems even when we think we're eating healthfully. My eating plan and suggested supplements offer a delicious and nutrient-dense program, with surprising modifications for particular problems.

But no matter how healthfully we eat, our bodies produce less and less of all hormones as we age. Our hormonal balance becomes mistimed, disproportionate, or slightly off-key. In isolated cases, we recognize this and try to compensate—with HRT at menopause, for example. But we're missing the forest for the trees. Rarely are the problem and solution found in one hormone alone. In fact, taking just one hormone can make the problem worse or cause new problems. Furthermore, most hormone prescriptions written today are for doses that are far too large, and they overwhelm rather than rebalance the system. Most are also synthetic versions that differ by a molecule or two from the chemicals the body makes and uses on its own. This might not sound so bad until you consider that the difference between testosterone and estrogen—some would say, the difference between a man and a woman—is also a matter of just a couple of atoms.

But with natural hormones in amounts as close as possible to what your younger body made for itself, you can re-create the same state of health and well-being you once enjoyed. I'll teach you the methods that have worked for me and for my thousands of patients. You'll find that when your hormones are balanced, perfectly in tune, and backed with strong nutritional support, you can look and feel vibrantly healthy at any age.

HORMONES IN MY BLOOD

*T*hat's just the kind of happy ending that lured me into medicine. But as for my chosen area of specialization, I've got the hormones in my blood to thank. As a fourth-generation physician experienced with hormone treatments whose father, grandfather, and great-grandfather talked about hormones, health, and aging at the dinner table, I learned the secrets of good health and longer life well before I even hit adulthood.

Still, I wasn't entirely sold on the idea of being a doctor and started medical school without much enthusiasm. I found the studies interesting enough but not inspiring. As I began working in the hospital—in my chosen field, psychiatry—I could not escape the feeling I was working with the wrong medicine. In many of the psychiatric patients, all I could see was signs of hormonal deficiencies. They were as clear as day to me but obviously had been overlooked by many medical professionals as the patient wound his way through the system before ending up with me.

Endocrinologists, the doctors "officially" in charge of hormones, seemed mostly to specialize in diabetes, only occasionally venturing into other therapies. Most of them were very traditional and spent their time on disease treatment rather than prevention. The specialization and sub-specialization of medicine today has left a lot of doctors with so narrow a focus that they miss even big flashing neon signs if they are outside of their area of expertise. I prefer to follow in my grandfathers' footsteps. The medicine I knew from my father and grandfathers was more holistic (not alternative, but truly holistic, meaning concerned with the whole person), more complete, and aimed primarily at achieving and maintaining total health.

I saw more of this kind of potential in family-practice medicine. There was room there, at least among some of my colleagues, for considering not just powerful drugs, but also nutrition (food, vitamins, and trace elements), environmental health, lifestyle choices, and even psychology when thinking about how to treat a patient.

So I finally switched over to general medicine, and the success I had with a surprising number of endocrinological cases finally lit a fire under me. Like Nicole, who was forty-nine and losing her hair. She'd also gotten flabby muscles and dry skin, felt tired and stress-sensitive all the time, and had bouts of nervousness, depression, and upset stomach—none of which had bothered her until she was closing in on fifty. We got her hormones balanced with natural estrogen, progesterone, cortisol, and DHEA (dehydroepiandrosterone), and a diet to support them, and she felt and looked better within two months. Her hair even stopped falling out—and grew back.

Or like Ken, about the same age as Nicole, who was losing his memory. He had poor concentration and muddled thinking. On top of that, he complained he was getting old—thinning hair, small wrinkles all over his face, a growing potbelly, loss of strength, back pain, and decreased sex drive and potency. But with growth hormone, testosterone (like half of men over fifty, though he had "normal" levels, much of the testosterone in his body was bound to excessively high levels of proteins in the blood that made it unavailable for regular use), thyroid hormone, DHEA, and cortisol—in natural forms and proper balance—along with vitamin and mineral supplements, Ken was soon bragging he felt like he'd gone back in time about fifteen years.

And like Wally, who I don't think would be alive today—or at least not leading a full, active life—if not for the thyroid hormone, growth hormone, testosterone, and cortisol he started taking. He had already survived two heart attacks and one triple bypass surgery by the time I met him. But his cholesterol remained stubbornly high no matter what he did, and depression and constant exhaustion were draining the life out of him. His body was prematurely old, with weakened muscles, low sex drive, thickening skin, weight gain around his belly, and a noticeable layer of fat under his skin. His surgeon and cardiologist were worried that even the surgery wouldn't protect his stressed heart for long. But once we got the full complement of hormones in him, with carefully adjusted small doses, he felt stronger and better than he had in years. And ten years later Wally was still alive and well and no longer convinced he'd meet his father's fate: death by heart attack before his son graduated from college.

Through cases like these, I discovered that I could help people understand what their bodies were telling them in order to zero in on the most appropriate treatment, and that gave me the sense of mission

I'd been missing. I realized it was a *gift,* not a burden, handed down to me through four generations.

The gift my great-grandfather, grandfather, and father gave to me was a truly holistic approach—treating the whole patient—and an understanding of the paramount importance of clinical symptoms. Every hormonal deficiency has a telltale group of physical and mental effects, and a careful history and physical will give you all the clues you need, *if* you know how to read them.

The final key came directly from my father, who recognized that particularly difficult cases were simply cases of deficiencies in not one but *many* hormones—what he called multiple deficiency syndrome. He discovered that filling in all the lacking hormones (as well as the nutrients that support them) could resolve seemingly intractable problems and even reverse the "inevitable" signs of age. There is no one miracle hormone for everyone. Each person needs different hormones, and always in combination, usually three to six at a time—rarely solo. Most of us could benefit from natural low-dose hormones, individually adapted and judiciously balanced, by the time we are thirty-five.

As my own practice developed, I saw that men's as well as women's hormones shift with age and that women's hormonal shifts start well before menopause (potentially accounting for many poorly understood clusters of symptoms). Furthermore, since women's bodies make small amounts of "male" hormones, they can have deficiencies of them, just as men can. All the rest of the many hormones in the body could become deficient as well and be equally problematic—and equally correctable.

To answer my many questions, I sought out the top experts in each hormone and pressed them on both the scientific mechanisms of action and practical applications. I learned at least as much by looking back at the way things were done in my grandfathers' time, when medicine was, by necessity, focused on clinical symptoms rather than lab values. Often all doctors had to go on at that time was what they could observe clinically, so they were extremely careful observers. I still believe that the interaction between doctor and patient is what is most useful in revealing the truly necessary information, and that while cold statistical values can be helpful confirmation of a clinically based hypothesis, they are limited in what they actually show. I'm glad to be practicing with all the resources of high-tech medicine available to me, but we can't afford to let the wisdom of the old school—a sort of high-*touch* medicine— get lost.

No matter how the problem gets diagnosed, however, the solution always follows the same pattern: the right hormones, in the right combination, at the right doses, with the right nutrients.

MY HORMONE PROFILE

I developed tools like these in pursuit of my own hormonal balance as well as for my patients. Since I'm forty-five, my glands aren't doing it on their own anymore. I started taking thyroid hormones to correct hypothyroidism when I was very young, thanks to my father. (This disease typically goes undetected in young people, and especially in young men.) I also take cortisol, DHEA, testosterone, melatonin, and growth hormone on a daily basis—and have for years. I depend on these supplements to maintain my mood, energy, and physical fitness. Of course, I also follow the basic principles of a healthful diet and use a handful of vitamin and mineral supplements to support the hormonal balance I'm after.

I started taking thyroid supplements as a child. As an adult I switched from a diet heavy in dairy products and meat to a diet moderate in protein and rich in fruit, and I was soon able to reduce the dose of thyroid hormone I took by two-thirds. I still do need the supplement, however; when I don't take it, I'm tired and stiff and cranky in the morning, and I don't think clearly.

Without supplemental cortisol, I have powerful sugar cravings. I need to eat absolutely anything put in front of me. I could put away an entire box of chocolates in one sitting. Maybe worse, I could eat all day long. You make more cortisol when you eat, so overeating was my body's way of getting the hormone balance I needed.

Without enough cortisol, I also feel drowsy and can't concentrate. Every stress feels like too much to handle. (Too much cortisol, on the other hand, leads to an unhealthy feeling of euphoria, so it's important to be vigilant about the doses.) I'm getting a cosmetic benefit from cortisol as well. On my father's side of the family, everyone's face thins out unattractively with age—a classic sign of insufficient cortisol. Thanks to my cortisol supplements, I've avoided that particular family trait.

Growth hormone is the supplement I'd be least willing to give up for any reason. I started taking it seven or eight years ago for reasons of vanity: I was starting to get jowly. Taking growth hormone stopped and reversed that process, but I found I also reaped other amazing benefits.

I'm now able to work more and sleep less, without any negative side effects. I'm cool, calm, and cordial even in the midst of heated conflict. I'm less anxious and more decisive. When half my house burned down—only days before a huge conference presentation—everyone thought I would lose it. But I was able to keep going, deal with the fire, comfort my wife, and deliver my speech without a hitch. Thanks to the growth hormone.

I started taking 0.35 mg daily of natural growth hormone in my thirties. As often happens, the supplement rejuvenated my own pituitary gland and I started to secrete more of the hormone. When my hands and feet started to swell slightly, I knew I had to cut back. Now I use 0.02 IU a day, which gives me all the benefits with no side effects. Unbelievable as it might seem, growth hormone is usually prescribed at *forty times* my current dose, though the young adult body normally only makes between 0.2 and 0.5 mg a day. To make matters worse, growth hormone is often prescribed on its own rather than in balanced combination with other hormones—the way I recommend it.

BALANCE IS EVERYTHING

Of course not everyone needs as many hormone supplements as I do. I have quite a few deficiencies, and given the pace of my life, I also need higher levels of some hormones than the average man my age. But there are usually at least three hormones involved in regaining anyone's natural balance. Standard hormone therapy is often ineffective or plagued by unpleasant side effects because only one or occasionally two hormones are given, and given without regard to context—which only serves to create further imbalance in the system as a whole.

Whether I'm treating myself or my patients, I always prescribe the smallest effective doses, in a plan carefully customized to the individual. Random or recreational pill-popping is never an option. Hormones are powerful medicine—which is why their appropriate use can improve your life so dramatically—and are not to be taken irresponsibly.

To create the right hormonal balance for your own body, fine-tuning and readjustment must be an ongoing process. I always encourage my patients to become aware of the signals and messages carried in their bodies. As you learn how to listen to your own biochemistry, you'll sense when doses need to be increased or decreased depending on circumstances on a particular day or season. For example, you might need more thyroid hormone when it's cold and less in warm weather. You might need increased doses of certain hormones, such as growth hormone and cortisol, in times of extreme stress. Or you might need to use a particular hormone only occasionally, the way I use aldosterone only when I have to sit or stand for a long time (to combat the negative effects of low blood pressure).

I am not recommending self-medication. I am, however, strongly suggesting that everyone can become more aware of his unique hormonal profile. Your body usually tells the truth. Listen carefully to what it is saying. But you must always talk to your doctor before making any changes in medication.

The delicate dance of hormones throughout your body is exquisitely designed to keep you in optimal health. But as you add more candles on your birthday cake, you need to give that system some active support to keep reaping all the benefits. The unique blend of low-dose natural hormones and nutritional balance I'll explain in this book restores your birthright: a strong, healthy, attractive body and a clear, quick, and powerful mind for nearly all of your life.

This book explores the entire spectrum of human hormones and their properties symptom by symptom. More important, it provides specific natural hormone and nutritional prescriptions proven to erase the negative signs of aging by balancing your unique hormonal profile.

SETTING LIFE IN MOTION

*T*he word *hormone* comes from the Greek, meaning "to set in motion." Hormones are made in the endocrine glands, then flow into the bloodstream and are carried to every part of the body to produce their varied effects. Some, like the thyroid hormones, act on practically every cell of the body. Others act in a more focused manner on just one or two organs, like aldosterone, which works in your kidneys to retain water and salt in your body, thereby maintaining blood pressure.

Hormones direct and coordinate the body's cells to ensure their proper functioning. From the blood they penetrate deeply into the cells, usually acting on the genes in the nucleus, unlocking a portion of the genetic code, accessing the information the cells need to do their jobs (including making hormones). With hormonal deficiencies, the cells simply won't—can't—function as well. Total absence brings total disorganization. To take just one example, the complete absence of thyroid hormones would turn a human being into an unconscious organism, incapable of forming the simplest thought or feeling the most basic emotion. In a sense, we wouldn't even be human without hormones.

TEAMWORK

When it comes to hormones, the brain acts more or less as project manager. The brain influences the production of hormones by most endocrine glands through two other small but powerful glands—the pituitary gland and the pineal gland—though the effects are not direct, but rather the result of chain reactions. Hormones secreted by other peripheral glands influence (usually by slowing down) the secretion of hormones by the pituitary and pineal, forming a system of checks and balances to make sure the body gets enough of what it needs, but not too much. In addition, one hormone might stimulate, or sometimes inhibit, the effect of another hormone on target cells.

Hormones are interactive, mutually pumping each other up or slowing each other down. If just one is missing or insufficient, many others will no longer act with the same effectiveness and the health of the body suffers. On the other hand, with a harmonious balance of levels the body functions properly and good health prevails. The effects of the various hormones are synergistic; combining them is a case of the whole being greater than the sum of the parts.

The complexity of all these systems accounts for the importance of proper dosage and multihormone balance when using supplemental hormones.

AGING

For years we enjoy hormonal abundance. But then, gradually, we all experience some degree of glandular deterioration and so some decrease in hormone secretion. Toxins from an ever more polluted environment accumulate in the glands and damage them. Additionally, our blood vessels—which carry the blood, which carries the hormones—get worn out or collapse over time, and blood circulation toward organs and endocrine glands gets more and more difficult. Oxygen and nutrients (and hormones!) end up arriving drop by drop rather than in a steady stream. Poor diet aggravates the situation, weakening the glands by depriving them of what they need to maintain themselves and what they need to create hormones. Repeated exposure to microbes, bacteria, viruses, parasites, and fungi destroys glandular tissue and function, either suddenly or gradually, depending on the situation.

But the major cause of low hormone production with age is the inevitable aging of the glands themselves. They simply get used up and worn out. They can no longer replace their own dead cells, and waste products build up and get concentrated in the remaining cells, which slows down their activity and reduces their effectiveness.

Deficiencies appear progressively, though the signs are not always noted or understood. They might become obvious only late in life, though by then there might already have been irreparable damage. That's why I advocate a proactive, preventive stance.

Most fifty-somethings have hormones that have tapered off to insufficient levels far below the ones they enjoyed in their twenties and into their thirties. No one with a normal life span will escape hormonal deficiencies without hormone replacement. In fact, most of us would benefit from it starting in our mid-thirties. Each person is unique, with an optimal hormonal and nutritional state all his own. If I ran the world, I'd have people get a baseline assessment of their hormonal and nutritional status when they are young and in optimal health, between eighteen and twenty-three for women and between twenty-one and twenty-five for men. At that age, people rarely show large deficiencies, and the hormonal levels can be considered (for that particular person) optimal. That would give us a target as to what is to be maintained through later hormonal supplementation as it becomes necessary.

From this good start, hormonal levels could be regularly monitored. If they were, we'd see the subtle shifts starting somewhere in the mid-twenties to mid-thirties, ahead of the signs becoming visible (at least to the perceptive observer), generally between forty and fifty years old. Under this plan, most people would probably start using supplemental hormones somewhere between thirty and forty-five years of age.

Of course, some people need to be treated with hormones at much younger ages—even from birth, in some cases—though they are clearly the exception. I believe the rest of us should do everything we can to optimize our hormonal levels through diet, supplements, and natural hormonal treatments from as young as possible.

Besides simply growing older, difficult periods in anyone's life can increase his need for vitamins, minerals, and/or hormones. Any long-term stress increases hormone consumption while decreasing production. Malnutrition, to take just one kind of long-term stress (as in anorexia, for example), causes a drop in hormone levels. The same goes for overeating, immoderate consumption of alcohol, smoking, drug use, infections and illnesses, exposure to pollution, and intense athletic training. All of these stress and strain the body, ultimately weakening it and wearing it out and influencing the pace at which it needs supplemental hormones.

BAD REASONS NOT TO USE HORMONE THERAPY

Hormones have been saddled with a somewhat scary public image. The big bogey monster is the threat of cancer. This is a myth that dies hard. I'm betting the widely known fact that estrogen, used alone, has been proven to increase the risk of endometrial and uterine cancer is to blame. But that is why estrogen must always be counterbalanced by progesterone—and when it is, the increased cancer risk disappears. Many studies have investigated the link between hormone use at menopause and breast cancer, but despite extensive trials, no definitive answer has emerged. In studies where the risk appears to increase with the use of hormones (and by no means do all studies indicate that), the risk is small and, in the vast majority of cases, outweighed by benefits.

What the estrogen example really demonstrates is the perils of single-hormone replacement. Hormones are not solo acts in the body, so using only one is often a direct route to new or worsened problems. It is also an object lesson in the dangers of large doses (like those most routinely used in contemporary medicine) and synthetic copies of actual hormones.

Other people worry that hormone therapy is somehow experimental or not thoroughly understood. While there are admittedly still gaps in our knowledge and useful questions remain to be answered, a quick check of Medline (the premier medical database) reveals a total of more than 350,000 studies mentioning in the title one of the hormones discussed in this book. No other substance or group of substances has been investigated more often than these hormones.

Estrogen tops the list with more than 42,000 studies. Even pregnenolone, apparently a poor cousin given its numbers so far below the others, can claim more than 1,200 studies. The most important things we need to know to use hormones safely, efficiently, and effectively are revealed in this work. No one doctor—and certainly no patient—would be expected to read up on more than a quarter of a million studies (in just this one area of practice!), but this book aims to digest the most important findings and share them in such a way that they are meaningful to lay readers and medical professionals alike.

Another popular objection comes from those who want only "natural" medicine and believe hormones to fall under the heading "unnatural." There are valid concerns around synthetic versions of hormones. But if by *natural* we mean not polluting the body with substances not already found there, hormone therapy, properly administered, is as natural as they come.

Drugs are medically defined as therapeutic substances whose structure and nature are foreign to the human organism. Hormones, then, are not drugs. Hormones are molecules produced by our own glands and so do not come with the undesirable side effects of traditional drugs—as long as the hormones prescribed are identical to those made by the body and are given in appropriate physiological doses in balance with other hormones.

A belief persists that using hormone therapy will make the endocrine gland sluggish. The truth is that as soon as one stops taking hormones, even after as long as thirty years, the endocrine gland almost always goes back to its usual (albeit insufficient) functioning. In fact, some studies show maintenance of initial performance of the endocrine gland after stopping hormone therapy, which is especially impressive when you consider that the endocrine normally slows down over time. All you need to do to ensure protection of the endocrine gland is to use low doses of natural hormones.

Finally, some patients are concerned that taking hormones will make them gain weight. This might be based on the experience many women have with birth-control pills. But hormones taken within the guidelines in this book (again, low doses, natural hormones, balanced treatment, appropriate forms of delivery) will not add an extra ounce to your frame (assuming you are eating right and getting some exercise). In fact, hormonal imbalance is often a cause of weight gain, and correcting it will help you slim down again, as with a correctly managed thyroid therapy.

A large part of the problem is that hormones have simply gotten a lot of bad press. It is not as if the newspapers, magazines, radio, television, and Internet are full of good news of any sort. It is the derailed train that gets covered, not the safe journeys and on-time arrivals. So it is with hormones—what gets coverage are the dangers and abuses. You've probably heard about (in no particular order) elite athletes doping with EPO (erythropoietin), hormonal additives in farm-animal feed, increases in cancer after treatment with synthetic products, and so on. Hormones, like any remedy, can be harmful if not used properly. Natural as they might be, hormones are not necessarily harmless if they aren't used correctly. When they are used correctly, they are as safe as can be. *Lack* of hormones is what is truly dangerous.

The real news—not that you're likely to see this on the front page anytime soon—is that hormones used properly are powerful forces for healing. The way hormones are used in contemporary mainstream medicine is often not the proper way but in doses many times greater than what the body itself makes and uses, commonly two to ten times physiological levels daily. From my perspective, that's an overdose, and not much different from the doping some renegade elite athletes have been caught doing, though then the doses run from five to *one thousand* times a normal dose.

THE LAY OF THE LAND

With this book you'll be able to access the positive power of hormones, understand the right doses of the right hormones, and work closely with your doctor to find your way back to optimal health. The chapters in the rest of this section look at each of the major hormones individually, along with the signs and symptoms of deficiencies and imbalances of each as well as the lab tests you need to assess your hormonal status, strategies for balancing your hormones naturally—both with proper nutrition and hormonal supplements—and how to work productively with your health-care professional.

The middle two sections of the book lay out the major groupings of problems associated with hormone deficiency, dividing them according to whether they affect primarily the body or the mind. Chapter by chapter, we'll look at everything from weight problems and the appearance of aging in your physical features to heart disease and cancer, from stress and fatigue to mood disorders and memory. In each case you'll get the hormones most responsible for the health of the relevant symptoms and how to make sure your body has the right amount in the right proportion to other hormones. I'll summarize the science underlying all this for you, so you can see for yourself you're getting the most up-to-date, authoritative information possible.

The last section of the book provides a specific diet plan and a program of nutritional supplements designed to create and support hormonal balance, along with strategies for adapting them to your specific situation.

Throughout the book I'll give you case studies from my patient files, so you can see how all this works for real people in real life. They are meant to underline the vast potential hormone replacement therapies hold for all kinds of people. Including you.

CHAPTER TWO

TEST YOURSELF

*T*o make your way on any journey, no matter the quality of the map you're reading or the guide you're following, you need to know where you are starting from as well as where you want to go. You're embarking on a journey to optimal health through hormone balance, so you've already got the second part of the equation in place. You know where you're going. So now I want you to take a few minutes to find out where you are right now.

To that end, this chapter consists of a series of self-tests that assess your level of each of the fifteen most important hormones. Later chapters will tell you all the specifics you need to know about each hormone and all the related health conditions, but for now, simply concentrate on how you feel. Just circle the numbers that describe your situation regarding each of the statements in the grids below, total each column, then add all the columns to get your total score for each hormone. The score key at the end of each test will help you focus on your particular areas of concern. (Of course, you'll need to confirm these results with some lab tests before beginning any kind of treatment, but more about that later.) I recommend keeping a list of your probable and possible deficiencies to guide your reading in the rest of the book and your discussions with your doctor. At the end of the chapter I've included a chart called Me and My Hormones that you can fill in to help you keep track.

That list will help you sort through the next chapter, focusing on the hormones you need to learn about. The end of this chapter then provides another list of questions to let you double-check that you've covered everything. The questions are divided by health concern (sleep, sex, memory, and so on), and a "yes" answer to any of them points you directly to the hormones you should read more about. Finding one or more "yes" answers in any given section will also clue you in to which chapters in Parts II and III will be most important for you. I'm sure you have a pretty good idea if you're more concerned about joint pain or weight gain or what have you. But taking the time to answer these questions will make sure you aren't overlooking something and guarantee we're literally on the same page when it comes to categorizing symptoms. Put your results from these questions, too, in the box on the last page of this chapter.

I hope you'll find this process interesting and enlightening. If you go no further than this, you'll still have a lot to discuss with your doctor on your next visit. But, of course, I hope it will also inspire you to continue through this book to understand how your hormone balance helps and hinders you, what you can do about it either way, and how to put The Hormone Solution into practice in your own life.

PART I

ACTH

Signs and Symptoms of Deficiency	No Never	Not Much Sometimes	In Moderation Regularly	A Lot Often	Tremendously Constantly
1. I have patches of hair loss.	0	1	2	3	4
2. I have a very pale complexion.	0	1	2	3	4
3. I sunburn easily.	0	1	2	3	4
4. I often have memory loss.	0	1	2	3	4
5. I'm stressed out. / I'm facing many difficulties.	0	1	2	3	4
6. My blood pressure has dropped.	0	1	2	3	4
7. My friends tell me I look thinner.	0	1	2	3	4

Total
Overall Total

SCORE:
7 or less: Satisfactory level.
Between 8 and 14: Possible ACTH deficiency.
15 or more: Probable ACTH deficiency.

ALDOSTERONE

Signs and Symptoms of Deficiency	No Never	Not Much Sometimes	In Moderation Regularly	A Lot Often	Tremendously Constantly
1. I urinate too many times a day.	0	1	2	3	4
2. I crave salty foods.	0	1	2	3	4
3. My blood pressure is low.	0	1	2	3	4
4. I feel dizzy when I stand up.	0	1	2	3	4
5. I feel much better lying down than standing up.	0	1	2	3	4

Total
Overall Total

SCORE:
5 or less: Satisfactory level.
Between 6 and 10: Possible aldosterone deficiency.
11 or more: Probable aldosterone deficiency.

CALCITONIN

Signs and Symptoms of Deficiency	No Never	Not Much Sometimes	In Moderation Regularly	A Lot Often	Tremendously Constantly
1. I have vertebral fractures (crushes)—compression fractures in my spine.	0	1	2	3	4
2. I've lost height.	0	1	2	3	4
3. My back hurts.	0	1	2	3	4
4. I'm very sensitive to pain.	0	1	2	3	4
5. I have thyroid problems (goiter, thyroid insufficiency, radiation applied to this area).	0	1	2	3	4

Total
Overall Total

SCORE:
5 or less: Satisfactory level.
Between 6 and 12: Possible calcitonin deficiency.
13 or more: Probable calcitonin deficiency.

CORTISOL

Signs and Symptoms of Deficiency	No Never	Not Much Sometimes	In Moderation Regularly	A Lot Often	Tremendously Constantly
1. My face looks thinner.	0	1	2	3	4
2. My friends call me skinny.	0	1	2	3	4

CORTISOL *(continued)*

Signs and Symptoms of Deficiency	No Never	Not Much Sometimes	In Moderation Regularly	A Lot Often	Tremendously Constantly
3. I have eczema, psoriasis, urticaria ("nettle rash"), skin allergies, or other rashes.	0	1	2	3	4
4. My heart beats quickly.	0	1	2	3	4
5. My blood pressure is low.	0	1	2	3	4
6. I crave salt or sugar (to the extent of bingeing).	0	1	2	3	4
7. I have digestive problems.	0	1	2	3	4
8. I have allergies (hay fever, asthma, etc.).	0	1	2	3	4
9. I'm stressed out.	0	1	2	3	4
10. I'm easily confused.	0	1	2	3	4

Total
Overall Total

SCORE:
10 or less: Satisfactory level.
Between 11 and 20: Possible cortisol deficiency.
21 or more: Probable cortisol deficiency.

DHEA

Signs and Symptoms of Deficiency	No Never	Not Much Sometimes	In Moderation Regularly	A Lot Often	Tremendously Constantly
1. My hair is dry.	0	1	2	3	4
2. My skin and eyes are dry.	0	1	2	3	4
3. My muscles are flabby.	0	1	2	3	4
4. My belly is getting fat.	0	1	2	3	4
5. I don't have much hair under my arm. (0=plenty of hair / 4=hairless)	0	1	2	3	4
6. I don't have much hair in the pubic area. (0=plenty of hair / 4=hairless)	0	1	2	3	4
7. I don't have much fatty tissue in the pubic area (flat "mount of Venus" in women). (0=padded / 4=flat)	0	1	2	3	4
8. My body doesn't have much of a special scent during sexual arousal.	0	1	2	3	4

DHEA *(continued)*

Signs and Symptoms of Deficiency	No Never	Not Much Sometimes	In Moderation Regularly	A Lot Often	Tremendously Constantly
9. I can't tolerate noise.	0	1	2	3	4
10. My libido is low.	0	1	2	3	4

Total
Overall Total

SCORE:
10 or less: Satisfactory level.
Between 11 and 20: Possible DHEA deficiency.
21 or more: Probable DHEA deficiency.

EPO

Signs and Symptoms of Deficiency	No Never	Not Much Sometimes	In Moderation Regularly	A Lot Often	Tremendously Constantly
1. I have a particularly pale complexion.	0	1	2	3	4
2. Prolonged physical effort leaves me breathless.	0	1	2	3	4
3. I'm anemic (diagnosed with a blood test).	0	1	2	3	4
4. "'A sense of well-being?' What's that?"	0	1	2	3	4
5. My blood test shows an increased BUN (blood uric nitrogen) level.	0	1	2	3	4

Total
Overall Total

SCORE:
5 or less: Satisfactory level.
Between 6 and 10: Possible EPO deficiency.
11 or more: Probable EPO deficiency.

ESTROGEN

Signs and Symptoms of Deficiency	No Never	Not Much Sometimes	In Moderation Regularly	A Lot Often	Tremendously Constantly
1. I am losing hair on top of my head.	0	1	2	3	4
2. I'm getting thin, vertical wrinkles above my lips.	0	1	2	3	4

ESTROGEN (continued)

Signs and Symptoms of Deficiency	No Never	Not Much Sometimes	In Moderation Regularly	A Lot Often	Tremendously Constantly
3. My breasts are droopy.	0	1	2	3	4
4. My face is too hairy.	0	1	2	3	4
5. My eyes are dry and easily irritated.	0	1	2	3	4
6. I have hot flashes.	0	1	2	3	4
7. I feel tired constantly.	0	1	2	3	4
8. I am depressed.	0	1	2	3	4
9. My menstrual flow is light. (0=moderate / 1–3=low / 4=none)	0	1	2	3	4
10. Women with periods: My cycles are irregular, too short (<27 days), or too long (>31 days).	0	1	2	3	4
11. Women without periods: I do not feel like making love anymore.	0	1	2	3	4

Total

Overall Total

SCORE:

10 or less: Satisfactory level.

Between 11 and 20: Possible estrogen deficiency.

21 or more: Probable estrogen deficiency.

GROWTH HORMONE

Signs and Symptoms of Deficiency	No Never	Not Much Sometimes	In Moderation Regularly	A Lot Often	Tremendously Constantly
1. My hair is thinning.	0	1	2	3	4
2. My cheeks sag.	0	1	2	3	4
3. My gums are receding.	0	1	2	3	4
4. My abdomen is flabby. / I've got a "spare tire."	0	1	2	3	4
5. My muscles are slack.	0	1	2	3	4
6. My skin is thin and/or dry.	0	1	2	3	4
7. It's hard to recover after physical activity.	0	1	2	3	4
8. I feel exhausted.	0	1	2	3	4
9. I don't like the world. I tend to isolate myself.	0	1	2	3	4

GROWTH HORMONE (continued)

Signs and Symptoms of Deficiency	No Never	Not Much Sometimes	In Moderation Regularly	A Lot Often	Tremendously Constantly
10. I feel continuously anxious and worried.	0	1	2	3	4

Total
Overall Total

SCORE:
10 or less: Satisfactory level.
Between 11 and 20: Possible growth hormone deficiency.
21 or more: Probable growth hormone deficiency.

INSULIN

Signs and Symptoms of Deficiency	No Never	Not Much Sometimes	In Moderation Regularly	A Lot Often	Tremendously Constantly
1. I crave sugar and sweets, and eat a lot of them.	0	1	2	3	4
2. I'm always thirsty.	0	1	2	3	4
3. I urinate a lot during the day as well as at night.	0	1	2	3	4
4. I have difficulty healing.	0	1	2	3	4
5. My stomach and buttocks are skinny.	0	1	2	3	4

Total
Overall Total

SCORE:
5 or less: Satisfactory level.
Between 6 and 10: Possible insulin deficiency.
11 or more: Probable insulin deficiency.

MELATONIN

Signs and Symptoms of Deficiency	No Never	Not Much Sometimes	In Moderation Regularly	A Lot Often	Tremendously Constantly
1. I look older than I am.	0	1	2	3	4
2. I have trouble falling asleep at night.	0	1	2	3	4
3. I wake up during the night . . .	0	1	2	3	4
4. and I can't get back to sleep.	0	1	2	3	4
5. My mind is busy with anxious thoughts while I'm trying to fall asleep.	0	1	2	3	4
6. My feet are too hot at night.	0	1	2	3	4

MELATONIN (continued)

Signs and Symptoms of Deficiency	No Never	Not Much Sometimes	In Moderation Regularly	A Lot Often	Tremendously Constantly
7. When I get up, I don't feel rested.	0	1	2	3	4
8. I feel like I'm living out of sync with the world, going to bed late and waking up late.	0	1	2	3	4
9. I can't tolerate jet lag.	0	1	2	3	4
10. I smoke, drink, and/or use a beta-blocker or a sleep aid.	0	1	2	3	4

Total
Overall Total

SCORE:
10 or less: Satisfactory level.
Between 11 and 20: Possible melatonin deficiency.
21 or more: Probable melatonin deficiency.

PREGNENOLONE

Signs and Symptoms of Deficiency	No Never	Not Much Sometimes	In Moderation Regularly	A Lot Often	Tremendously Constantly
1. I have memory loss.	0	1	2	3	4
2. My joints hurt (fingers, wrists, elbows, feet, ankles, knees).	0	1	2	3	4
3. I'm feeling a bit drained and I have a hard time handling stress.	0	1	2	3	4
4. I don't see colors as brightly as before.	0	1	2	3	4
5. I have lost interest in art; I don't appreciate art as much anymore.	0	1	2	3	4
6. I don't have much hair under my arms or in the pubic area. (0=plenty of hair / 4=hairless)	0	1	2	3	4
7. My muscles are flabby.	0	1	2	3	4
8. I have abundant, light-colored urine during the day.	0	1	2	3	4
9. I have low blood pressure.	0	1	2	3	4
10. I crave salty foods.	0	1	2	3	4

Total
Overall Total

SCORE:
10 or less: Satisfactory level.
Between 11 and 20: Possible pregnenolone deficiency.
21 or more: Probable pregnenolone deficiency.

PROGESTERONE

Signs and Symptoms of Deficiency	No Never	Not Much Sometimes	In Moderation Regularly	A Lot Often	Tremendously Constantly
1. My breasts are large.	0	1	2	3	4
2. My close friends complain I'm nervous and agitated.	0	1	2	3	4
3. I feel anxious.	0	1	2	3	4
4. I sleep lightly and restlessly.	0	1	2	3	4

The following questions are for women who have not yet reached menopause, and menopausal women who are taking hormone replacement therapy (estrogen or estrogen and progesterone).

	No Never	Not Much Sometimes	In Moderation Regularly	A Lot Often	Tremendously Constantly
5. My breasts are swollen and tender or painful before my period . . .	0	1	2	3	4
6. and my lower belly is swollen . . .	0	1	2	3	4
7. and I'm irritable and aggressive . . .	0	1	2	3	4
8. and I lose my self-control.	0	1	2	3	4
9. I have heavy periods . . .	0	1	2	3	4
10. and they are continuously painful.	0	1	2	3	4

Total
Overall Total

SCORE:
Post-menopausal women *not* treated with hormone replacement therapy (estrogen or estrogen and progesterone):
4 or less: Satisfactory level.
Between 5 and 8: Possible progesterone deficiency.
9 or more: Probable progesterone deficiency.
Menstrual women and menopausal women taking hormone replacement therapy (estrogen or estrogen and progesterone):
10 or less: Satisfactory level.
Between 11 and 20: Possible progesterone deficiency.
21 or more: Probable progesterone deficiency.

TESTOSTERONE

Signs and Symptoms of Deficiency (MEN AND WOMEN)	No Never	Not Much Sometimes	In Moderation Regularly	A Lot Often	Tremendously Constantly
1. My face has gotten slack and more wrinkled.	0	1	2	3	4
2. I've lost muscle tone.	0	1	2	3	4

TESTOSTERONE *(continued)*

Signs and Symptoms of Deficiency (MEN AND WOMEN)	No Never	Not Much Sometimes	In Moderation Regularly	A Lot Often	Tremendously Constantly
3. My belly tends to get fat.	0	1	2	3	4
4. I'm constantly tired.	0	1	2	3	4
5. I feel like making love less often than I used to.	0	1	2	3	4

Total
Overall Total

Signs and Symptoms of Deficiency (MEN ONLY)	No Never	Not Much Sometimes	In Moderation Regularly	A Lot Often	Tremendously Constantly
6. My breasts are getting fatty.	0	1	2	3	4
7. I feel less self-confident and more hesitant.	0	1	2	3	4
8. My sexual performance is poorer than it used to be.	0	1	2	3	4
9. I have hot flashes and sweats.	0	1	2	3	4
10. I tire easily with physical activity.	0	1	2	3	4

Total
Overall Total

SCORE FOR WOMEN:
5 or less: Satisfactory level.
Between 6 and 10: Possible testosterone deficiency.
11 or more: Probable testosterone deficiency.

SCORE FOR MEN:
10 or less: Satisfactory level.
Between 11 and 20: Possible testosterone deficiency.
21 or more: Probable testosterone deficiency.

THYROID HORMONES

Signs and Symptoms of Deficiency	No Never	Not Much Sometimes	In Moderation Regularly	A Lot Often	Tremendously Constantly
1. I'm sensitive to cold.	0	1	2	3	4
2. My hands and feet are always cold.	0	1	2	3	4
3. In the morning my face is puffy and my eyelids are swollen.	0	1	2	3	4
4. I put on weight easily.	0	1	2	3	4

THYROID HORMONES (continued)

Signs and Symptoms of Deficiency	No Never	Not Much Sometimes	In Moderation Regularly	A Lot Often	Tremendously Constantly
5. I have dry skin.	0	1	2	3	4
6. I have trouble getting up in the morning.	0	1	2	3	4
7. I feel more tired at rest than when I am active.	0	1	2	3	4
8. I am constipated.	0	1	2	3	4
9. My joints are stiff in the morning.	0	1	2	3	4
10. I feel like I'm living in slow motion.	0	1	2	3	4

Total
Overall Total

SCORE:
10 or less: Satisfactory level.
Between 11 and 20: Possible thyroid hormone deficiency.
21 or more: Probable thyroid hormone deficiency.

VASOPRESSIN

Signs and Symptoms of Deficiency	No Never	Not Much Sometimes	In Moderation Regularly	A Lot Often	Tremendously Constantly
1. I'm thirsty at night.	0	1	2	3	4
2. I get up at night to urinate.	0	1	2	3	4
3. I bleed a lot when I get hurt.	0	1	2	3	4
4. I'm losing my memory.	0	1	2	3	4
5. I have a hard time thinking straight.	0	1	2	3	4

Total
Overall Total

SCORE:
5 or less: Satisfactory level.
Between 6 and 10: Possible vasopressin deficiency.
11 or more: Probable vasopressin deficiency.

PART II

ENERGY

- Do you have a hard time getting up in the morning? When you take a break during the day, does resting only seem to make you more tired?

Read more about . . .
thyroid hormones

- Do you always feel tired, no matter what you do? Do you avoid brief physical efforts because they leave you breathless and tired, and it's hard to recover?

   Read more about . . .
   estrogen
   testosterone
   DHEA

- Does the least amount of stress leave you weak and even trembling?

   Read more about . . .
   cortisol

- Do you feel light-headed and shaky while standing?

   Read more about . . .
   aldosterone

- Do you hesitate to start on sustained physical efforts for fear of not being able to finish?

   Read more about . . .
   EPO

- Do you have difficulty recovering from any effort? Do you have difficulty getting over your fatigue? Can you no longer tap into your former vigor? Do you feel exhausted?

   Read more about . . .
   growth hormone

- If you have any type of diabetes or the tendency to it, do you lack energy for tiring work? Do you tend to be extremely thin?

   Read more about . . .
   insulin

- Do you have a hard time getting started in the morning after having slept poorly?

   Read more about . . .
   melatonin

SEX

- Do you lack sexual desire? Do you have a lack of body hair and sexual odors?

   Read more about . . .
   testosterone

DHEA

estrogen (women only)

- Does your penis or clitoris seem less sensitive? Do you have trouble getting or maintaining an erection?

  Read more about . . .

  testosterone

- Are your erections not firm enough?

  Read more about . . .

  testosterone

  cortisol

  DHEA

  growth hormone

  vasopressin

- Do you have difficulty calming down and relaxing?

  Read more about . . .

  melatonin

  progesterone (women only)

  growth hormone

- Have you lost your attraction toward your partner? Do you lack vaginal lubrication?

  Read more about . . .

  estrogen

- Are you unable to fantasize? Do you have problems with erection or ejaculation?

  Read more about . . .

  testosterone

- Do you have a hard time getting aroused? Do you have a hard time turning desire into action?

  Read more about . . .

  cortisol

- Do you have a weak erection? Is your clitoris difficult to stimulate?

  Read more about . . .

  vasopressin

- Do you lack endurance? Is your erection—penile or clitoral—weak or short-lasting?

  Read more about . . .

  growth hormone

- Do you no longer feel fulfilled, relaxed, and drowsy after sex?

Read more about . . .
progesterone
- For you, does deep sleep no longer follow sex?
  Read more about . . .
  melatonin

SLEEP

- Do you sleep poorly? Wake up frequently? Rarely dream? Are you jet-lagged or prone to jet lag?
  Read more about . . .
  melatonin
- Do you dream only infrequently?
  Read more about . . .
  estrogen
  progesterone
  testosterone
  DHEA
  melatonin
  growth hormone
- Do you sleep for long periods of time but still not feel restored?
  Read more about . . .
  growth hormone
  thyroid hormones
  cortisol
  melatonin

MEMORY

- Are you unable to trust your memory?
  Read more about . . .
  testosterone
  DHEA
  estrogen
  pregnenolone
- Do you have trouble concentrating?
  Read more about . . .
  thyroid hormones
  ACTH
  cortisol

aldosterone

melatonin

- Is your thinking slow or are your thoughts unclear?

    Read more about . . .

    thyroid hormones

- Do you want to stimulate your memory? Are you unable to remember a list of items without writing them down?

    Read more about . . .

    pregnenolone

- Do you feel light-headed in stressful situations?

    Read more about . . .

    cortisol

- Do you feel light-headed when standing up?

    Read more about . . .

    aldosterone

- Do you suffer from short- or long-term memory loss?

    Read more about . . .

    vasopressin

SKIN AND HAIR

- Do you have large wrinkles that cover the face or are on both sides of the nose and mouth, with fallen, flabby cheeks (the bulldog look)? Do you have smile lines, droopy eyelids, forehead creases, and/or a double chin?

    Read more about . . .

    growth hormone

- Do you have little wrinkles around the eyes and crow's feet at the corners of the eyes?

    Read more about . . .

    testosterone

    estrogen

- Do you have age spots?

    Read more about . . .

    cortisol

    melatonin

    DHEA

- Have you had skin cancer or are you prone to it or at risk for it?

Read more about . . .
thyroid hormones
- Do you have excessively dry skin?
	Read more about . . .
	thyroid hormones
	growth hormone
	estrogen
	testosterone
	DHEA
- Do you have thin skin?
	Read more about . . .
	growth hormone
	estrogen
	testosterone
- Do you have pale skin?
	Read more about . . .
	estrogen
	testosterone
	thyroid hormones
- Is your skin very wrinkly?
	Read more about . . .
	growth hormone
	testosterone
	estrogen
- Is your skin dehydrated? Do you have sharp-edged wrinkles?
	Read more about . . .
	aldosterone
	vasopressin
- Are you sensitive to sunlight?
	Read more about . . .
	ACTH
	testosterone
	growth hormone
- Does your skin heal slowly? Do you bruise easily? Is your skin easily abraded?
	Read more about . . .
	growth hormone
	testosterone

- Are you losing (or have you lost) your hair? Is your hair dry, thick, brittle, and/or slow-growing? Is your hair lusterless?
  Read more about . . .
  thyroid hormones
- Is your hair lacking body and highlights? Is your hair no longer as wavy as it once was? Is your hair thinning all over your head?
  Read more about . . .
  growth hormone
- Men: Is the hair disappearing from the top of your head? Are you losing hair on your abdomen (between the pubic area and the belly button), legs, or chest? Is your beard sparse?
  Read more about . . .
  testosterone
- Women: Is the hair disappearing from the top of your head? Or do you have too much hair in general?
  Read more about . . .
  estrogen
  progesterone
  cortisol
- Women: Do you have hair loss in the pubic area and under your arms?
  Read more about . . .
  DHEA
- Is your hair disappearing in circular patches?
  Read more about . . .
  ACTH
  cortisol
- Is your hair totally disappearing? Do you suffer from total alopecia?
  Read more about . . .
  ACTH
  thyroid hormones
  And, secondarily:
  growth hormone
  DHEA
  testosterone
  estrogen
  progesterone
- Is your hair turning gray?
  Read more about . . .
  ACTH

testosterone

growth hormone

WEIGHT CONTROL

- Are your calves too big? Are your legs and ankles swollen in the morning? Is your face bloated in the morning?

    Read more about . . .

    thyroid hormones

- Is your face swollen? Do you have a face like a full moon?

    Read more about . . .

    cortisol

- Do you have thick folds of unsightly skin? Are you cellulite-prone? And (men only) are your breasts enlarged?

    Read more about . . .

    growth hormone

    testosterone

- Women: Are your breasts too large? Do they get larger before your period?

    Read more about . . .

    progesterone

- Do you have a "buffalo hump" of fat on your upper back?

    Read more about . . .

    cortisol

    growth hormone

    testosterone

    thyroid hormones

- Is your abdomen too plump? Is it distended?

    Read more about . . .

    growth hormone

    thyroid hormones

    testosterone

    DHEA

- Are your buttocks and thighs too well padded? Are you pear-shaped?

    Read more about . . .

    thyroid hormones

    growth hormone

    testosterone

- Are you underweight because you lack muscle mass?

    Read more about . . .

growth hormone
testosterone
DHEA
insulin
estrogen
- Are you underweight because you lack body fat?
  Read more about . . .
  insulin
  cortisol

STRESS

- Do you have gray hair?
  Read more about . . .
  testosterone
  growth hormone
- Do you have wrinkles and tiny lines?
  Read more about . . .
  growth hormone
  testosterone
  estrogen
- Are your muscles slack?
  Read more about . . .
  growth hormone
  testosterone
- Are your muscles tense?
  Read more about . . .
  growth hormone
  progesterone
  melatonin
- Do you suffer from constant fatigue?
  Read more about . . .
  testosterone
  estrogen
  progesterone
  DHEA
  growth hormone
- Do you feel tired, particularly when you are resting?
  Read more about . . .
  thyroid hormones

- Do you feel tired, particularly when stressed?
  Read more about . . .
  cortisol
- Do you lack endurance? Do you have a hard time recovering from exerting yourself? Do you feel exhausted?
  Read more about . . .
  growth hormone
- Do you get anxious?
  Read more about . . .
  testosterone
  growth hormone
  progesterone
  melatonin
- Do you sleep poorly?
  Read more about . . .
  melatonin
  growth hormone
  testosterone
  estrogen
  progesterone
- Do you have memory problems?
  Read more about . . .
  thyroid hormones
  testosterone
  DHEA
  estrogen
  pregnenolone
  vasopressin
  growth hormone
  ACTH
- Do you have low blood pressure?
  Read more about . . .
  aldosterone
  cortisol
  vasopressin
- Do you have high blood pressure?
  Read more about . . .
  thyroid hormones
  estrogen

testosterone
melatonin
DHEA
growth hormone

MOOD

- Are you anxious while resting and/or upon waking in the morning, but not while active? Do you feel depressed in the morning? When you are at rest?

    Read more about . . .

    thyroid hormones

- Are you frequently nervous, irritable, ill at ease, easily excitable, afraid, and/or worried?

    Read more about . . .

    testosterone

    DHEA

    progesterone

    growth hormone

- Are you anxious to the point where it interferes with your ability to get or keep a job or relationship? Do you withdraw as a way of coping with your anxiety? Do you lack self-confidence? Do you feel fragile? Excessively vulnerable to stress? Do you easily collapse in even minor stress situations?

    Read more about . . .

    growth hormone

- Do small things set you off? Are you unable to see how to confront or escape a situation? Do you have difficulty organizing your ideas, especially in stress situations? Are you confused? Distracted? Can even the littlest thing make you feel pessimistic and defeated? Would you always rather flee than fight?

    Read more about . . .

    cortisol

- Do you have nighttime anxiety and/or sleep problems?

    Read more about . . .

    melatonin

- Women: Are you anxious in the second half of your menstrual cycle? Or irritable, worried about trivialities, aggressive for no reason, nervous, or irrational?

Read more about . . .

progesterone

- Women: Are you constantly depressed?

  Read more about . . .

  estrogen

  testosterone

- Men: Are you constantly depressed?

  Read more about . . .

  testosterone

- Does your depression affect your sexual desire?

  Read more about . . .

  estrogen

  testosterone

  DHEA

- Do you feel better lying down than standing up?

  Read more about . . .

  aldosterone

CIRCULATION (HEART AND STROKE)

- Do you have heart disease? Do you have high blood pressure, with the diastolic (the bottom number in a written reading, the second number when you hear it said aloud) being too high or with the diastolic and systolic readings being too close together? Are you at risk for stroke? Heart failure?

  Read more about . . .

  thyroid hormones

- Do you have clogged or damaged arteries or damaged heart muscles? Are you in menopause—or, for men, midlife—and have high blood pressure, with both the systolic and diastolic readings being high?

  Read more about . . .

  estrogen

  testosterone

  melatonin

- Have the arteries or your heart gotten less healthy as you've gotten older? Do you have high blood pressure related to poor kidney function?

  Read more about . . .

  growth hormone

- Is your blood cholesterol too high?

  Read more about . . .

  thyroid hormones

  DHEA

  testosterone

  estrogen

  growth hormone

  melatonin

- Do you have low HDL ("good cholesterol") and high LDL?

  Read more about . . .

  estrogen

  testosterone

  growth hormone

  DHEA

- Is your cholesterol high from a fatty diet? Heredity? Aging? Medications? Do you have a high systolic and diastolic reading in your blood-pressure measurement? Do you have blood clots? A high platelet count? Men: Do you have angina?

  Read more about . . .

  melatonin

- Is your cholesterol high because of diabetes? Do you have atherosclerosis related to diabetes? Is your risk of stroke elevated because of diabetes?

  Read more about . . .

  insulin

- Do you have poor kidney function? Low red blood cell count?

  Read more about . . .

  EPO

- Do you have atherosclerosis? Damage to or blockage of your coronary arteries? Angina? Arteriosclerosis? Leg ulcers? Gangrene? Intermittent claudication (calf pain when walking)? Men: Do you have blood clots?

  Read more about . . .

  testosterone

- Do you have arterial hypertension? Arteriosclerosis? Angina? Heart disease? Men: Are you at increased risk of heart attack?

  Read more about . . .

  DHEA

- Do you often get woozy? Do you sometimes feel faint when standing up?

  Read more about . . .

  aldosterone

  vasopressin

- Do you have little or no resistance to stress? Do you have a weak or rapid heartbeat, especially when you are under stress or that is more pronounced when you are standing up?

  Read more about . . .

  cortisol

- Do you have a weak heartbeat?

  Read more about . . .

  thyroid hormones

  growth hormone

  testosterone

  cortisol

- Women: Are you in menopause?

  Read more about . . .

  estrogen

  progesterone

- Have you had ruptured blood vessels? Severe hemorrhaging after physical trauma?

  Read more about . . .

  vasopressin

- Do you have low-blood-pressure problems?

  Read more about . . .

  cortisol

  aldosterone

- Have you had a stroke?

  Read more about . . .

  estrogen

  progesterone

  testosterone

- Have you been diagnosed with ischemia (lack of blood supply to tissue, like the heart or brain)?

  Read more about . . .

  estrogen

  testosterone

• Do you have cerebral edema from trauma?
  Read more about . . .
  progesterone

JOINTS

• Do you have rheumatoid arthritis?
  Read more about . . .
  cortisol
  ACTH
  testosterone (for men)
  estrogen
  progesterone (for women)
  melatonin
  pregnenolone
  thyroid hormones
  growth hormone
• Do you have lupus?
  Read more about . . .
  cortisol
  DHEA
• Do you have fibromyalgia?
  Read more about . . .
  DHEA
  estrogen
  testosterone
  growth hormone
  cortisol
  thyroid hormones
  melatonin
• Do you have osteoarthritis?
  Read more about . . .
  testosterone
  estrogen
  cortisol
  thyroid hormones
  growth hormone
• Do you have osteoarthritis in the hip?
  Read more about . . .
  growth hormone

- Women: Are you in menopause?

  Read more about . . .

  estrogen

- Do you have joint pain when you get out of bed in the morning? Or do you have pain when you are resting that decreases when you are active? Are you stiff early in the morning? Is your pain aggravated by cold? Do you have carpal tunnel syndrome (tingling sensation in the fingers)? Gout (arthritis in your thumbs and big toes)?

  Read more about . . .

  thyroid hormones

BONES

- Have you lost muscle mass, tone, and strength? Do you feel depressed and fatigued throughout the day? Have you had bone loss in your spine and hips?

  Read more about . . .

  testosterone

  DHEA

  growth hormone

- Women: Do you have bone loss in your spine?

  Read more about . . .

  estrogen

  testosterone

  DHEA

  growth hormone

- Do you have bone loss in the spine, hips, and extremities (hands, wrists, ankles, feet)?

  Read more about . . .

  growth hormone

- Does your stomach sag, pushed forward by curvature of your spine? Is your spine asymmetrical?

  Read more about . . .

  thyroid hormones

  growth hormone

- Are your bones visibly thinner, especially in your jaw and fingers?

  Read more about . . .

  growth hormone

- Do you have osteoporosis in which the cause is "idiopathic" (unknown)?

    Read more about . . .

    estrogen

    progesterone

    testosterone

    growth hormone

- Women: Are you in menopause?

    Read more about . . .

    estrogen

    growth hormone

    calcitonin

- Do you have osteoporosis from excessive cortisol and/or other steroids?

    Read more about . . .

    DHEA

- Do you have bone loss in the spine and premenstrual syndrome with excessive nervousness?

    Read more about . . .

    progesterone

- Are you experiencing accelerated bone loss from immobilization or advanced age?

    Read more about . . .

    calcitonin

    growth hormone

- Do you have vertebral fractures or crushes? Pain from fractures?

    Read more about . . .

    calcitonin

- Did you grow slowly? Do you have shorter legs and arms?

    Read more about . . .

    thyroid hormones

- Do you have scoliosis?

    Read more about . . .

    melatonin

    thyroid hormones

    growth hormone

- Do you have bone cysts in your arms or legs?

    Read more about . . .

    cortisol

- Do your muscles sag? Do you have thin skin? Thin hair?

    Read more about . . .

    growth hormone

IMMUNE SYSTEM (FOR DEFENSE AGAINST INFECTIONS AND CANCER)

- Have lab tests indicated you have a low ratio of CD4 to CD8 (indicators of immune strength)?
  Read more about . . .
  thyroid hormones
  growth hormone
  DHEA

- Do you have a low number of antibodies? Do you have cancer or a viral, bacterial, or parasitic infection? Are you at increased risk of those things?
  Read more about . . .
  DHEA

- Have you had radiation therapy? Do you have problems with your thymus or spleen?
  Read more about . . .
  melatonin
  DHEA
  growth hormone

- Do you have cancer?
  Read more about . . .
  estrogen
  progesterone
  thyroid hormones
  melatonin

- Are you at risk for breast, endometrial, or ovarian cancer?
  Read more about . . .
  progesterone

- Do you have or are you at risk for prostate cancer?
  Read more about . . .
  DHEA

- Are your white blood cell levels low? Do you have a bacterial or viral infection? Do you have terminal cancer and want to maintain your quality of life and length of survival?
  Read more about . . .
  melatonin
  thyroid hormones

- Do you want to maintain body weight and muscle tone?

Read more about . . .

growth hormone

- Do you have pain from spinal fractures due to cancer metastases of the bone?

  Read more about . . .

  calcitonin

- Do you have or are you at risk for viral infections? Do you have inflammation, fever, pain, or loss of appetite related to cancer treatment? Do you have leukemia, lymphoma, or myeloma?

  Read more about . . .

  cortisol

HEALTH AND HORMONES SUMMARY

	Weight Control	Skin and Hair	Joints	Bones	Circulation	Immune System	Sex	Sleep	Memory	Mood	Stress	Energy
ACTH		✓	✓						✓		✓	✓
Aldosterone										✓	✓	✓
Calcitonin				✓	✓							
Cortisol	✓✓*	✓	✓	✓	✓	✓	✓		✓	✓	✓	✓
DHEA	✓	✓	✓	✓	✓	✓	✓	✓		✓	✓	✓
EPO					✓					✓		✓
Estrogen	✓✓*	✓	✓	✓	✓	✓	✓	✓	✓	✓	✓	✓
Growth Hormone	✓	✓	✓	✓	✓	✓	✓	✓	✓	✓	✓	✓
Insulin	✓✓*	✓ (skin)	✓		✓	✓	✓	✓	✓	✓		✓
Melatonin		✓ (skin)	✓	✓	✓	✓	✓	✓	✓	✓	✓	✓
Pregnenolone			✓					✓	✓			
Progesterone	✓	✓ (hair)	✓	✓	✓	✓		✓	✓	✓	✓	✓
Testosterone	✓✓*	✓	✓	✓	✓		✓	✓	✓	✓	✓	✓
Thyroid Hormones	✓	✓	✓	✓	✓	✓		✓	✓	✓	✓	✓
Vasopressin					✓		✓	✓	✓			

*"✓✓" indicates that the hormone is useful for cases of low weight as well as overweight.

ME AND MY HORMONES

Check off your results from this chapter in this chart, so you have one easy place to refer back to as you read on.

	Possible Deficiency	Probable Deficiency	Read More About
ACTH			
Aldosterone			
Calcitonin			
Cortisol			
DHEA			
EPO			
Estrogen			
Growth Hormone			
Insulin			
Melatonin			
Pregnenolone			
Progesterone			
Testosterone			
Thyroid Hormones			
Vasopressin			

CHAPTER THREE

THE TOP FIFTEEN

*T*his chapter covers all fifteen of the major hormones in detail, including their sources and primary functions and the effects of deficiency. I realize this big pile of facts can be a bit overwhelming. Don't worry, you don't have to memorize it all now. There won't be a test. Anyway, you can always turn back to it later. There will be cross-references in all the chapters in Parts II and III, which look at specific health issues related to hormones and hormonal deficiency and imbalance, to help you do that. Think of this chapter as necessary background for those upcoming chapters and as a guide to help you identify which of the remaining chapters are particularly relevant for you. Anyway, armed with the results of your self-tests, you already know which parts of this chapter you need to pay attention to and which parts you might be able to skim.

ACTH (Adrenocorticotrope Hormone) controls adrenal secretion of antistress hormones. It makes you more attentive, vigilant, focused, and resistant to stress. It clarifies thoughts and stimulates memory, especially visual memory. It is calming and makes you less anxious, more sociable, and more joyful, and it maintains your energy level. ACTH helps tan the skin and helps fight hair loss all over the body. It can even grow hair in cases of total baldness.

ACTH is made and distributed principally by the pituitary gland, though certain brain neurons also make it for use as a neurotransmitter (a substance used as a messenger between nerve cells). The pituitary gland uses ACTH to stimulate secretion of other hormones from the adrenal cortex.

Without sufficient ACTH, your skin and face will be pale, you'll have patches of hair loss, you'll sunburn easily, and you'll probably be thin. You might be slow to focus and have difficulty concentrating. You'll have a low tolerance for stress and feel a general lack of panache. You might be prone to fainting and even, in the most severe deficiencies, risk falling into a coma.

ALDOSTERONE controls blood pressure when you are standing. It energizes and stimulates you and raises blood pressure in stressful situations just enough to help you cope.

Aldosterone comes from the adrenal glands, which are just above the kidneys. It is secreted mostly during the day. Its primary job is to maintain your blood pressure when you are standing up. It also improves blood pressure when you are upright, and in all your arteries, especially in your head. Aldosterone also energizes and stimulates you (making your blood pressure rise just a bit) to help you handle stressful situations. It fights drowsiness and absent-mindedness (which can come with low blood pressure).

With insufficient aldosterone, your blood pressure will be too low, with readings often under 100. You'll look sort of dried out and listless, especially when standing. Your face will often look thinner, as if deflated. You'll need to urinate frequently during the day and immediately after drinking, and you'll produce abundant, clear, almost colorless urine. Yet you'll feel thirsty and dehydrated all the time and will crave salt and salty foods. You'll tire quickly when standing and may have dizzy spells or feel woozy when standing. It might seem that you need to lie down to feel really well.

CALCITONIN strengthens the bones, makes stress easier to bear, protects against migraines and stomach ulcers, and fights inflammation.

Calcitonin comes from the thyroid gland, at the base of the neck. It protects the bones by maintaining their minerals and slowing the natural cycle of bone-cell breakdown. It can decrease the risk of osteoporosis as well as bone pain, as in fractures, spinal compression, or cancer metastases to the bone. Because it regulates the level of calcium in the blood, calcitonin also protects the nerves. It can prevent or relieve migraines.

If you don't have enough calcitonin, you might develop osteoporosis, including losing height, a "dowager's hump" curving the top of your spine forward, and a propensity to easily fracture bones, including vertebrae. Paget's disease, a bone deformation, can also be countered by calcitonin, as can intense pain in the bones with vertebral fractures (spinal compression). Ulcers, frequent migraines, and low resistance to stress all point a finger at calcitonin deficiency.

CORTISOL helps the body respond quickly and constructively to stress. It also stimulates appetite, boosts energy levels, improves digestion, eases movement in the joints, eases inflammation and pain, soothes allergies, fever, and reactions to toxins, and enhances the immune system (though at excessive doses cortisol actually depresses the immune system). Assuming the correct balance with androgens ("male" hormones like testosterone) is maintained, cortisol might help you live longer.

Cortisol, sometimes called hydrocortisone, comes from the adrenal glands. Casual investigation might lead you to associate cortisol with stress—and, indeed, cortisol levels soar when you are under a great deal of stress. But it is really the *anti*stress hormone. It rises under stress because it is actually helping your body handle stress, trying to give you a way to get rid of it. Cortisol frees up your energy reserves at opportune moments. At times of stress, cortisol makes the heart beat faster, increases blood pressure (and so the supply of oxygen and nutrients to all parts of the body), and boosts blood-sugar levels to provide strength and energy. Cortisol drives blood toward strategic parts of the body, including the head, shoulders, trunk, pelvis, and hips—basically preparing you for "fight or flight." These are all short-term responses you need in the moment of greatest stress, though this hormone also works over the long term. Cortisol helps keep you ready for anything and eager for action.

Cortisol stimulates the brain, muscles, heart, and circulatory and respiratory systems. It fights certain forms of cancer (at reasonable doses), like leukemia and certain lymphomas. It also fights jet lag, fatigue, confusion, hypoglycemia, sugar cravings, anxiety, irritability, low mood, "burnout," and low blood pressure. It stimulates the immune system, helping ward off the flu and other viral, bacterial, or parasitic infections as well as cancer.

Humans cannot live without cortisol. Even mild deficiencies can wreak havoc in the body, resulting in hair loss, emaciation, low blood pressure, rapid pulse and/or palpitations in response to the least stress, painful and inflamed joints, and skin problems including eczema, psoriasis, hives, allergies, vitiligo, or spots of excessive pigmentation (melanoderma). Insufficient levels of cortisol can also cause flu-like fatigue that gets worse under stress, cravings for sweets and/or salty and spicy foods, a dazed feeling and confused thoughts or empty-headedness, inability to handle stress, loss of appetite, nausea, digestive problems (including colitis), allergies and asthma, medication intolerance, rheumatoid arthritis, and regular spiking of fevers.

DHEA (Dehydroepiandrosterone) is made into several different active substances by the body, including testosterone and estradiol (estrogen). It strengthens muscles, keeps mucous membranes soft and moist, promotes hair growth under the arm and in the pubic area, stimulates immunity, boosts energy levels, fights anxiety and depression, improves mood, increases libido (in women), enhances memory, and (at least in animal studies) fights cancer, diabetes, and heart disease. It also relieves joint pain.

Over a lifetime, you'll secrete more DHEA than any other hormone. In young adults, its concentration in the blood is almost twenty times higher than any other hormone. Tissues, including the brain, may also have high levels. Just the production of DHEA would keep the adrenal glands plenty busy.

A great part of what DHEA does, however, is achieved after it is converted into a variety of different substances. These derivatives, or active metabolites, include several androgens, including testosterone, and estrogen. As powerful as DHEA can be, its derivatives pack an even bigger wallop. For example, the metabolite androstenediol stimulates immunity one hundred times more than the original DHEA—and androstenetriol three hundred times.

One final important benefit to DHEA is its ability to control some of the negative effects of excess cortisol.

Without sufficient DHEA, your face will look strained, your eyes will be dry and lackluster, and your hair dry and lifeless. You'll have scant hair under your arms and in the pubic area, dry and delicate skin, a tendency to a pot belly, cellulite on the thighs, and even a flattened pubic mound. You'll tend to feel insecure, anxious, gloomy, and sad. If you are female, your libido will flag. You won't have enough energy; one idiosyncratic way a lack of DHEA may manifest itself in people over sixty-five is in difficulty climbing stairs.

EPO (Erythropoietin) increases the production of red blood cells, the cells that transport oxygen in the blood and allow the lungs to better absorb oxygen, improving physical performance and providing a sensation of well-being. It gives you endurance, especially for long-term efforts like cross-country running, and lets you recover from physical exertion better and more quickly. The increased production of red blood cells might reduce the risk of cardiovascular disease and stimulate the immune system. EPO prevents anemia and the fatigue that comes with it.

Without enough EPO, your face and skin would be pale. You'd get winded easily and lose some of your capacity for physical exertion. You would be constantly fatigued and slow to recover from any sort of ordeal, whether it be a strenuous workout or a long day or an injury or surgery.

If you have heard of EPO before, it might well have been in the context of abuse. It is EPO that some athletes use for doping. Given the benefits described, you can see why. I want to be very clear that the levels of supplementation I am recommending are meant only to supply what your own body normally would. In cases of doping, EPO is administered at twenty to thirty times the normal dosage and can have grave consequences.

ESTROGEN creates the female shape (breasts, hips, pelvis, and even face) and controls the menstrual cycle. It keeps skin smooth and unwrinkled, prevents excess hair growth, and keeps the vagina moist. It enhances sexual desire, increases physical endurance, and contributes to a positive mood. Estrogen keeps the eyes and mouth moist and the eyes shining. It produces a positive mood—happiness, enthusiasm, and zeal—and prevents depression. Estrogen prevents menstruation-related migraines. Estrogen develops sexual desire and the desire to love. It fights fatigue, reduces the risk of heart disease, retards osteoporosis, protects the brain, keeps the joints healthy, and supports immune function.

Estrogen is actually a family of "feminine" hormones. Though many have similar effects, for the most part when I say *estrogen* I am referring specifically to estradiol, the most common (and potent) natural form used in supplements. Men's bodies need estrogen, too—without it, they are infertile and might have a low libido—but men are not actually treated with supplements because they can cause prostate problems.

At puberty, the ovaries start producing significant amounts of estrogen, with a helping hand from the pituitary gland, which stimulates the ovaries with other hormones (FSH, follicle-stimulating hormone, and LH, luteinizing hormone). Some estrogen is made in fat cells by metabolizing other hormones originating in the adrenal glands. At menopause, as the ovaries dramatically decrease production, fat tissue becomes the predominant source of estrogens. Either way, estrogen is a very powerful hormone. Consider that a woman's body typically produces 80 mcg (micrograms) of it each day, which is enough to balance the 25,000 mcg of androgens (male hormones) it also produces.

Levels of this hormone in the body vary cyclically. Every month, estrogen builds up a mucous membrane on the walls of the uterus, preparing it to receive a fertilized egg. In the absence of such an egg, estrogen levels drop toward the end of the cycle and the uterine lining sloughs off as menstruation. If there is a fertilized egg and pregnancy occurs, there's a nine-month hiatus from the regular cycle, during which several hormones alter their patterns, including estrogen, which skyrockets.

If you are a woman without sufficient estrogen, you'll have hair loss on the top of your head; plentiful small, fine wrinkles around the eyes and mouth and especially above the lips; and dry, irritated eyes. Your breasts will shrink and/or sag, and you'll lose some of the plumpness that adds the curves to your figure at the chest, hips, and pelvis. You'll experience vaginal dryness and lack of sexual desire and possibly painful intercourse. You might have excessive hairiness or hair growth patterns similar to men's. A deficiency of estrogen can make you tired all day long, give you a tendency toward depression, and encourage feelings of discouragement. And of course it would cause a host of menstrual problems: inadequate, nonexistent, or protracted (more than five days) flow, painful periods with severe cramps, and/or cycles that are irregular (either too short or too long).

Lowered estrogen levels are the source of many of the familiar symptoms of menopause, most famously hot flashes. Younger women might also get hot flashes during menstruation if their estrogen levels are too low.

GROWTH HORMONE is necessary throughout childhood to help us grow up, but even once we've reached our adult size, we need it to maintain muscle tone. It helps keep the spine straight and decreases fat, provides energy and endurance, makes sleep more restorative, lessens anxiety, and provides a feeling of serenity and security.

Growth hormone is produced by the pituitary gland. It determines the ultimate size of the adult body, strengthening it and developing the nose, chin, jaw, and shoulders in particular. It also tones and firms the muscles, develops strong bones, keeps the joints healthy, and protects the kidneys, heart, and other organs, including the digestive system. It keeps the arteries clear and flexible and supports the immune system. Growth hormone helps prevent obesity and in particular slims the stomach, firms up the thighs, and makes the knees thinner. It reduces the severity of heart disease and the risk of osteoporosis and, at least in animal studies, certain cancers. All that, and it keeps the skin from thinning and major wrinkles from forming, too. For all these reasons, growth hormone is apparently the most important hormone when it comes to helping you stay young-looking.

During the day, growth hormone provides energy and endurance. At night, it shortens how long you sleep while at the same time making the sleep you do get more restorative. It helps you recover from any sort of stress or strain, particularly in the hours after midnight.

Growth hormone makes us more assertive, strong-minded, decisive, and calm—which is why it might be considered the "leader's hormone." It provides a deep feeling of serenity and security, reducing anxiety and making you resistant to stress.

Without sufficient growth hormone, you'll have thin, limp hair, droopy eyelids and cheeks, thin lips and jaw, and receding gums—basically, a sagging face. You'll get large and deep wrinkles. You'll have thin, dehydrated skin, less muscular shoulders and buttocks, sagging triceps, jiggly inner thighs—a generally flaccid body with loose, hanging muscles and weak bones. You'll carry extra weight all over. Telltale signs are an overhanging belly, little cushions of fat above the knees, and, on men, "breasts" almost like a woman's.

Your mental state will sag along with your body, producing negative attitudes, insecurity, fatigue, anxiety, depression, lack of self-esteem, and an excessive need for sleep. You'll have a hard time controlling your emotions. You'll be exhausted after physical activity and slow to recover from anything that upsets you or demands extra effort. You won't be able to easily stay awake after midnight, and you'll generally have a low resistance to stress. You'll have a hard time asserting yourself, and you will tend to feel incompetent. You might have an excessive need to isolate yourself socially and find yourself making curt conversational replies and rude retorts.

INSULIN, which is made by the pancreas, has the primary job of controlling your blood-sugar levels. It prevents (and treats) diabetes, and works against hyperglycemia (high blood sugar) symptoms including excessive thirst and urine loss. Insulin protects against heart disease, strengthening the heart and arteries. It also strengthens muscles and fortifies the immune and digestive systems. It creates energy reserves and stores fats, which can cause weight gain (usually in the sense of preventing excessive thinness, not causing obesity), and helps fill out the stomach, hips, and thighs. Insulin energizes you and increases endurance.

In one of the clearest cause and effect relationships in the world of hormones, if you don't have enough insulin, you get diabetes. You'd have symptoms including a ravenous need for sugar, sleepiness all day long, and excessive thirst, and you'd make lots and lots of clear urine, night and day.

Without insulin you'd be like a stick figure, with no fat on the stomach and thighs (as happens in type I diabetes). With excess insulin you tend to be overweight, particularly on the stomach and thighs (as

THE TWO TYPES OF DIABETES

Type I diabetes: The pancreas is unable to make insulin, or make normal amounts, so there is a real lack of insulin in the blood. It can occur in younger people, including children, and used to be known sometimes as "juvenile diabetes." In many already rather thin older people (generally over 70), insulin starts to decrease, and there is progressive weight loss as a result.

Type II diabetes: Despite an excess of insulin in the blood, its action is less and less effective. What action it does manage is directed at the fat cells. This type is common in overweight people, and older people with this type gain rather than lose weight, as the fatty tissue continues to react well to insulin.

happens in type II diabetes). You'd be dehydrated, with a dry mouth and skin that stays creased a long time after it's been pinched.

MELATONIN is the sleep hormone; it functions primarily in helping you fall asleep at night; sleep well, soundly, and deeply; and wake up in the morning. It is what makes you yawn and want to go to bed at night, and (by activating thyroid hormones) it's what prompts you to arise—if you have the luxury of not handing that job over to an alarm clock. Melatonin creates your body's day/night rhythm, including the timing with which other hormones are released. It is helpful with sleep problems, including those from shift work, and jet lag.

Melatonin is a powerful antioxidant and captures potentially damaging free radicals. It protects the heart and arteries and reduces the risk of cardiovascular disease. Its antioxidant properties might explain why it might reduce the risk of cancer; in the lab melatonin has also been shown to slow down the growth of cancer cells. It has also been shown to inhibit the proliferation of the AIDS virus. Furthermore, melatonin protects the pancreas and the organs of the immune system (another anticancer angle and perhaps the explanation of its effect with AIDS).

Melatonin also relaxes muscles, relieves tension, reduces stress and anxiety (especially at night), and lowers blood pressure. It calms you and provides a sense of serenity.

You can thank the pineal gland for most of your melatonin, though other tissues, including the intestines and the retina, are also capable of producing it.

Without enough melatonin, you'll get poor, superficial sleep deprived of dreams and full of agitation and brooding. You'll be quite the night owl, because your body won't know when to go to bed. You'll have a hard time getting to sleep and going back to sleep when you wake up during the night. You'll feel tired when waking up and will never feel well rested, so you'll often be in a bad mood. You'll be hard hit by jet lag.

If you don't have sufficient melatonin, you'll often feel tense, anxious, irritable, and aggressive. You'll look older than your age, thanks in part to prematurely graying hair and bags under your eyes. No one looks his best when not well rested, and few of us hide it very well.

PREGNENOLONE I think of as the memory hormone. In animal studies it improves memory one hundred times more than even DHEA in the same dose. It enhances memory at least in part because it clarifies think-ing and stimulates concentration (which are benefits all on their own, of course) and prevents memory loss. In addition, pregnenolone at higher doses might reduce fatigue, fight depression, protect the joints, relieve arthritis, and speed healing. Perhaps its most unusual effect is that, according to some patients' experiences, it might intensify the way you see colors.

Produced in the adrenal glands and the brain, pregnenolone is a precursor of all the adrenal and sex hormones. It is the most abundant hormone in the brain, where you'll find two to four times the amount of DHEA, which already has a brain concentration double that of its very high blood concentration. Pregnenolone's concentration in the brain is seventy-five times higher than in the blood.

Without enough pregnenolone, you're sure to have memory prob-lems and poor concentration. You'll be vulnerable to stress and depres-sion and at risk for chronic fatigue and reduced capacity for physical exertion. You might have joint pain and produce excessive urine.

Because pregnenolone feeds production of so many other hormones, if you don't have sufficient levels of the one, you'll create a domino effect with the others—with a host of other symptoms following. For example, you might get the slack muscles and lack of hair under your arms and in the pubic area that signify low DHEA, or the low blood pressure and weight loss linked to low cortisol levels, or the low blood pressure and dizzy spells when standing up related to insufficient aldosterone.

PROGESTERONE is dominant during pregnancy and otherwise regulates the menstrual cycle. Its main job is to prepare the uterus for a fertilized egg by relaxing it while closing the cervix. Progesterone production reaches 40 mg per day in the second half of a regular menstrual cycle, skyrocketing to 500 mg a day during a normal pregnancy. That's a hor-mone world record—thousands of millions of billions of new hormone molecules created every day! During pregnancy progesterone acts as a "serenity hormone," lessening worry and bringing a sense of peace and sometimes even a little laziness.

In women progesterone is secreted mainly in the second half of the menstrual cycle. It prevents PMS, including bloating, irritability, anxi-ety, breast tenderness, and migraine, by balancing the estrogens that can promote these things. It also tones down heavy flow and eases painful periods.

Progesterone protects the heart and bones and has anticancer effects, particularly against endometrial and breast cancer. It can also help prevent endometriosis. Finally, progesterone relaxes and calms, reduces worry and nervousness, and provides better and deeper sleep. It can trigger a sense of deep tranquillity and inner peace.

Progesterone is made primarily in the ovaries as well as by the placenta during pregnancy. The adrenal glands produce small quantities in both men and women, and the testicles also make a small amount.

The most common sign of progesterone deficiency is painful, tender, swollen breasts before your period. Other signs include anxiety, aggression, irritability, bloating, bad headaches, and a tight and painful lower stomach before your period, painful periods with a hard and swollen belly and back, and extremely heavy periods. Without enough progesterone, your face, hands, and feet will be bloated as you retain water. Your facial muscles will be tense, and you'll have a nervous, aggressive look as if you are under a lot of pressure. Obesity in the lower half of the body, with a ballooning stomach, is another telltale sign. Your breasts can provide other clues to progesterone deficiency, including being too large and developing cysts. Ovarian cysts can also indicate insufficient progesterone, as can uterine fibroids.

TESTOSTERONE is often thought of as the hormone of virility. And while that's not wrong, it is important to realize its importance to both men and women. Testosterone stimulates the libido in both sexes. For men, testosterone is necessary for erections, ejaculations, and fertility; it prevents impotence. Testosterone stimulates love—sexual and otherwise—across the board.

Testosterone protects the heart and arteries and reduces the risk of heart disease. It can also counter high cholesterol and angina. Testosterone also protects the pancreas, kidneys, and digestive organs. It prevents joint and muscle pain, osteoporosis, and, in men, obesity. And men take note: Testosterone stops those outbursts of excessive sweat that in fact correspond to hot flashes in women.

Testosterone builds muscle and increases muscle tone, preserves bone mass, and reduces fat, including cellulite, firming up the body's contours (in men). It tightens and tones the skin, preventing dryness and small wrinkles. Testosterone keeps mucous membranes moist. It stimulates growth of hair, especially on the head—though a derivative, dihydrotestosterone, stimulates hair loss.

Testosterone increases your ability to withstand stress and reduces anxiety, depression, and excessive emotionality; provides energy and endurance; and contributes to a positive mood. With testosterone you have plenty of self-assurance, but also a desire for others' recognition. It helps you take initiative and makes you assertive, audacious, and mentally tenacious. It helps you face and surmount difficulties and helps put the petty annoyances of everyday life into perspective. In men it tends to spur "macho" behavior.

In men, the testicles produce most of the testosterone, though the adrenal glands also produce some. In women, the adrenal glands and ovaries produce testosterone, and estrogen is manufactured directly from testosterone.

Without enough testosterone, you'll suffer a loss of sexual desire. Men will have weaker erections and ejaculations, and women will lose clitoral sensitivity. Men's penises will get flabby and sometimes develop hardening that could lead to a deforming curvature during erection (Peyronie's disease). In addition, the foreskin might be too big and soft, the testicles soft and/or smaller, and the prostate thick, soft, irregular, and/or infected.

When testosterone is low, you feel fatigued day and night. You lose self-confidence and tend toward depression, anxiety, and excessive emotionality. Your sleep might be agitated. Your memory suffers. You lose your sense of creativity and become rigid in your attitudes, actions, and decisions. Men might experience hot flashes and more frequent outbursts of excessive sweat.

In testosterone deficiency, you'll get flabby cheek muscles, a pale face and skin, dry eyes, tiny wrinkles around the mouth and on the cheeks and at the corners of the eyes, and a listless expression. Lack of testosterone causes a "soft" appearance, with a hunched back, loose stomach, and fatty hips. Men will have poorly developed mustaches or beards and a lack or loss of hair on the torso.

THYROID HORMONES are made by the thyroid gland, situated at the base of the neck. What it secretes is primarily (90 percent) thyroxine (T_4). The secondary thyroid hormone, about 10 percent of what the thyroid gland secretes, is triiodothyronine (T_3). The pituitary gland is part of the act, too, as it releases a hormone (called, appropriately enough, thyroid stimulating hormone, or TSH) that stimulates the thyroid to release its hormones.

Since the greater part of thyroxine is converted into triiodothyronine in the liver, when I write about thyroid hormone, I am usually referring to triiodothyronine. It is the one that is truly active—between three and five times as active as thyroxine.

Thyroid hormones speed up metabolism and help control weight, thinning the face, torso, and calves in particular. They boost blood circulation, thereby increasing the supply of nutrients, oxygen, water, and hormones to cells all over the body. They keep the skin soft, flexible, and warm thanks to a good blood supply and improved production of sweat by the sweat glands. Thyroid hormones also keep muscles and joints supple and pain-free with this increased blood supply. They prevent dry hair, hair loss, puffy faces, and swollen eyelids. They prevent memory and concentration problems. Thyroid hormones are important in keeping you looking and feeling young and healthy.

Thyroid hormones energize all the cells and organs by stimulating the mitochondria—the cells' little powerhouses—freeing heat and energy. Thyroid hormones warm the body (and especially the extremities) and prevent excessive sensitivity to cold. They prevent morning fatigue, fatigue at rest, low mood (particularly in the morning), and general slowness. Thyroid hormones provide a certain quickness of mind. They protect not only the brain, but also the kidneys and the digestive and immune system organs, among other body tissues—the heart and arteries prime among them. They stimulate fat-burning and dissolve cholesterol, thereby opening up the arteries and moderating blood pressure as they encourage the elimination of waste from the cells and around the cells of the arterial walls, making them more supple. They prevent constipation by activating the smooth muscle cells of the intestinal walls and eliminating the swelling, and they help you avoid diffuse headaches, also by eliminating swelling and improving blood flow through the brain. Thyroid hormones reduce the risk and severity of heart disease, cancer, and other conditions with otherwise high mortality rates.

Without sufficient thyroid hormones, the body bloats. You'll have a particularly swollen face, with puffy eyelids and thicker lips—especially the lower lip. If that's not enough to make you want to ensure proper levels, you might also want to know that that effect is thanks to waste materials that accumulate between the cells.

You'll also have dry, rough, brittle, and sparse hair, lifeless eyes, a pale face, cold hands and feet, constipation, and dry skin. You'll have problems with memory and concentration. You'll get fat, without changing anything about the way you eat or how you exercise. You'll feel tired, especially in the morning and when you are resting. You'll feel cold, especially in the evening and when you are resting. You'll have stiff and painful joints, especially in the morning and after resting. Some people get slowed down in their movements and their thoughts, while others get agitated, hyperactive, and hyperkinetic, moving constantly, probably in an unconscious attempt to accelerate blood circulation and so the supply of nutrients and hormones to the tissues. In any event, you'll feel better when you are on the move than when you are still.

VASOPRESSIN sharpens attention and concentration, keeps you active, supports various memory functions, and creates a feeling of well-being.

The pituitary gland makes most of the body's vasopressin, but some brain neurons produce it for use as a neurotransmitter. It is secreted mostly at night. I think of it as another "memory hormone" since some of its most important functions are in that area. Vasopressin improves visual memory, recognition, and recall. It sharpens attention and concentration. It can even wake up failing memories, fighting memory loss.

Vasopressin's main roles are to keep us from losing too much water (in the form of urine), particularly at night, and to prevent excessive bleeding in case of injury. It can also reduce drug dependency.

If you don't have enough vasopressin, you are likely to experience memory loss and perhaps moments of confusion. Many people describe it as being unable to clearly see the difference between what is essential and what is incidental. You'll need to urinate too frequently and with urgency, especially at night. You'll often wake up to go to the bathroom. All that will be because your kidneys are producing too much urine, and the resulting water loss will give you the symptoms of dehydration: dry skin that stays folded for a while after being pinched; sharp wrinkles; excessive thirst; and thin, almost colorless, urine. In addition, you'll have low blood pressure and might experience heavy bleeding (if you have surgery or are injured, for example).

CHAPTER FOUR

WORKING WITH YOUR DOCTOR

*T*his chapter is all about how to get yourself the medical assistance you need and understand your doctor's approach. But before we get into that, I want to make sure you understand the key premise this chapter is built upon, which is that the doctor-patient relationship must be that of a team. Then we'll move on to finding a doctor, the steps to diagnosis, the available tests, how to interpret test results, and the limitations of tests.

No matter how many specialists you consult, you will always be the best expert on your own body. One thing I hope you learned from the self-tests, perhaps the most important fact they can reveal, is just how much you can tell about what's going on in your own body once you know how to tune in and really listen to what your body is telling you. Still, you don't have the clinical experience of objective education. You and your doctor have different skills and so different responsibilities, but working together is the most effective way to go.

Your doctor will start with a thorough history, and the more specific you can be in answering the questions and describing your symptoms, the more revealing that history will be. Be as precise as you can about how you feel and where, and when, and under what circumstances. Your job isn't done with the history, though. You need to monitor yourself just as closely as you embark on treatment, being equally observant of the changes you undergo as you were of your initial state in order to monitor your progress and fine-tune your program.

FIRST, FIND A DOCTOR

The first step to getting the best health—via the best health care—you must take on your own. That is, you must find the right health-care practitioner for you. Your internist or family practitioner or even psychiatrist might be able to guide you, as long as he or she is familiar with the techniques of multiple-hormone therapy. You could also ask for a referral to an endocrinologist, as they officially specialize in hormones. Either way, you want to make sure your doctor has plenty of clinical experience with all hormone deficiencies and multiple-hormone treatments. The only way to know that is to ask. (Even though an endocrinologist—the majority of whom focus on diabetes—might have learned about all the hormones in this book in theory, in practice he or she might not ever have used two-thirds of them.) Though there are fewer of them, most doctors who specialize in anti-aging medicine (not to be confused with gerontology, the medicine of aging) work with hormones, too, and might have some better experience in the hormones the endocrinologists aren't usually working with, like growth hormone, DHEA, and melatonin. See the Resources section at the back of the book for an organization that can help you find a doctor.

SEVEN STEPS TO
IDENTIFYING DEFICIENCY

Your doctor will go through a seven-step process in diagnosing you. To be a valuable part of the doctor-patient team, you should have a basic understanding of the process yourself, which is why I'm including it here. The thing to remember is that what is really important is the effect any given hormone is having (or not having) in your body, in its target cells. If the desired effect is insufficient, your most likely diagnosis is deficiency. Using the seven steps presented here, you can nail down a diagnosis so that you can move on to treatment.

1. Complete history, including all complaints and reported signs of deficiency. A detailed, in-depth review will allow your doctor to appreciate your real hormonal activity. Your doctor should cover with you all the possible complaints linked to the suspected hormone deficiency or deficiencies, including your current and past complaints—and your fam-

ily members' health issues, too. Your comments help the doctor confirm (or not) a deficiency, as well as give an idea of its importance.

2. Thorough physical exam, looking for signs of deficiency. A careful examination of your body will either support or dispel the symptoms described in the history—and the tentative diagnosis. It is also important to rule out any other, nonhormonal causes of your symptoms, as well as to clear you for treatment at the end of this process.

A good screening for hormone deficiencies should include a head-to-toe examination. Much of it might not even require touching, but your doctor should be *looking* at you quite carefully. As you'll see while reading through the various signs and symptoms, the details matter.

In addition to the tests discussed below, aimed at specific hormone levels, your physical should include, at least, a check of blood pressure and pulse, which can give clues to the status of various hormones, and a prostate check for men, and a breast exam for women.

3. Blood, saliva, and/or twenty-four-hour urine tests. Despite the problems we've discussed above, technical tests are always useful, and particularly so in borderline cases. These tests can help find the origin of the deficiency (and so help in choosing a treatment). They indicate the seriousness of the deficiency and whether it is likely to be reversible or correctable (as it almost always is with appropriate treatment). (See below for specifics about testing for particular hormones.)

4. Your age. The amount of hormone your body needs and makes shifts as you age, so your doctor should be factoring your age into any evaluation. By the time you are seventy, chances are you won't have enough melatonin, growth hormone, testosterone, estrogen, DHEA, and pregnenolone, just to name the most likely candidates. But levels don't just drop off as if over a cliff when you reach some predetermined age. They decline gradually over time, and the age when you'll start feeling the effects, and how, vary from one individual to the next. The sooner you pinpoint any deficiencies and take action, the easier the transition will be on you, the less damage your body will suffer, and the slower the aging process will appear to be. You rack up your birthdays at exactly the same rate, of course, but most of the negative signs and symptoms we think of as part of getting older are actually signs of hormone imbalance or deficiency and so are preventable and often even correctable if addressed in time.

5. Your doctor's clinical experience. Extensive experience with

patients and the effects of hormones (and the effects of not enough hormones) gives the best experts a kind of sixth sense. Good doctors' painstakingly developed intuition and knowledge allow them to have a good idea what to investigate most closely about you just about as soon as you walk into the room—when no other doctor you've seen has even suspected it. Your face, your hands, your body silhouette, the way you walk, how you look—all of these can reveal signs of one or more hormone deficiencies, pointing the experienced physician in the right diagnostic direction. This finely honed clinical sense can then be confirmed by the other steps discussed here, but your doctor's extensive experience in this area is an undeniable advantage to you.

6. Tests to rule out other conditions. Depending on which symptoms you are experiencing, it is crucial to undergo any necessary tests to rule out nonhormonal conditions. Hormones can do many things, but solving nonhormonal problems isn't one of them.

7. Your reaction to treatment. When your doctor makes a treatment recommendation, you might think the diagnosis part of the process is over. But really your reaction to the treatment is the final step in confirming or undermining the diagnosis. If the treatment works and your health improves, the diagnosis was correct. If it doesn't, the choice of treatment or the dose or form might need to be adjusted. If adjustments don't produce the desired effect, then the diagnosis must be refined or even changed. In some cases, when no other objective, technical test is available—as is often the case with melatonin—this kind of "therapeutic test" might be used early in the process.

TYPES OF TESTS

The history and physical, like the self-tests, will reveal the avenues that need further exploration. Your doctor should then order the appropriate tests.

Most doctors use two types of tests to evaluate hormonal levels: blood tests and urine tests. (Though you still can't get what many patients need at every lab, you can certainly find a lab that suits.) The best urine test for hormones is not the single sample you might be used to, but the twenty-four-hour urine analysis, which involves, as the name implies, collecting all your urine for an entire day and night and measuring the amount of a given hormone present. The good things about this are that it is not influenced by the many fluctuations in hormone levels throughout the day, confirms that the cells are using (and then needing to excrete derivatives of) the hormone, and tracks the active, free, bioavailable hormone (as opposed to one affixed to a blood protein and therefore not immediately available to the target cells). The drawback is that you get no idea of the daily rhythm of activity (and so can't pinpoint if there's a particular phase causing the problem).

On occasion, a twelve-hour, overnight urine test will suffice for hormones like melatonin or growth hormone that are secreted almost exclusively at night. The twenty-four-hour urine test is *not* a good option for anyone with kidney disease.

I always use urine analysis with a new patient, because it covers several hormones. Blood tests are easier, though. There are basically two types of blood tests. The first and most common is the simple measure of levels of hormones present. The second entails first injecting a substance that stimulates secretion of a particular hormone, then checking the resulting levels in the blood. The first tells you how much the body is making and using on its own; the second tells you basically that the body is still capable of producing the hormone, given the proper stimulus (though it might well not, in point of fact, be producing it on its own).

THE PROBLEMS WITH TESTS

Of course, rarely is it that straightforward. Consider, for example, what happens to the thyroid hormones starting with the nerve signal to secrete them until they manage to actually act on your cells. Just to get to the final active form of the hormone (T_3) is a multipart high-wire act involving various parts of the brain, several glands, the blood, the liver, and a team of precursor hormones. After that, the T_3 still has to get to the target cells, which it does by hitchhiking on large transport molecules in the blood. Then it has to extricate itself again from the fierce bindings those molecules make to reach its ultimate destination, whereupon it is dependent on the existence of special receptors, in sufficient quantity, to allow it to dock. Then and only then can it affect the target cells. Or, *begin* to affect the cells. The thyroid hormone still requires the presence of certain building materials and fuels to complete its projects. It needs amino acids, the building blocks it uses to make proteins, as well as the fuel from carbohydrates that it uses to activate the cellular machinery to do the job. Poor nutrition or bad digestion creates short-ages of these materials, short-circuiting the positive effects of the thyroid hormone.

I'm telling you all this so you understand just how many opportunities there are in this process for things to go awry. Even if you are tested and found to have low thyroid hormone levels, that test tells you nothing about where the actual problem is. In fact, all current blood tests can account for only two to four steps of the whole long chain. And they entirely overlook the most important point of all—the ultimate thyroid effect on your cells.

The point is, these are imperfect tests, even when perfectly executed and perfectly interpreted, which of course they aren't always. Perhaps their worst fault is that they don't uncover unobtrusive borderline hormonal deficiencies, deficits that are intermediate, and not yet catastrophic. By their very nature—beyond some line in the sand, you are deficient, otherwise you are not—these tests are "all or nothing." But when it comes to hormones, it is almost never a matter of "all or nothing." Most of us are neither grievously ill or in perfect health. Rather, we inhabit one of the many, many intermediate stages reflecting subtle glandular breakdowns.

Furthermore, those lines in the sand are somewhat arbitrary. Start with this fact: Every laboratory has its own set of "normal" values. Send the same blood to two different labs, and you might well be labeled deficient by one and normal by the other. Since each lab has its own equipment and techniques, it is to some degree logical for each to have its own values.

But there are problems with this system, the first of which is how they arrive at these "normal" values, deriving them from an analysis of (for large labs) thousands of blood samples they process. But most people who get tested for any given hormone are motivated by health problems. The lab doesn't go out and get a large group of people in excellent health to get their veins jabbed in the name of science (or another large group of people who are deathly ill, for that matter, either). The lab takes what comes to it, calculates the extremes, and—voilà!—everything in between them is "normal."

According to the laws of statistics, 95 percent of the studied group should fall into "normal" range. Only 2.5 percent of patients are slotted into "below normal," and another 2.5 percent into "above normal." But these levels have little or no relationship to those patients' actual states of health or the effects on their bodies of their current hormone levels. Almost everyone in the studied group was initially suspected of having hormone deficiencies or dysfunction. Why else were they being tested? One thing I can tell you for sure is that more than 2.5 percent to 5 percent of the general population would benefit from appropriate treatment for hormonal problems. I don't have the exact numbers, but I'd say the vast majority of adults seeing the signs of aging feel the effects of insufficient hormone levels.

Officially, *normal* means nothing more than "that which is frequently found," according to a leading scientific reference. But how many of us, including doctors interpreting test results, truly understand that? Personally and professionally, I always take "normal" with a huge grain of salt. Taking lab values together with what I observe in my patients clinically drives home the point that what "normal" really means is that we've gotten to the point where deficiencies are actually normal.

Furthermore, hormone levels change with age. Many labs will account for this, setting new "normal" levels for different age groups. This might sound meticulous, but often it can actually make the problem worse. Take, for example, estrogen, perhaps the most famously declining hormone, which plunges at menopause. In women sixty years old or older, the "normal" range is often between 10 and 40 pg/ml—the values obtained in 95 percent of women that age who are not taking hormone supplements. But that is, in point of fact, a deficiency. Even 55 pg/ml, a large margin above that usual upper limit of "normal," does not suffice. At that level, bones decalcify (soften and weaken), fatigue sets in, aging accelerates, and so on. Optimal levels of estrogen are actually between 70 and 180 pg/ml (the wide range accounting for the range of individual physical condition).

Normal values do not in any way define good health. All they do is give you an idea of the average hormonal levels of the other patients tested by that laboratory. They are often referred to as "reference values," which is at least better-sounding than "normal," though of course a semantic change doesn't compensate for the inherent problems. Either way, the thing to remember is that what you should strive for are *optimal* levels, and no current lab test can tell you that on its own. To top it all off, the optimal level of a hormone varies from one individual to another.

I'm grateful for every last advance of modern technological medicine. But as the issues surrounding these lab tests—relatively low-tech though they are—show modern technological medicine is not, and never will be, the be-all and end-all. If you had to rely only on the technology, statistics, and cutting-edge techniques, even if you could always trade up for the latest and greatest, you'd be missing out on the most powerful weapon we have when it comes to hormones: detailed histories and physical exams. When you interpret lab results within the context of what is observable to the observant patient and the experienced clinician, you're getting the best of both worlds. Lab tests alone can miss deficiencies that are clinically detectable or even obvious. The numbers might come back "normal" across the board, but a quick visit and a good dose of common sense tell you otherwise.

TESTING, TESTING

Here is a summary of the recommended testing for all the hormones discussed in this book, with the results that indicate deficiency.

ACTH

Your doctor will confirm a deficiency with a CRF (corticotropin-releasing factor) test. After taking a baseline reading, he or she will inject CRF into your veins to stimulate the secretion of ACTH. You have a deficiency if levels of ACTH and cortisol in your blood do not double in thirty to sixty minutes.

ALDOSTERONE

Your doctor can verify a lack of aldosterone in one of two ways. One choice is comparing two blood tests, taken when you are at rest, lying down, and then after you've been active. If the level is low or there is little or no increase in aldosterone with activity, you have a deficiency.

The other option is a twenty-four-hour urine analysis to detect low aldosterone levels (less than 5 mcg [micrograms] over twenty-four hours). That's likely to appear alongside too little potassium and too much sodium in the urine, despite a low-salt diet.

CALCITONIN

Verify a deficiency via blood test. Very low or undetectable calcitonin levels after stimulation with 3 mg of calcium (taken intravenously or orally to stimulate secretion of the hormone) means you are deficient.

CORTISOL

Your doctor can check your cortisol levels by analyzing blood or urine.

The free cortisol level in your blood measures the proportion of hormone that is active, ready to enter into the cells; a morning measurement of less than 10 ng/ml (or less than 5 ng/ml in the afternoon) indicates deficiency. That might be confirmed by checking the level of total cortisol (some of which might not be immediately available to the cells), which should be above 100 ng/ml in the morning and above 30 ng/ml in the afternoon. A final option might help pinpoint where your problem lies: ACTH test. Cortisol levels *should* double following an injection of 25 units of ACTH, and a failure to do so indicates deficiency. ACTH levels might be very high when adrenal glands (which secrete cortisol) are failing, while the pituitary gland (which frees ACTH) remains intact.

The level of free cortisol in a twenty-four-hour urine analysis measures how much cortisol the adrenal glands are producing; less than 20 mcg/dl indicates a deficiency. To measure how much cortisol is being used—not just how much is being produced—I prefer the more precise technique of gas chromatography to measure the level of 17-hydroxycorticosteroids (metabolites, or cortisol-derived molecules) found in the urine after cortisol has been used. For women, under 3.5 mg per twenty-four hours indicates deficiency. For men, the cutoff is 5 mg per twenty-four hours.

DHEA

Your doctor can verify a deficiency using a blood or urine test. The most reliable is the DHEA sulfate level in your blood. Average values in young people range between 150 and 450 mcg/dl. For women, levels under 150 indicate a deficiency; for men, the cutoff is 200. (And here's an extra bit of motivation for correcting a deficiency: A study of men over fifty found that levels below 140 increased the risk of heart disease and death two to three times.)

In a twenty-four-hour urine analysis, a DHEA level below 0.10 mg per day in women and below 0.50 mg per day in men indicates deficiency. To be safe, the sum of all DHEA derivative metabolites, called the 17-ketosteroids, should be at least 4 mg per day in women and 8 mg per day in men (using a 17-ketosteroid chromatography test).

EPO

A deficiency is indicated by EPO levels under 500 mU/l in the blood and by anemia (lack of red blood cells).

ESTROGEN

What you are looking for depends on whether or not you are menopausal, and, if you are not, when in your menstrual cycle you perform the test (with day one being the first day of your period). We'll look at blood tests first: In menopause, you want estrogen levels to be at least 70 to 80 pg/ml, especially to avoid osteoporosis. Before menopause, on the seventh day of your cycle, less than 50 pg/ml indicates deficiency; on the thirteenth day, less than 170 pg/ml; and on the twenty-first day, less than 100 pg/ml.

High FSH levels can indicate an estrogen deficiency—in general, more than 13 mIU/ml, though at ovulation mid-cycle it might climb to 25 mIU/ml. Only levels above 25 mIU/ml should concern you.

You can also check estrogen levels through urine tests, using a twenty-four-hour analysis (that is, using all your urine collected for one entire day). In menopause, total estrogen levels under 25 mcg indicate a deficiency. Before menopause, from urine collected in the second half of your cycle and definitely not during your period, total estrogen under 20 to 30 mcg indicates a deficiency.

GROWTH HORMONE

Confirming a deficiency isn't as simple with growth hormone as with many other hormones. Growth hormone levels are generally undetectable in the blood in men during the day, so there is no simple test. Levels are often checked after stimulation by substances that increase its secretion, like insulin or arginine, when less than 10 mcg/1 indicates deficiency. A better option is to check the levels of somatomedin C (or IGF-1), a close partner to growth hormone, which is released when the liver is stimulated by growth hormone. Somatomedin C levels under 150 mcg/1 indicate a deficiency in growth hormone. You can also ask to have your level of insulin-like growth factor binding protein 3 (IGF-BP-3) measured; if it is high (above 4,000 mcg/1), too much of the somatomedin C is bound to the IGF-BP-3, its blood transporter, and you probably don't have enough somatomedin C available, and so not enough growth hormone activity.

Alternatively, you can have a twenty-four-hour urine analysis. However, there is great variability in how much growth hormone a person secretes into urine as well as in lab analysis techniques and so results vary, and there is currently no consensus about what healthy levels should be. For now, the guideline I use is that if you find less than 2.5 ng a day—or none at all—you have a growth hormone deficiency.

INSULIN

The most basic way to verify a diagnosis of inadequate insulin is looking for glucose (sugar) in the urine. Any level detected in a simple urine analysis indicates a lack of insulin.

In the blood, a high glucose level (over 100 mg/dl) on an empty stomach indicates an insulin deficiency. You could also look for insulin levels on an empty stomach (less than 3 mcU/ml indicates deficiency). Too high, over 25 mcU/ml, or more than 10 mcU/ml on an empty stomach, marks the onset of, respectively, type II diabetes or simply insulin resistance. A high glycosylated (bound-to-glucose) hemoglobin HbA1 level (over 7 percent) indicates high blood glucose levels.

MELATONIN

Acceptable melatonin levels in the blood fluctuate between 15 and 35 pg/ml during the day and go above 100 pg/ml at night. If your levels are lower than that, you have a deficiency. In urine collected for twelve hours you could check for 6-sulfatoxymelatonin, the main derivative of melatonin. If it is low (under 25 mcg), your melatonin levels in the target cells are no doubt also low.

PREGNENOLONE

Pregnenolone testing is not available at all labs, in which case testing for hormones derived from pregnenolone might tell you what you need to know. Less than 1 ng/ml (100 ng/dl) of pregnenolone sulfate in your blood indicates a deficiency, which can also be indicated by low levels of cortisol, DHEA, aldosterone, and/or progesterone. You can also check the urine for low levels of the pregnenolone metabolites 17-ketosteroids (less than 4 mg in women, or 8 in men), 17-hydroxysteroids (less than 3.5 mg in women, or 5 in men), cortisol (less than 10 mcg/l free cortisol in the morning), and aldosterone (less than 5 mcg/24 hours).

PROGESTERONE

Progesterone levels in your blood under 10 mg/dl seven days before your period indicates deficiency. In a twenty-four-hour urine analysis, what is measured is actually pregnanediol, which is what progesterone is metabolized into. Levels under 2 mg per day in women during the second phase of the cycle indicate progesterone deficiency.

TESTOSTERONE

The best way to confirm a testosterone deficiency is via a blood test. The total testosterone levels should be above 6,000 pg/ml in men and above 200 pg/ml in women. Alternately, the free testosterone level should be above 120 pg/ml in men and above 4 pg/ml in women. You could also test for SHBG (sex hormone binding globulin). The higher the level of SHBG, the more testosterone is bound up and unavailable to the cells. Testosterone lowers the production of SHBG. Men's SHBG levels should be low, under 35 to 40 nmol/l—and optimally 25—and women's should be higher, above 55 and under 75 nmol/l—optimally, 65.

THYROID HORMONES

In the blood, *high* levels of TSH (above 4 mIU/ml and, in some cases, even above 2 mIU/ml) can indicate low thyroid activity. You'd also want to make sure you keep your free triiodothyronine level above 1.8 ng/l, and your free thyroxine above 0.8 or even 1.2 ng/dl. If your numbers fall below those, supplements are indicated.

In a twenty-four-hour urine analysis, watch out for low levels of triiodothyronine (under 1,500 pmol/24h) and/or thyroxine (under 1,800 pmol/24h).

VASOPRESSIN

A blood vasopressin level under 2 ng/ml indicates a deficiency. You get a less exact measure with a twenty-four-hour urine collection after seriously restricting liquids. The inability to raise the urine concentration—meaning your urine remains clear and abundant—suggests a deficiency.

PART II

BODY

CHAPTER FIVE

WEIGHT PROBLEMS

ola was a fat child. Her parents always had her on one diet after
another, but the weight was always very hard to lose—and immediately regained. That pattern repeated countless times, right through
adolescence and young adulthood, and Lola suffered a personal low point
when she started taking birth-control pills and put on an additional
twelve pounds. Fat accumulated everywhere: her belly, her breasts, her
hips, her thighs. She carried 229 pounds on her 5'7" frame. She developed high blood pressure before she turned thirty, and, by the time I met
her, was chronically depressed.

She was also totally discouraged. Her grandmother had fought the
same battle against obesity (unsuccessfully) her whole life, though the
rest of her family was of normal weight, and Lola was convinced this was
to be her fate, too. On top of that, she felt lousy much of the time.

As I listened to her complaints, I heard one after another that were
classic signs of low thyroid function, beginning with her depression and
the type of high blood pressure she had, with the diastolic ("bottom")
number being too high, more so than the systolic. She also had fatigue
that was most intense in the morning, daytime sleepiness, headaches,
cold hands and feet, exquisite sensitivity to cold, and swollen face and
feet. She also told me her father and grandmother had goiters, which are
a swelling of the thyroid gland that can be caused by low levels of thyroid hormone.

My exam backed up the theory I had created from her history. Lola
had a slow, weak pulse, dry skin, cold feet, and slow Achilles tendon
reflexes when I checked with a rubber hammer, all of which are signs of

thyroid insufficiency. Lab tests later confirmed the deficiency. In all of her years of going from doctor to doctor looking for a solution to her weight problem, no one had ever mentioned this possibility before.

Lola also complained of PMS, especially the bloating in her belly and breasts. That is often an indication of progesterone deficiency, and she had other clinical signs that pointed in the same direction, including overdeveloped breasts, swollen legs, hip and thigh obesity, and premenstrual sugar cravings. Blood tests confirmed this, too.

Lola told me that no matter what she ate, she never felt satisfied. She had a weakness for chocolate, but otherwise considered her diet reasonably healthful: lots of dairy products, whole-grain cereals and breads, and pasta. What she didn't know was that all of those foods not only stimulate weight gain in people with thyroid problems, but also promote hormonal *im*balance. I recommended a high-protein, moderate-calorie diet rich in vegetables and some mineral and trace element supplements to complement the hormones I prescribed (thyroid hormone and, in the second half of her menstrual cycle, progesterone). In the interests of sorting out which approaches were successful, I suggested she wait to change her diet until her body had a chance to adjust to the hormone supplements, which takes about two months.

Lola was the kind of patient doctors call "compliant." She followed my directions to the letter, and within two months her symptoms cleared up. Pleased with her newfound wellness and energy, Lola diligently set about changing the way she ate. After another two months, she'd lost nine pounds. But she seemed to be stuck at that level. And her complaints stemming from low thyroid levels, which had disappeared with hormone treatment alone, started to reappear—and they seemed to be even worse. She was back to being cold, slow to wake up, and tired in the morning. She also developed dry skin (again), which, like a stubborn weight-loss plateau, can indicate thyroid deficiency.

In some people, a high-protein diet can actually slow down thyroid activity. Fortunately, the solution was simple: Just a bit more thyroid hormone made a world of difference. Her symptoms went away, permanently this time, and she lost forty-four pounds over the next five months, and thirty-one more the five months after that. Her muscles firmed up, and she was free of fatigue, depression, PMS, high blood pressure—and, at 145 pounds, obesity. Hormones alone couldn't peel off all the weight—and you wouldn't expect them to—but rebalancing her hormones in conjunction with a hormonally supportive diet did allow her to finally control her weight in a way no diet alone had ever allowed her to do before.

IF NOTHING ELSE GETS YOU, MIDDLE-AGE SPREAD WILL

*I*t's one of the most common complaints I hear from my patients, both men and women. No matter what you do, the needle on the scale keeps moving up. You need to buy new pants once your old ones can't be let out anymore. You give up wearing sleeveless tops because of that wiggly thing that happens on your upper arms. More than half of Americans are overweight. After the age of fifty, make that 75 percent. (I get complaints of underweight, too, and we'll get to that next.)

The fact is, over the years, the human body tends to go soft. It loses muscle mass. It loses water. Fat builds up. Everything sags. Rolls of fat start to hang down over various parts of the body, distorting its contours and exacerbating the visual effects of the decrease in muscle tone. Whether you've always been heavy, like Lola, or whether weight-watching is a new concept for you, unless you take action, the numbers on the scale are going to creep up even faster than the number of candles on your birthday cake.

It usually seems to happen despite the attention we pay to what we eat and the time we devote to exercise. Or fighting it off requires more attention and time than we gave before. Even if you're lucky enough to have your weight stay the same, the loss of muscle mass means you won't look as trim as you did before. It's enough to make most of us throw up our hands, accepting the gradual buildup of unwanted pounds as part of getting older, as if it were inevitable.

It's not.

There are plenty of other books to advise you on what to eat and how to exercise to lose weight. There are even plenty of medically sound ones mixed in with the unrealistic quick fixes and questionable fads. And you will need to learn to regulate your calories through both what you eat and how active you are. That's a necessary start. But it is not enough.

You must also address the hormone deficiencies that underlie almost all accumulation of excess weight. Any diet that doesn't take hormones into account won't provide lasting results. When certain hor-

---

ON THE WEB

The best way to determine the healthiest weight range for you is to calculate your body-mass index (BMI), which takes into account not just height and weight, but also frame size and body fat content. You can do it by hand, but it takes a little bit of math (BMI=704.5 × weight in pounds/height in inches). So let your computer do it for you. Go to http://www.thusness.com/bmi.t.html.

---

mone levels drop with age, they not only encourage the body to store up extra pounds, but also trigger compensatory reactions from other hormones, creating a vicious cycle. Lola had weight problems all her life, but they seemed to get more stubborn as she got older. And her body seemed less and less able to handle either the excess weight or the stress of trying to get rid of it. She had hormone deficiencies to thank. The deficiencies she most likely had all along got worse when her body's hormone levels began to drop as she got older.

Even with balanced hormones, permanently losing weight takes time and effort. There is no magic-bullet hormone. But pairing well-balanced natural hormone therapy with better nutritional choices (like those described in chapter 17) tailored to your specific hormonal health should allow the loss of between nine and thirty-five pounds over one to four months. In all but the most serious cases of obesity, that's all you should need. Best of all, those pounds will come off just where you most want to lose them, where the fat "hangs over." Diet and exercise alone can't do that. In fact, losing weight that way sometimes has disappointing results: You don't *look* much different.

Losing larger amounts of weight will take a more concerted effort, including exercising at least three times a week and following an organized diet plan that's right for you. Psychological and emotional support, as in learning (and using!) stress-reduction techniques and fully expressing emotions, will also play an important role. Depending on your individual situation, you might need to abstain from certain foods (coffee, sodas, alcohol, simple carbohydrates, sugar, and dairy products being the most common bad guys). Finding the proper balance of hormones will allow even those who have fought this battle unsuccessfully before to achieve, at last, a healthful, stable weight—and tone up besides.

DETECTING AND DECODING YOUR DEFICIENCIES

To find the hormonal balance that will allow you to keep your weight steady, even as you age—winning the battle of the bulge once and for all—you need to figure out exactly where your imbalance is coming from. There are ten usual suspects: deficiencies in cortisol, aldosterone, DHEA, growth hormone, progesterone, testosterone, and thyroid hormones, and excesses of insulin, estrogen, or cortisol. But the specific answers are different for everyone. Running through the following series of questions will allow you to pinpoint the problem.

Is your face puffy in the morning? Are your cheeks swollen and puffed up? Are your eyelids swollen, forming heavy bags under your eyes, especially in the morning?

If so, your thyroid gland is probably not quite up to snuff. Talk to your doctor about getting the necessary tests to confirm the diagnosis and about taking **thyroid hormone** supplements. Your face should slim down within several months.

Is your face swollen like a full moon? Your adrenal glands are probably releasing **too much cortisol,** the stress hormone. That can happen when you are under intense or prolonged stress. Actually, the cortisol is useful to you, allowing you to handle even intense stress. It's just that the more intense the stress, the more cortisol you make—and the greater the likelihood of the unwanted side effect of a bloated face.

The "moon face" also often indicates **growth hormone and testosterone** insufficiency, which makes you more susceptible to stress. It creates a state of anxiety and perpetual agitation, so you perceive danger too often and too quickly. In response, your body releases a lot of cortisol in an attempt to cope with whatever stress you're facing (real or imagined).

The excess cortisol can also give you a sluggish thyroid gland and so perhaps a deficiency in **thyroid hormones.**

Talk to your doctor about testing and supplements. The correct natural hormones will not only firm up and slim down your face, but also calm your overstimulated state, restoring a more realistic outlook on life. In addition to the treatments you'll read more about, an important complementary approach is to take regular relaxing vacations, leaving all your stress behind. Doctor's orders!

Do you have a "buffalo hump"? The mound of fat that accumulates on the nape of the neck and upper back is caused by **excess cortisol.** Just as in the case of a moon face, lack of **growth hormone, testosterone,** and **thyroid hormones** is to blame—with stress being a contributing factor.

Talk to your doctor about testing and supplements, and cut way down on animal proteins and fats to reduce cortisol production. The fatty deformity should melt away.

For women: Are your breasts disproportionately large, especially before your period? Have they increased in size since they originally stopped growing at the end of adolescence? If a woman's **progesterone** levels drop too low, especially in relation to estrogen, her breasts can become tender and painfully swollen before menstruation. After years of deficiency, her breasts will become too heavy throughout her cycle. She's also likely to have premenstrual bloating in her belly; heavy, painful periods; and irritability and anxiety. On top of that, the excessive weight of her breasts can cause a stooped posture and back problems.

Talk to your doctor about taking progesterone. **Testosterone** and **growth hormone** might also be lacking, and supplements can, in addition to correcting a deficiency, tone up the muscles and skin on the chest and back, lifting the breasts.

For men: Are your breasts enlarged? Do they look like a woman's? Men's breasts begin to develop when they are not getting enough **growth hormone** and/or testosterone, as well as when they are overweight.

Talk to your doctor about supplements, including a **testosterone** cream (with dihydrotestosterone) that can be applied directly on the chest. The misplaced fatty tissue should melt away. This particular form of testosterone is important here. It is one of the two normal products of the breakdown of testosterone. This one can help decrease the size of

EAT TO HEAL

Animal proteins and fats can help increase both the male and female sex hormones. Women should avoid dairy products, however, as they too often contribute to yeast infections, which interfere with the delicate balance of estrogen and progesterone.

Unfortunately, many cooking techniques raise the temperature of the protein and fat high enough to change their molecular structure. Steaming, boiling, pressure-cooking, and slow cooking in a pan without butter or oil is more healthful and, with the right spices, tastier as well.

breasts. The other, estradiol—a form of estrogen—increases breast size. Sometimes, small doses of chrysin (100 mg/day) or anastrozole (0.25–0.5 mg/day) can be used, as they block the conversion of testosterone to estradiol.

Lowering your alcohol and coffee consumption, reducing your fat intake, and eating more meat should help.

Is your fat concentrated around your abdomen? Is your belly distended?

Low levels of **testosterone** might be to blame, in both men and women, though you'll need diet and exercise as well as a prescription for testosterone. **DHEA** might also be helpful for distended abdomens, though the proven results (impressive success within four months when used with targeted exercise) come from the experience of some (not all!) women with excess weight on their stomachs either after pregnancy or with aging. **Growth hormone** might be even more effective than testosterone.

Are your hips and thighs too well padded? Are you pear-shaped but overweight? Do you crave sweets or carbs? Are you a yo-yo dieter?

You are most likely producing too much insulin. One of insulin's jobs is to create a reserve of energy for the body, which it does by storing fat on the abdomen, hips, and thighs. This is basically preparation for famine. That's very rare in developed countries—we certainly have

SCIENCE SAYS

A deficiency in the newly discovered hormone **leptin** can create an enormous appetite—and particularly an appetite for fattening foods like simple carbs and dairy products. Obviously, big eaters gain weight, and all diets are doomed to fail if you feel hungry no matter what.

Experiments with mice and rats produced spectacular results proving that leptin curbed hunger pangs and prevented obesity. Trials in humans have just begun, and their progress will be well worth following closely.

the feast but no longer much real risk of famine. But insulin remains vigilant. Too much insulin results in too much fat.

Insulin's other job is to break down sugar in the body. High levels of insulin create hypoglycemia—severely low blood sugar—and the fatigue that comes with it. Most people then instinctively pounce on foods that will provide a burst of sugar, like sweets, pasta, bread, pretzels, soft drinks, and alcohol. That certainly increases blood sugar levels but provides extremely short-lived relief because it also spurs even more insulin production, creating a vicious cycle.

One clear way to break out of this self-destructive and self-perpetuating cycle is to stop eating sugar (including the simple carbohydrates that quickly convert to sugar, like pasta, bread, and cereal). But it's no wonder it is so hard to summon the willpower to do this: You are getting powerful biological messages from your body that this is a matter of survival (even though you know intellectually it is not).

Getting enough of four other hormones that, when present in sufficient quantities, help the body regulate insulin and sugar levels provides the missing link. They are cortisol (more slowly released in overweight people even in times of stress), thyroid hormone (often low in overweight people), growth hormone (often severely lacking in obese people), and testosterone (low particularly in overweight men, but also in some women).

Talk to your doctor about identifying and correcting any of these deficiencies you might have. Your sugar cravings will disappear because your physiological need for sugar disappears. You will need to follow a sugar-free diet (including avoiding the simple sugars of bread, pasta, and even dairy products) as well for at least three weeks to get back into balance, but then your body should be able to handle the moderate amounts of sugars contained in a healthful, well-rounded diet.

This combination is particularly effective for people who have struggled through many different weight-loss attempts, especially starvation diets (which are a very efficient way to initiate an excessive insulin problem because they lead to deficiencies in the four above-mentioned hormones).

In addition to helping control sugar and insulin, growth hormone and testosterone will help tone up the muscles of the abdomen, trimming the "pear" shape a bit.

Do you have "love handles"? Thick folds of skin and fat on the upper arm and under the shoulder blades? One important measure doctors use to assess whether someone is overweight is the "skin-fold" test—pinching the skin with a special instrument called a sphyngometer to measure the fat layer under the skin. The usual suspects are the back of the arm, halfway up the triceps muscle, under the shoulder blades, and along the sides (the "love handles"). I'm betting that, with the possible exception of the shoulder blades, you didn't need me to tell you that. If that test reveals too high a percentage of fat or if the signs above tell you all you need to know, talk to your doctor about growth hormone. With my patients, I have found up to a 70 percent reduction in skin-fold measurements with growth-hormone therapy, though something in the range of a 20 to 35 percent decrease is more usual. To get good results, you need to use it in conjunction with a well-tailored diet.

Testosterone can also reduce skin-fold measurements, in part because it raises the level of growth hormone (and somatomedin C) in the body, so you might want to look into taking both. Filling in any deficiency of testosterone is the best way to maximize results from growth hormone.

Do you have cellulite? Testosterone helps firm up the muscles of the thighs, and growth hormone rehydrates the shriveled "orange peel" skin, both of which reduce the appearance of cellulite. It can take several months, but even without diet and exercise, these two hormones can help you firm up your thighs.

An optimal diet can also give excellent results without hormones. Here again the goal is to reduce insulin, which is busily storing fat on your thighs. Eat mostly fruits and vegetables (make the fruit a separate meal or snack, and don't mix it with other types of food), along with meat and healthful fats to reduce insulin secretion. Avoid other carbohydrates (especially bread and pasta) and sweets. Coffee, tea, alcohol, and caffeinated sodas all stimulate the release of insulin, so they should be avoided too.

Exercise is another good way to reduce cellulite. The best results come, of course, from combining these methods.

Are your calves too heavy? Disproportionately so?

That's a sign of thyroid insufficiency. Talk to your doctor about testing and supplements. Treatment will diminish this symptom.

Are your legs and ankles swollen? Edema—swelling—in the legs is another sign of low thyroid levels. Talk to your doctor about testing and supplements.

It can also indicate an excess of aldosterone, which retains water and salt in the body. Taking 1 to 3 g of potassium daily should relieve the swelling. Resting during the day—especially lying down with the legs elevated—will also help.

If you have heart or kidney problems, which often come with leg swelling, consult your doctor about the possibility of adapting hormone therapy to the appropriate course of cardiac or renal medication.

EAT RIGHT

You'll get a detailed eating plan in chapter 17, but the main thing to keep in mind is to, like Lola, make sure you get the animal proteins and fats you need (a warning mostly to people who have been trying to avoid them—moderation is still in order) and to eliminate dairy products to support hormonal balance.

NUTRIENTS FOR WEIGHT LOSS

VITAMINS

Vitamin C: 1 g three times a day
Niacin: 10 mg daily
CoQ10: 100 mg daily
Vitamin D: 10 mg/day

MINERALS

Zinc: 10 mg daily

TRACE ELEMENTS

Chromium: 0.2–2 mg daily

AMINO ACIDS

L-glutamine: 500–2,000 mg daily
5-HTP (5-hydroxytryptophan): 10–50 mg one or two times a day
on an empty stomach at least a half-hour before a meal, and 25–50
mg one hour before bedtime
Tryptophan*: 500–2,000 mg four times a day one hour before
meals and at bedtime

FATTY ACIDS

Evening primrose oil: 2–8 g daily

*no longer available over the counter, but available by prescription

NUTRITIONAL SUPPLEMENTS

Sound diet and physical exercise are both essential to good health in
general and losing weight in particular. They are also important in creating hormonal balance—with and without taking hormone supplements—and retaining the vibrancy of youth.

Vitamin C and niacin lower blood lipid (fat) levels. In a study comparing vitamin C against placebo in patients following the same diet,

patients taking 3 g of C a day lost five and a half pounds in six weeks, compared to two pounds for those getting the placebo.

The coenzyme Q10 (CoQ10) and the amino acids L-glutamine and 5-HTP (similar to tryptophan, but FDA-approved in this country) also improve the results of weight-loss diets. Glutamine can blunt carbohydrate cravings, while tryptophan, which is generally low in obese people, and 5-HTP reduce sugar cravings. In one study of patients deficient in CoQ10 who took 100 mg of it a day for eight to nine weeks, patients lost an average of thirty pounds—compared to nine pounds in patients who were not deficient to begin with.

But the most important nutritional therapy for weight loss, particularly when excess insulin is the issue, is the trace element chromium, which lowers insulin levels in the blood. You get a bonus, too: Chromium lowers total cholesterol levels and increases the proportion of HDL ("good") cholesterol to LDL ("bad") cholesterol. At high enough doses—2 mg a day—chromium can reduce sugar cravings.

In patients needing to lose more than 10 percent of their body weight, omega-6 fatty acids can help. Evening primrose oil is one choice, and it reduces the appetite.

Many overweight people are deficient in zinc and vitamin D, so you might want to get yourself tested for those and take supplements to correct them as necessary.

YOU CAN BE TOO THIN

Weighing too little is most common in people over seventy, though it can happen to anyone, even young adults, teenagers, and children. A related complaint I get is, "I've gained weight all over, except where I *wanted* to."

A lot of people start to shed pounds unintentionally heading into their eighth decade. At first, their faces thin out. Then they lose weight in the arms, thighs, and legs. Then the hands and feet start to look bony. Usually the skin and hair thin out as well. Finally, weight is lost around the stomach. (Wouldn't you know that's the last to go! I've seen plenty of patients you might call spindly—but still with that old spare tire.) The culprit is, of course, hormonal imbalances.

People who are simply slim don't, of course, complain about their situation. Less popular (and assuredly less healthful) is the "just skin and bones" look, losing weight without meaning to, and being bent over even when you stand up "straight"—all signs of decreasing muscle mass. (Often decreasing bone mass and even organ volume—liver, kidneys, lungs—come right along with it.) That's one type of excessive thinness. The other is lacking in body fat (instead of or, most commonly, in addition to lacking muscle mass). Although both are most common in old age, either can occur as early as young adulthood—and even, occasionally, in children. Your particular signs and symptoms will point you toward which hormones you should be concerned about.

Are you underweight? Do you have muscle loss that is particularly noticeable in the biceps and triceps (arms), calves, pectorals (chest), and abdominals? Low levels of testosterone are probably to blame if the results are showing up especially in the areas of the body that are most different in men and women.

Have your shoulders and/or hips narrowed? Are your jaw and lips thinner? Are your hands and feet smaller and more delicate-looking? Are your hair and skin thinning, too? Have you developed a slump? You are most likely looking at a lack of growth hormone if you have lost muscle mass, particularly in the shoulders, pelvis, thighs, hands, feet, and jaw. The growth hormone provides volume to the muscles as well as supporting bone volume.

Lack of insulin, estrogen, and testosterone can add to the problem, as they stimulate production of a key component of growth hormone.

Have you lost weight all over your body? Have your cheeks thinned out? Have you lost fat even around your stomach? Have your buttocks lost their shape? Insulin is the hormone most responsible for fat production and it, too, tends to decline with age.

Have you lost your appetite? Do you have no cravings, with the exception of sweets? Do you tend to pounce on sweets? Blame cortisol—or rather lack thereof. If cortisol deficiency is severe, even excessive consumption of sweets won't make you gain any (or much) weight.

Prudent replacement therapy with the proper hormones can correct an underweight problem.

SUMMARY: WEIGHT-PROBLEM HORMONES

Hormone Deficiency	Symptoms	See also pg.
Cortisol	underweight; loss of appetite with sweets cravings (excess cortisol: moon face; thick neck; swollen shoulders; abdominal obesity)	26
DHEA	fat abdomen	27
Estrogen	narrowed hips; small or droopy breasts (excess estrogen: swollen face; large breasts; fat belly)	28
Growth Hormone	bloated face; lack of muscles; buffalo hump; large breasts (man or woman); fat hips and thighs; love handles and other skin folds; cellulite; narrowed hips and shoulders	29
Insulin	narrowed hips and shoulders; all-over weight loss/ lack of body fat (excess insulin: fat hips and thighs; cellulite; fat face)	30
Progesterone	large breasts (woman)	32
Testosterone	bloated face; lack of muscles; large breasts (man or woman); fat abdomen; fat hips and thighs; love handles and other skin folds; cellulite; underweight/muscle loss	32
Thyroid Hormones	puffy face in the morning; bloated face; fat hips and thighs; heavy calves; swollen legs and/or ankles	33

CHAPTER SIX

THE BEAUTY PRESCRIPTION: CARING FOR YOUR SKIN AND HAIR

There are all kinds of ailments that get more and more common with age, including America's number one and two killers—heart disease and cancer. But what do you worry most about? I don't have any official statistics, but I'd say we've already covered the big one—weight gain. The subject of this chapter follows closely behind: wrinkles and gray hair. We can rail all we want to about impossible standards of beauty and an ageist society that idolizes youth. But to tell the truth, this is what really gets to us—our skin and hair. We think it's what makes us look old.

And we're right. Not only about looking old—*unnecessarily*—but also, as it turns out, about putting our energy into worrying about them. The immediate problem is superficial. But these aesthetic problems signify hormone deficiency and imbalance. They are a message from our bodies that all is not well, so there are more reasons than vanity to pay attention to them. Any hormone deficiency is going to be causing more problems than just what you see in the mirror. Correcting any imbalance isn't just a matter of improving the way you look; it will address physical problems, perhaps stopping them before they impact your quality of life or even before you notice them. You'll be reading more about that in upcoming chapters. For now we'll focus on maintaining healthy hair and skin—erasing wrinkles, fighting fine lines and thin skin, reversing hair loss, maintaining hair color, and so on. Just remember, beauty might be only skin deep, but health and hormones are total-body experiences.

Take Nicole, for example. She was nearing fifty when she came to see me. She had a list of complaints to share with me, but the thing that finally convinced her to make an appointment wasn't how she was tired even when she was at rest and especially in the morning. It wasn't the host of digestive problems, including constipation, nausea, and stomach pains. It wasn't that she was often depressed or anxious or that her hands and feet were swollen or that she had terrible PMS, with particularly bad bloating of her belly. No, what ultimately brought her into my office was that her hair was falling out. What was left was thin and flat. She'd been losing it slowly over the last few years. Lots fell out every time she washed it. By now Nicole estimated she had only half the hair she started out with.

Apparently, Nicole had learned to live with a lot of bothersome things. But she did not want to live with balding anymore! She was afraid she was going to have the Telly Savalas/Michael Jordan look before long, and while it worked well for those guys, Nicole just didn't see it for her. She was, of course, glad to hear that proper treatment could not only stop the hair loss, but also reverse the condition—and that the same treatment would also likely clear up her other nagging symptoms, as the underlying problem (hormonal imbalance) was the same.

I suspected low thyroid function because of her fatigue, depression, swollen hands and feet, cold feet, dry skin, and the fact that she was slowly gaining weight, especially on her abdomen, and losing hair all over her head (and what was left was thin and dry). On exam I could see her extremities were bluish red because of lack of oxygen and she had a slow Achilles tendon reflex, typical signs of a sluggish thyroid.

Nicole also had symptoms of low cortisol levels: the stomach troubles and nervousness I mentioned as well as frequent sugar cravings, drowsiness, and sensitivity to stress. On top of that, her fatigue combined with an excessive need for sleep, dry mouth, droopy breasts, and above-average weight—along with hair loss predominantly from the top of the head—suggested estrogen deficiency. Nicole's PMS and nervousness suggested low progesterone, although she was taking birth-control pills (estrogen and progesterone), as she had since she was a young adult. Finally, I thought Nicole was most likely low in testosterone, as her muscles seemed loose, especially on the belly, and so much of her weight gain was in the abdominal area.

After lab tests confirmed all these deficiencies, Nicole started taking natural thyroid hormones (derived from dried pig thyroid glands), moving slowly up to 120 mg a day. She kept taking the Pill, and also added DHEA and cortisol (in the form of hydrocortisone). This natural cortisol has to be taken in divided doses because the body uses it up so quickly, so Nicole took small doses three times a day. Within two months she felt much better in almost every respect, and she had begun to lose weight. Ironically, the first thing that brought her in for a consultation was the last thing to respond to treatment. Her hair loss slowed soon enough, but reversing it took longer. (While most patients feel a difference very quickly, it is not unusual for hormone therapies to work their full effects slowly.) Within two years, new hair had grown in, and Nicole was sporting a full head of hair.

WHY WE WRINKLE

Not every bare head is going to sprout a new thicket of hair, and you are never going to get rid of every last line on your face. While hormone deficiencies cause both hair and skin problems, they aren't the only contributing factors. Correcting the imbalance, then, can fix only what's attributable to the hormones in the first place.

Wrinkles, like scarring, damage tissue and can't be undone. (Another argument for prevention over treatment.) More important is the contribution of free radicals to the signs of aging. Free radicals, the inescapable product of our bodies' use of oxygen, are unstable molecules

---

SKIN-CARE ALERT

Strategies for keeping your youthful looks don't get any simpler than this: Avoid excessive sun exposure. That means staying out of the sun, particularly during the peak hours of the day (10 A.M. to 3 P.M.), and wearing liberal amounts of full-spectrum sunscreen (blocking UV-A *and* UV-B rays). The sun's ultraviolet radiation effectively creates a vitamin A deficiency—which, in practical terms, means the toughening and wrinkling of the skin. It also causes skin cancer.

WHAT THE FUTURE HOLDS: HORMONE FACELIFT

Theoretically, you could achieve nearly total disappearance of wrinkles with the proper combination of large numbers of hormones. Ten to twenty hormones used as a team in places where blood supply is poor, part of them injected locally during the earlier stages of treatment, could almost totally renew the skin and surrounding tissues. I believe that time is coming, though two important pieces of groundwork have yet to be laid—the ability to buy all the hormones in pharmacies, and the ability to balance all the hormones against each other and against those already in the body.

that cause minimal but continuous deterioration of our cells. Given enough time—that is, as we get old enough—the deterioration starts to show. That's what we see as the signs of aging. Although wrinkles might indicate acquired wisdom and confer a different kind of attractiveness, most of us would rather have fewer of them—and not so soon!

The good news is that, to the degree aging skin is the result of hormonal deficiencies, we can slow, stop, and sometimes reverse the process by filling in the deficiencies. The right combination of hormones can firm up the tissue, skin, and muscles of your face in a kind of nonsurgical face lift. Growth hormone is the most powerful in most cases, followed by estrogen and testosterone.

HAIR TODAY, GONE TOMORROW?

We lose, on average, one hundred hairs a day. We also grow one hundred hairs a day. When we're young, we have about 100,000 hairs on our heads. Even if no new hair grew, which is rare, it would take almost three years to lose all your hair. So, you have time. Within that time, you can find and correct any hormonal deficiencies that are causing the loss and the lack of growth. Even if your hair is coming out more quickly—by the handful—you can often slow, stop, or reverse the process by properly balancing your hormones.

If any of this applies to you, you will no doubt recognize the powerful fear losing your hair can inspire. You might be interested to know that that kind of fear (of losing your looks, your youth, your health) itself comes, at least in part, from a lack of the hormones that provide calm and self-assurance—often the very same hormones behind the hair loss. Addressing any imbalance will not only improve the situation on top of your head, but within it as well. Then, even if your hair situation remains less than perfect, you might well care much less about it.

Right up there with hair loss on the list of concerns about aging is hair that's going gray or white. Hair gets its color from the pigment melanin, which is produced by small cells at the base of the hair follicles. The number of these cells—between 1,000 and 2,000 per square millimeter—decreases with age, and the activity of those that remain declines as well. As a result, the hair receives less and less melanin and progressively loses its color. Gray hairs have lost a lot of pigment; white hairs have lost practically all of it. Though there is not yet a proven, direct hormonal treatment for this situation, restoring hormonal balance does seem to help prevent the appearance of gray and white hairs. Many of my patients taking hormones for various reasons experience some recoloring of their hair as a kind of bonus side effect. ACTH in particular seems to be useful in this way, though I wouldn't prescribe it for hair color alone.

Even male pattern baldness, at least if it is recent, might reverse with hormonal treatment. I experienced this personally when my hair started to fall out a few years ago. In my mother's family, all my uncles are almost completely bald, with just a little hair left near the ears and at the back of the head. My brother is equally bald. I felt lucky to have kept my hair so long, but as I reached forty, it began to fall out quicker and quicker. After nearly two years of trying different products, I found what worked for me: increasing my deficient testosterone levels with a transdermal testosterone combined with a tablet of finasteride, which blocked the conversion of testosterone into dihydrotestoerone, which is associated with balding, and a nightly application of polyunsaturated fatty acids (vegetable oil). I don't know who was happier, me or my wife, to see that within six to twelve months my hair grew back much as it was before, at least three times denser and thicker than in the worst period of hair loss.

WHAT THE FUTURE HOLDS: GOOD-BYE GRAY

Leaving aside hair dyes, there is no 100 percent effective treatment for gray hair on the market right now. I think there will be one some day and that it will be based around the hormone MSH (melanocyte-stimulating hormone), secreted by cells at the base of the hair follicles that release melanin—the melanocytes. Produced by the pituitary gland, this hormone stimulates the production of melanin. One (albeit unproven) explanation about why hormone therapy recolors some patients' hair is that the hormones that help give more color to the hair actually boost the production or effectiveness of MSH. It should also be noted that ACTH is structurally quite similar to MSH, which might one day end up explaining why ACTH seems to be particularly good in this area.

Studies using MSH alone in elderly people have not produced satisfactory results. On the other hand, one researcher experimenting on himself regained color in his hair after taking MSH together with large doses of B vitamins. As work continues, two things seem clear: MSH will ultimately play a role in maintaining our natural hair color, and it will work best in conjunction with excellent nutrition.

NOURISH YOUR SKIN

No matter what your hormone levels, there are important ways you can nourish your body, and specifically your skin, to keep it as healthy and young as possible. At the very least, make sure you are not deficient in the nutrients covered here. Better yet, look into high-quality supplements.

You already know that you need to avoid overexposure to the sun to protect your skin from aging and particularly from skin cancer. What you might not know is the mechanism by which sun exposure brews up trouble, which is that the sun's UV radiation effectively creates a **vitamin A** deficiency. Furthermore, vitamin A is an antioxidant, meaning it neutralizes free radicals, making it an important weapon in the battle to maintain your skin in general. Vitamin A is particularly good at countering liver or age spots.

The **B vitamins** are just as important. A general deficiency leads to easy bruising, so a B complex is a good idea. The individual B vitamins help with particular conditions as well. **Riboflavin** can heal small cracks on the edges of your lips as well as the oily or greasy skin inflammation known as seborrheal dermatitis on the sides of the nose, the earlobes, and/or the edges of the eyebrows. Insufficient **niacin** can cause redness of exposed skin, as on the face, neck, and hands, or skin that reddens seemingly at the drop of a hat. **Pantothenic acid** helps heal sores, burns, and cracks in the skin; lack of it can cause brittle, poorly growing nails, loss of hair, and skin ulcers. **Folic acid** deficiency brings on eczema-like lesions, cold sores, and acne.

Vitamin C is another powerful antioxidant and so an important addition to your arsenal. In addition, it speeds healing of wounds. Deficiency results in scurvy, which manifests as, among other things, purplish patches where blood is leaking into the skin, and small reddish spots under the skin.

Vitamin E, too, fights free radicals as an antioxidant, so it is good in general for keeping your skin healthy. It is particularly useful if you are dealing with liver or age spots.

The trace element **selenium** is another antioxidant and should also be at the top of your list for protecting your skin against aging. It is beneficial just in general, and in particular for liver or age spots. The foods richest in selenium are meat and fish and vegetables. But note that garlic, onions, and mushrooms contain essentially none, so use them to enhance your meat, fish, and vegetable dishes, but don't expect any added selenium. **Manganese, copper, zinc,** and **iron** should fill out the list. Manganese deficiency can cause eczema; insufficient zinc can cause acne; and if you don't have enough iron you might develop split ends in your hair and brittle nails. Lack of copper can cause eczema, psoriasis, and gray hair. It is particularly indicated if you are extremely sensitive to the sun.

Finally, one hormone and two enzymes round out the group of best antioxidants: The hormone is melatonin, and the enzymes are **superoxide dismutase** and **catalase,** which can slow down the aging of the skin.

NOURISH YOUR HAIR

*H*ealthy hair also requires good nutrition, whether or not you end up using hormones. If you are losing your hair, and what hair you have is untamed and full of split ends, suspect an **iron** deficiency. If you are losing your hair, and what hair you have is dry and unmanageable, you might not be getting enough polyunsaturated fats. When hair loss is accompanied by dandruff and itching (mycosis of the scalp, actually a yeast infection), try avoiding milk products, bread, and other foods with yeast and refined carbohydrates and sugar.

As for hair that's losing its color, make sure you supply it with plenty of the nutrients necessary for melanin creation: **cysteine, copper, thiamine,** and **vitamin B$_6$,** all of which are less well absorbed as you age, meaning you have to take in more to get the same effect you used to.

DECODING YOUR DEFICIENCIES

SKIN

Do you have large wrinkles that cover your face, especially on either side of your nose and mouth? Do you have flabby, fallen cheeks (giving you a "bulldog" look)? Do you have drooping eyelids or forehead creases? Growth hormone can decrease or erase these signs if you are deficient.

Do you have little wrinkles around your eyes (crow's feet) or smile lines? These signs will soften and at least partially disappear when you correct any deficiencies in testosterone and estrogen.

Have tiny vertical wrinkles appeared around your lips? In women, lack of estrogen is a cause; in men, it's lack of testosterone that should be suspected.

Do you have a double chin? A double chin or wrinkled skin that hangs in large vertical folds under the chin indicates a combination of hormonal deficiencies, the main one being growth hormone.

Are your cheeks crumpled like old paper? Do you have thinning or furrowed eyelids? You'll regain a more appropriate tone if

NUTRIENTS FOR HEALTHY HAIR AND SKIN

VITAMINS

Vitamin A: 1–10 mg daily
Thiamine: 5 mg daily
Riboflavin: 5 mg daily
Niacin: 10 mg daily
Pantothenic acid: 15 mg daily
Folic acid: 1 mg daily
Vitamin B_6: 20 mg daily
Vitamin C: 300–500 mg daily
Vitamin E: 10–50 mg daily

MINERALS

Zinc: 10 mg daily
Copper: 0.7 mg daily
Iron: 25 mg daily
Manganese: 6 mg daily

TRACE ELEMENTS

Selenium: 25 mcg daily

AMINO ACIDS

Cysteine: 80 mg daily

ENZYMES

Superoxide dismutase: 25 mg daily
Catalase: 20 mg daily

you correct any growth hormone deficiency. Lack of testosterone causes a more moderate form of aging skin (for men and women both).

Do you have age spots? Do you have brown folds on your palms? Scars that are hyperpigmented? Irregular brown spots on the skin? These excessive colorations of the skin are just the accumulation of a pigment known as lipofuchsin, which is made up of oxidized fats. Deficiencies of melatonin, growth hormone, and DHEA favor them. So does excessive ACTH, which stimulates melanin production. Cortisol also has a role. In cortisol deficiency, many people make excessive amounts of ACTH in a desperate attempt to spur cortisol production; excess ACTH leads to spots of hyperpigmentation.

In addition to correcting any hormonal imbalances, make sure you are getting enough vitamin A, vitamin E, and selenium.

Do you have skin cancer? Have you had any precancerous growths removed?

Over time, some skin cells become irregular, predisposing you to getting skin cancer. Limiting your sun exposure helps prevent this, but you should also make sure you are getting sufficient thyroid hormones and melatonin. These hormones might boost the immune system and protect the skin against cancer.

Do you have dry skin? With a lack of thyroid hormones and growth hormone, the sweat glands, which secrete water, atrophy, and without enough estrogen, testosterone, and DHEA, the sebaceous (oily) glands atrophy. With either or both, the outer layer of your skin gets less hydrated.

Do you have thin skin? The inner layer of skin thins over time, particularly when there isn't enough growth hormone, estrogen, testosterone, and DHEA.

Have you gotten paler? Deficiencies in estrogen, testosterone, and thyroid hormone lessen the blood flow to the skin, which makes the skin paler.

Do you have a lot of wrinkles? Insufficient growth hormone and testosterone interfere with the interconnection of the layers of the skin, creating wrinkles.

Are you sensitive to the sun? After you pass thirty, the number of pigment cells in the skin diminishes. Deficiencies of ACTH, testosterone, and growth hormone can stimulate this effect. Besides correcting your hormone balance, you should make sure you're getting enough copper.

Is your skin slow to heal (from burns, cuts, scrapes, insect bites, etc.)? Cells rebuild themselves more slowly as you grow older, particularly in the outer layer of the skin. A deficiency in growth hormone or testosterone can be behind it. You should also take zinc, the trace element most important to wound healing.

Do you bruise easily? That happens when your capillary walls get thin and fragile, which is a result of growth hormone and testosterone deficiency. That can also make your skin less sensitive, and less reactive, which increases the risk of the sort of accident that would leave you bruised. Besides hormone supplements, you should look into getting plenty of B vitamins and vitamin C.

Do you have bruises and minor skin wounds? First, fat thickens and accumulates under the skin, and then the tissue thins out and becomes fragile, thanks to insulin deficiency (or lack of efficiency of insulin). The subcutaneous fat acts as a shock absorber. Without enough insulin, there is not enough shock absorption.

Is your skin easily abraded? Low levels of testosterone and growth hormone can cause a flattening of the sometimes chaotic network under the top layer of skin, which toughens it somewhat.

Does your skin emit fewer and less intense sexual odors than it once did? Don't underestimate how important this is to your sex drive and your sex life. Look for deficiencies in testosterone and DHEA.

HAIR

Do you have dry, brittle, thick, slow-growing hair? Are you losing the hair all over your head bit by bit? Appropriate treatment with thyroid hormones (at least four months' worth) will get you back to normal.

Has your hair lost its shine, waves, body, or natural highlights? Is it thin and wispy? Is it thinning out all over your head? Growth hormone deficiency is the likely cause.

Is your hair disappearing from the top of your head? Blame a lack of testosterone and an excess of dihydrotestosterone, men. As your hair has been vanishing, your testosterone level has most likely been decreasing, too. The resulting imbalance in male hormones is behind the hair loss—not, as popular mythology holds, an *excess* of male hormones. The good news is that correcting the deficiency and slowing down the conversion of testosterone to dihydrotestosterone will stop the hair loss and maybe even restore hair. Men under twenty-five with this pattern often have lower than average testosterone levels, and supplements in physiologic doses usually allow them to regain a full head of hair. After twenty-five, the best result expected is no further hair loss with testosterone alone, but improvement with assistance from a blocker of the testosterone-to-dihydrotestosterone conversion. The latest findings suggest an excess in dihydrotestosterone, which is responsible for body-hair growth, is to blame for male pattern balding, and my personal experience suggests there is a link between that and a lack of testosterone.

Women with this type of hair loss do often have high levels of male hormones, but that's not the most important fact. More to the point is that they are also often low in female hormones—estrogen and progesterone. So they also have irregular periods, difficult or unusual periods, and PMS. Restoring the balance will restore the hair.

Low cortisol might also be at fault for women. That spurs an increase in DHEA and testosterone in an attempt to compensate, which suppresses the production of female hormones. Taking supplemental cortisol calms the overly excited adrenal glands and reactivates the ovaries. Testosterone will fall, estrogen and progesterone will rebound, and (given enough time; results always take at least three to four months) the hair grows back completely.

Is your hair disappearing in circular patches? You might have a deficiency of ACTH or cortisol. Correcting them, along with supplements for any other deficient hormones, particularly thyroid, will restore a full head of hair. Don't expect major improvements until you've been on treatment for four months.

If this pattern of loss is accompanied by dandruff and itching, you might have a fungal or yeast infection known as mycosis of the scalp, and you should try a fungicidal shampoo (ask your pharmacist) together with a diet devoid of yeast, sugar, and dairy products to clear it up.

HAIR-LOSS ALERT

If you're serious about restoring a full head of hair, skip the temptation to try a wig in the meantime. Wearing a wig slows down the blood flow to the scalp, preventing full effectiveness of the helpful hormones.

Are you entirely bald (or getting there)? You should suspect deficiencies in a series of major hormones. Pituitary gland secretions have dried up, and most of the other endocrine glands, which are essential for hair—and dependent on the pituitary glands (adrenals, thyroid, ovaries, and testicles)—have weakened. Discuss with your doctor ACTH, growth hormone, DHEA, thyroid hormones, testosterone, and/or estrogen (together with progesterone).

Women: Are you losing hair in your pubic area and/or armpits? You probably have a deficiency of DHEA.

Men: Are you losing hair on your abdomen (between your pubic area and your bellybutton), legs, or chest? Is your beard sparse? These are signs of testosterone deficiency.

Women: Do you have unwanted hair? Hair under the nose, on the chin, breasts, lower abdomen (between the pubic area and the bellybutton), thighs, legs, and arms is often blamed on excess male hormones, but in reality it is more likely to occur in women low in estrogen. They are likely to also have soft, weak muscles and be tired and depressed. They might also be low in testosterone but have at the same time greater deficiencies in the female hormones estrogen and progesterone. Sometimes a lack of cortisol is to blame, as it triggers an increased secretion of male hormones to compensate. Taking hormone supplements lessens—or even erases—the growth of undesirable hair. To get good results, you must make sure you are eating enough calories and address any digestive problems. It takes six months of treatment to start noticing a decrease in unwanted hair, and one to four years to have complete results, because a body-hair follicle stays about four years in the skin.

KURT

Kurt was at the end of his college career when he came into my office. He was completely bald—and not just on his head. He had no hair anywhere on his body. Nothing in his armpits or in the pubic area or covering his arms or legs, no beard, nothing. The problem had appeared quite suddenly two years before after an otherwise minor infection. He'd been to various experts in an attempt to get his hair back, all to no avail. Nothing helped, and all the doctors he consulted eventually told him there was nothing more they could do and he should learn to live with it.

Simple blood and urine tests showed Kurt had low levels of ACTH and thyroid hormones. Thyroid hormones are known to help with diffuse hair loss and ACTH treatment with total loss of hair, so Kurt started right away on a program of two injections a week of a slow-release ACTH formula and a daily dose of thyroid hormones. After two months, the hair on the top of his head was nearly completely restored. After the addition of testosterone to the regimen, the hair on the sides of his head, around his ears, grew in thickly, and hair sprouted all over his body in the expected places—including a decent beard.

We experimented once with stopping the ACTH injections, though all we succeeded in doing was verifying their importance: He lost his hair again, then regained it when he resumed the injections. Ten years later, continuing his multiple-hormone therapy, Kurt is a triathlete with a full head of hair. He shaves every day.

Is your hair turning gray or white? Treatment with testosterone and growth hormone (and perhaps ACTH, though it is not easy to use and so rarely is) sometimes spurs repigmentation of hair that has gone gray or white. Fading hair does not necessarily indicate a deficiency, and you shouldn't take hormones just to address hair color. But if you have a confirmed deficiency and take the hormones for another reason, this might be one of your side benefits. In any event, you might find cysteine, copper, thiamin (vitamin B_1), vitamin B_6, and sulfur to be useful supplements.

SUMMARY: BEAUTY HORMONES

Hormone Deficiency	Symptoms	See also pg.
ACTH	losing hair on head in circular patches; sun sensitivity; entirely bald; hair turning gray or white	25
Cortisol	hair loss in patches; in women: hair disappearing from top of head; unwanted body hair	26
DHEA	age spots; dry skin; loss of sexual odors; balding all over the head; in women: losing hair in pubic area and/or armpits	27
Estrogen	tiny vertical wrinkles around lips; dry skin; thin skin; pale skin; balding all over head; in women: hair disappearing from top of head; unwanted hair; little wrinkles around eyes; smile lines	28
Growth Hormone	lots of wrinkles; large wrinkles on sides of nose and mouth; small wrinkles around eyes or mouth; creased forehead; double chin; dry skin; thin skin; slow healing; easily bruised or scraped; hair that has lost its waves, body, highlights; thin, wispy hair; hair thinning on top of head; balding near the ears; gray hair; thin eyelids; cheeks look crumpled	29
Insulin	bruises or minor skin wounds; gangrene; skin infections; insensitivity or tingling of skin on the feet	30
Melatonin	age spots; skin cancer	30
Progesterone	balding on top of head; in women: hair disappearing from top of head; unwanted body hair	32
Testosterone	lots of wrinkles; small wrinkles around eyes or mouth; creased forehead; dry skin; thin skin; pale skin; sun sensitivity; slow to heal; easily bruised or scraped; loss of sexual odors; balding on top of head (with excess dihydrotestosterone); gray hair; in men: losing body hair on abdomen, legs, chest; sparse beard	32
Thyroid Hormones	skin cancer; dry skin; pale skin; dry, brittle, slow-growing hair; balding all over the head	33

CHAPTER SEVEN

SMOOTH JOINTS

A certain number of aches and pains come with aging . . . or so it seems. Unchecked, they can eventually interfere with your normal activities, right down to getting out of bed, going up or down stairs, walking, even getting dressed. But none of that is inevitable or necessary.

You'll need to get sufficient appropriate exercise, of course, and, in some cases, physical therapy, although that is beyond the scope of this book. What *is* covered here are the hormonal and nutritional strategies that can lessen pain, revitalize damaged joints, and even get at and eliminate the causes of some conditions.

I couldn't cover every kind of chronic pain in one book, let alone in one chapter. Here you'll find the symptoms most associated with hormones, which include rheumatoid arthritis, osteoarthritis, carpal tunnel syndrome, gout, lupus, and fibromyalgia. I spend the most time on arthritis (which itself refers to more than one hundred conditions) because it is incredibly common: About forty-three million Americans have it—about 18 percent of the population. More women are affected than men (another clue that hormones might be at play); about 62 percent of cases are in women. Arthritis is the leading cause of disability in this country, seriously restricting activity for about eight million people. And that's just the people limited in very basic ways and doesn't take into account those who have had to give up "optional" things, like their beloved tennis or knitting or piano or skiing or weekend hikes with grandchildren, and so on.

DIANE

*I*t was obvious what ailed Diane as soon as she walked in. She moved so slowly, so excruciatingly carefully, calculating every gesture to cause the least pain, it was almost hard to believe she had once been a talented and versatile athlete. Only in her mid-forties, she should still have been hitting the track and the slopes whenever she wanted. Instead, the pain in her joints had gotten so intense that not only was she no longer physically active, but she had had to quit her job, and even daily household tasks were often beyond her.

Though Diane was pleasant and friendly, she looked pale and tense. And no wonder: Nearly all her joints, from her feet to her neck, were sore and provided a sharp pain with any sudden movement. Both her hands were becoming deformed by the inflammation. Every time she got any type of infection, be it the flu or bronchitis or just an average cold, it brought on a severe rheumatoid crisis (severe inflammation of the joints to the point she could walk only with difficulty) that took weeks to months to recover from—at the end of which the baseline state of her joints would be even worse.

This had been going on for five years. She'd tried many different treatments with several different doctors—anti-inflammatory medications, painkillers, high doses of steroids, vitamins, psychotherapy, even injections of gold—to no avail. Nothing stopped or slowed down the progression of the severe rheumatoid arthritis. Finally, she found a degree of relief from a diet focused on vegetables, fruits, and meat, fish, or poultry cooked at low temperatures (by steaming, pressure-cooking, or nonstick pans for sautéing without oil or butter). Grains, dairy products, sugar, and citrus fruits exacerbate rheumatoid arthritis, so she avoided them.

Still, Diane was in pain and kept seeking solutions, which is what brought her to my office. Basic blood and urine tests showed that she had dramatic deficiencies in thyroid hormones, estrogen, progesterone, testosterone, cortisol, and DHEA. Her vitamin and mineral levels (with the lone exception of magnesium), on the other hand, were excellent.

Since Diane was already on the diet I would recommend, and obviously her body was getting all the nutrients it needed that way, together we focused on hormone therapy. The centerpiece was low-dose natural cortisol, because people with insufficient cortisol get inflammation all over their bodies, and particularly in their joints, just as Diane had. (The digestive tract is often inflamed as well in such cases, though Diane had escaped that particular problem.) I also prescribed DHEA, estrogen, progesterone, and testosterone. Estrogen can considerably decrease rheumatic pains; in some women, DHEA and testosterone perform even better. Thyroid hormone deficiency can also cause diffuse joint and muscle pains.

The combination brought dramatic improvement. In just one week, Diane estimated her level of pain had decreased 50 percent. After a month, she was helping her husband around the house and providing him some professional assistance as well. A month later, although her pain had not completely retreated, she was able to resume all her normal daily activities. She continued to improve after we made a change in her regimen, substituting a synthetic form for the natural cortisol she started with, as her ankles were swelling with the natural cortisol, and to take advantage of the synthetic's full-day effectiveness. Six months after she began hormone treatment, Diane was again swimming, skiing, running, and biking!

Diane has maintained these spectacular results for more than eight years now, thanks to strict adherence to the program she created for herself. Of course, she wasn't perfect. But her body responded loud and clear to deviation. Any change in her diet (splurging on sugary treats, for example) or in her hormone therapy (like the time we tried to lower her cortisol and thyroid doses) brought a resurgence of her joint pain. The detours taught Diane the importance of staying on the path.

ANITA

So that you don't think I can't see beyond arthritis, I'd like to tell you about another patient in chronic pain. When I met her, Anita had been suffering for more than a year from intense and disabling—but unexplained—pains, and had been diagnosed with fibromyalgia and, for good measure, chronic fatigue syndrome. She was tired all the time and had such a collection of minor, nagging problems that even on the rare occasions when the pain let up for a while, she felt unwell. With her whole body aching, she'd eventually had to stop working as a nurse.

"It's like I hit the big 4-0 and my body just started to betray me," Anita confided. Like so many of my patients, she wondered aloud why things couldn't just go on as they had in her twenties and thirties. "I always thought of myself as a healthy person," she said. "But these last few years it's been one thing after another. Is it really going to be like this for the rest of my life?"

Anita was careful about what she ate, and, before the pain made it impossible, she'd exercised regularly. Her doctor's only solution at this point had been to slap a label on the problem (fibromyalgia), then declare it untreatable.

He also prescribed an antidepressant, which only served to make Anita sleepy during the day (this on top of her exhaustion!). No doubt he wanted to make her feel better about her condition—chronic pain and fatigue can certainly get you down. But the prescription did not treat the pain itself, much less the underlying cause of the pain. Since her regular doctor had nothing more to offer, Anita made an appointment with me.

WHAT'S REALLY GOING ON

When I questioned her, Anita admitted to a number of complaints she dismissed as secondary but that set off alarm bells for me about possible thyroid deficiency: cold hands and feet, poor circulation, puffy eyes and face, dry skin, and brittle nails. She told me she was constantly exhausted but that her fatigue peaked each morning and again in the evening. On exam, I found she had a slow, weak heartbeat and slow Achilles tendon reflexes.

I also saw she had symptoms of low ovarian function: pale face, drooping breasts, little wrinkles above her lips, dry eyes. Most likely she wasn't getting the female hormones in sufficient amounts. Progesterone particularly was lacking, I guessed, based on her PMS (featuring bloating, particularly of the belly), nervousness, excessive emotionality, and cystic breasts. We all know that women's hormones shift at menopause, usually around age fifty, but we still tend to think of it as one dramatic change, as if a switch somewhere were suddenly turned from on to off. In reality, women's hormones change gradually over many years, starting as early as the mid-thirties. So I wasn't surprised Anita was feeling the effects already.

Another cluster of symptoms—excess weight (especially on the belly and thighs), cellulite, loss of muscle tone and muscle strength (especially in the biceps, abdominals, and legs), and pain in her lower back—made me suspect Anita had low levels of male hormones, too.

TURNING BACK THE CLOCK

Lab tests confirmed these deficiencies, and Anita started on low-dose natural supplements right away, via pill, patch, and cream. At the same time, she made changes to her diet. While she'd been a vegetarian for years and followed a low-fat diet, she did eat a lot of dairy products and not much fruit (fearing the sugar). I thought dairy products might be exacerbating her symptoms, particularly the bloating but also her dandruff and white-coated tongue, and so I recommended she eliminate them. Fruit, on the other hand, though I recommend against mixing it with any other foods, is full of valuable nutrients and fiber.

After just a few months, not only had most of the annoying symptoms cleared up, but also her fibromyalgia was gone! Her energy was back and she delightedly reported that now when someone asked her "How are you?" she could honestly smile and say with conviction: "Fine, thanks!" Since she still had a tendency to put on weight before her period, I increased the amount of progesterone she took and added a potassium supplement to reduce swelling.

Anita was back at work and had joyfully resumed juggling her many activities. She said it was like getting her old self back—her old *young* self.

NUTRITION

A balanced diet, moderate in protein, is the best foundation for fighting pain, particularly from arthritis. You should focus on vegetables, fruit, and moderate amounts of lean meat protein, and cut back on or eliminate grains, dairy products, and sugar.

Beyond a solid diet, several supplements can be helpful. (At the very least, make sure you don't have any deficiencies in these areas.) For example, **vitamin C** is often too low in women in menopause who aren't using hormone replacement therapy—especially those whose bone density is low, which often causes pain, particularly in the spine.

Vitamin D is crucial for metabolism of phosphorus and calcium, which is in turn crucial for healthy joints and bones. When combined with calcium, it also helps prevent painful small fractures in the spine and potentially devastating hip fractures. **Vitamin K** also supports bone density by binding calcium in the blood, thereby allowing it to be used in the body rather than excreted.

NUTRIENTS FOR JOINT PAIN

VITAMINS

Vitamin C: 500–2,000 mg daily
Vitamin D: 20 mcg daily (800 IU)
Vitamin K: 300–600 mcg daily

MINERALS

Calcium: 1,000 mg daily
Magnesium: 1,500–2,000 mg daily
Potassium: 1,000–1,200 mg daily
Copper: 0.8 mg daily

TRACE ELEMENTS

Phosphorus: 500–600 mg daily
Silicon: 90 mcg daily

Calcium (in combination with vitamin D) protects against fractures, including those in the spine, which can be a source of severe pain. **Magnesium, potassium, copper,** and **phosphorus** are useful in cases of osteoarthritis or other joint pain associated with muscular pain. Some doctors have found copper and phosphorus to be particularly good in cases of sudden severe inflammation. **Silicon,** as in the herb meadowsweet as well as in standard supplements, helps prevent bone loss and the associated pain.

DECODING YOUR DEFICIENCIES

Do you have osteoarthritis? Stiff or painful joints? The most common form of arthritis is osteoarthritis, afflicting more than sixteen million Americans. It is essentially the result of years of wear and tear on the joints. Just about all of us get at least a touch of it as we get older, and once we have it, it generally gets worse over the years. Hips, knees, fingers, and the spine are particularly susceptible. When the cartilage lining the joint cracks and flakes, it can no longer work to smooth the action of the joint, and movement can become painful. The bone underneath can also thicken or get distorted, making movement still more difficult, painful, and restricted.

This sort of arthritis is painful (to varying degrees) when you move the joint even the slightest bit, though the feeling dies down rapidly at rest. Aging is the most common underlying cause, though osteoarthritis can also stem from being overweight, having poor posture, injury, and/or repetitive strain (usually from work or a favorite hobby). It can be quite debilitating, though the most common symptoms are pain and stiffness.

The standard treatment is anti-inflammatory drugs, but though they often work well, all too often they provide little or no relief. Even in the best case, the drugs are intended to relieve the pain of the condition but do nothing to repair the damage or prevent the pain. Hormonal treatments, on the other hand, are 70 to 90 percent effective, including reversing harm done and preventing new pain.

Thyroid hormones can calm arthritic pain. They speed up blood circulation by making the heart beat faster and increase total blood volume. That increases the blood supply to all the tissues, especially the joints, and makes sure it consists of fresh, well-oxygenated blood. Because the thyroid gland weakens and secretes fewer hormones as you get older, the joints get less fresh blood. Without oxygen, nutrients, and water, the joints get swollen more easily. Thyroid hormones also activate metabolic reactions, freeing up energy and heat, and joints without enough of those resources wear out faster.

Osteoarthritis patients are often low in DHEA. In those who are deficient, hormone supplements can decrease pain.

Calcitonin seems to decrease inflammation and rebuild bone.

Testosterone rebuilds different parts of the joint, making healthier bones, muscles, tendons, membranes, and cartilage. Without enough of it, everything thins out and gets fragile and can't resist even normal wear and tear. Taking testosterone fights inflammation and can decrease the pain of arthritis. (Excessive doses, however, can cause fluid retention and joint pain.) Growth hormone acts similarly.

Do you have osteoarthritis in your hips? Osteoarthritis of the hip responds particularly well, in my patients' experience, to growth hormone. The condition is most common in elderly people, and with hormone therapy I've seen improvement of mobility and reduction and even disappearance of pain. The positive anabolic effect of the growth hormone seems to lead to a sort of regeneration of the hip.

Do you have rheumatoid arthritis? Rheumatoid arthritis affects more than two million Americans, two-thirds of them women. Unlike osteoarthritis, which generally begins with age, rheumatoid arthritis, which is harder to control and capable of damaging the joints more severely, usually shows up in twenty- to fifty-year-olds (though it can start at any time). It attacks many joints, though the most common targets are the hands. The primary symptom is inflamed, painful, and swollen—and eventually deformed—joints. The inflamed joints are swollen and warm, and painful even at rest. The skin around them tends to get a reddish tint. A host of other symptoms often come along for the ride, including general weakness, fatigue, and loss of appetite. Rheumatoid arthritis can flare up suddenly or suddenly go into remission; it is unpredictable. It can be extremely disabling.

Cortisol was one of the first hormones discovered to be helpful with rheumatoid arthritis. People with rheumatoid arthritis tend to have low blood cortisol levels. Furthermore, their immune systems tend to have fewer than normal receptor cells for cortisol, which even at normal blood levels could give you, effectively, a deficiency—the cortisol that was there would have no way of getting its whole job done. Finally, people with severe arthritis often don't have the expected daily fluctuations in cortisol levels (which normally are high early in the day and low in the evening).

Cortisol prevents the production or release of substances in the joints that can inflame them, like nitric oxide or destructive enzymes. It combats or even prevents sclerosis (fibrous tissue that replaces cartilage, interfering with joint mobility) by controlling the excessive production of two of its major components, collagen and hyaluronic acid. Cortisol also alleviates joint inflammation by blocking the inflammatory cells and liquid (from the blood) that make it swell. Finally, cortisol slows the action and production of inflammatory agents such as histamine, prostaglandins, and dilating blood vessels.

Because of all these beneficial effects, cortisol and its synthetic derivatives have been used for a long time in treating rheumatoid arthritis and other inflammatory conditions. The most basic way, perhaps, is injections directly into the affected joint to relieve both inflammation and pain.

Injections have a reasonable safety record and so are frequently used in children as well as adults. Using cortisol orally is another long-used technique, and in fact Dr. Philip Hench won the Nobel Prize in 1950 for his early studies on its effects with rheumatoid arthritis. But the misuse of the hormone—using it in overdoses—after the pharmaceutical companies brought it to market too quickly has cast a long shadow.

Fifty years later, many doctors still prescribe doses that are much too high, and mistrust of the hormone and its artificial derivatives remains strong. In the initial euphoria over its discovery, the basic principle of hormone therapy—give only the required dose to fill in the hormonal deficiency, no more and no less—seems to have gone right out the window. The medical literature is full of reports of the ravages of cortisol—swollen face, thin skin, easy bruising, high blood pressure, bone loss, osteoporosis. But those are rightly considered the ravages of cortisol *overdoses*. The truth is that too little cortisol is equally harmful, causing more frequent infections, malnutrition due to lack of appetite, arthritis, and more. Physiological doses of 20 mg of natural cortisol or 1 to 4 mg of pharmaceutical preparations of potent synthetic cortisol derivatives, like methylprednisolone (which is five times more powerful than natural cortisol) do not cause any bone loss in patients with rheumatoid arthritis, for instance, although bone loss is observed starting at 5 mg per day of methylprednisolone.

In my experience, the best way to use cortisol, besides in physiologic doses, is to pair it with hormones that balance its catabolic, or energy-producing, effects—which can cause tissue breakdown in the process. These anabolic hormones, including growth hormone, DHEA, testosterone, estrogen, and progesterone, covered in the following paragraphs, construct and rebuild tissue, keeping cortisol's potentially negative effects in check, allowing higher doses of cortisol or a synthetic derivative without bone loss or other adverse effects. They all have specific arthritis-fighting effects.

DHEA is the most important cortisol counterbalance. A Swedish study has shown that patients with rheumatoid arthritis who *don't* take the cortisol derivative glucocorticoids, which diminish natural cortisol secretion, already have little DHEA in the tissue of their inflamed joints (60 percent below normal) and even less in the blood (75 percent below normal). But the patients who do take the glucocorticoids, suppressing their own body's production of cortisol, have even less.

Patients (men and women both) with rheumatoid arthritis are more frequently low in blood levels of testosterone. In male patients taking the synthetic cortisol derivative prednisone, the blood testosterone level is lower than that of nontreated patients. So it is important to check your testosterone levels when you are using any synthetic cortisol and to fill in any deficiency. Women in menopause should do the same, as testosterone counteracts bone loss around the joints, including the hips, that are affected by rheumatoid arthritis but also susceptible to osteoporosis.

Rheumatoid arthritis occurs two to four times as often in women as in men, a difference that is most likely due to the significant drop, with age, of those hormones that decrease more rapidly in women than men, most notably estrogen. Estrogen has been used to prevent, relieve, or cure some types of rheumatoid arthritis, particularly cases in women whose ovaries are not producing enough hormones (and especially estrogen). Just regular oral contraceptives (synthetic estrogen and progesterone) reduce the incidence by two-thirds. Women who have taken noncontraceptive estrogens in the past are two-thirds less likely to get rheumatoid arthritis. Women currently taking them are seven times less likely to get it. Animal studies on mice indicate that estrogen is protective against osteoarthritis in males, too.

Progesterone is helpful, too, although it is often overlooked. Injection of natural progesterone into a swollen joint diminishes the inflammation in much the same way cortisol does, and the effect lasts up to two months. Though the exact effect of progesterone used for rheumatoid arthritis deserves to be better studied, it is clear that for adults it builds up the joints in healthful ways. It is also worth noting that progesterone at high doses, taken orally, has anesthetic effects.

Growth hormone (and its working partner somatomedin C) can limit or reverse the development of rheumatoid arthritis. It is particularly important in children who develop the disease. A study of children with rheumatoid arthritis showed they had 40 percent less somatomedin C than kids without rheumatoid arthritis. These kids also had other signs of growth hormone deficiency, chief among them being the fact that they were relatively short for their age.

In addition to the importance of cortisol and the anabolic hormones, treatment of rheumatoid arthritis must also take into account the fact that patients with rheumatoid arthritis often have low levels of several other hormones, including calcitonin, melatonin, pregnenolone, and thyroid hormones—precisely the hormones that have anti-inflammatory (antirheumatoid) properties.

Calcitonin, a hormone secreted by the thyroid gland, is most widely known for its bone-building properties. But it also has significant anti-inflammatory action and can be useful for arthritis, though I use it primarily for pain relief in cases of vertebral fractures or crushes.

A study of patients with rheumatoid arthritis revealed that their average level of blood melatonin during the day was four times lower than normal for their age. People with idiopathic pain have little melatonin in their blood or urine. Furthermore, melatonin has an analgesic effect (it relieves pain, like that other famous analgesic, aspirin, to name just one). The pain-relief effect is stronger at night, because melatonin is secreted primarily at night. This explains why pain sensitivity is heightened during the day (peaking four hours after sunrise) and decreases at night (with the low point two hours before waking). My rheumatoid arthritis patients sleep better with melatonin and experience less pain at night. They tend to be taking other hormones as well, however, and we're awaiting studies that look specifically at melatonin for arthritis pain relief in humans. Studies in mice show that melatonin does decrease pain (at night).

However, some studies of mice with rheumatoid arthritis induced by collagen injections show that melatonin can aggravate the arthritis. In my opinion, this is due to a decrease in cortisol caused by melatonin, which calms everything down, including cortisol production. So patients with rheumatoid arthritis and a known cortisol deficiency should take melatonin only in conjunction with cortisol supplements. Anyone with rheumatoid arthritis who uses melatonin should do so only in low doses.

Pregnenolone counters rheumatoid arthritis, though it takes fairly large, but apparently nontoxic, doses, around 500 mg per day.

Thyroid hormones are also effective against rheumatoid arthritis symptoms, as well as osteoarthritis, as described earlier. Many patients with serious thyroid insufficiency have swollen, painful joints. Low levels of these hormones, or hypothyroidism, often result in motion-caused pain with early-morning stiffness. The joint pain is worse in the morning and when starting to move again after resting, and it decreases during the day and when active. (Activity speeds up the blood flow, supplying the joints with fresh, warm blood, which revives them.) It is aggravated by cold and humidity. It generally does *not* come with inflammation, erosion, and sclerosis of the joint and the surrounding tissue, as is the case with rheumatoid arthritis. Joint pains related to thyroid deficiency are caused by an accumulation of waste products swelling the joints. In any event, correcting the deficiency can improve or even remove all these symptoms. If it does, then the symptoms indicate hypothyroidism, not true rheumatoid arthritis, though the symptoms are so similar the conditions can be difficult to tell apart.

Which thyroid hormone preparation you use might make a crucial difference in how effective you find it to be in any case, particularly with arthritis symptoms. Early studies (one major one published in 1970) show close to 100 percent of low-thyroid patients improved, with joint pain eradicated, when they took thyroid hormones. Other similar studies over the years since have shown effectiveness, but at a seemingly steadily declining rate. By 1992 a major published study reported 50 percent of patients improving, but only 9 percent got rid of their joint pain altogether.

It isn't possible that the condition itself changed so drastically in just two decades. The mystery is explained, rather, by a closer look at just what hormones were actually being used. The first researchers were using either thyroid powder (a mixture of the main thyroid hormones T_3 and T_4), or T_3 alone. More recent scientists have used today's standard treatment, synthetic T_4, thyroxin, which the body converts into T_3, triiodothyronine, the active thyroid hormone. T_4 is practically inactive by itself, and while the assumption is that the body will convert supplemental T_4 into T_3 as needed, many patients' bodies no longer make that conversion efficiently. As we get older, most of us don't make the switch easily anymore. In patients taking T_4, their blood T_4 levels are generally abnormally high, while their T_3 levels remain rather low. This is an instance in which medical progress is no progress at all. The old-fashioned treatment is still available, and I recommend it to most of my patients, and particularly to those who haven't had ideal responses to standard T_4 treatment.

Do you have fibromyalgia? Fibromyalgia is a syndrome with diffuse pain in the muscles and tendons all over the body, usually paired with chronic fatigue, characterized by a pattern of at least thirteen of sixteen to eighteen "tender points" of unusually strong pain, generally where muscles and tendons meet. Simply put, it hurts when you press on these points. The pain of fibromyalgia is often severe enough to make working extremely difficult. Yet because the disease is poorly understood and its exact cause remains unknown, and because there are no lab tests to prove the disease is really there, and because a lot of patients actually look as if they are quite well, friends and family and even doctors sometimes think it is all in the patient's mind, obviously adding to the difficulty of the situation.

Fibromyalgia strikes ten times more women than men. Not surprisingly, estrogen plays an important role. Women with fibromyalgia tend to have lower levels of estrogen than healthy women of the same age. Although there are no scientific studies of estrogen treatment for fibromyalgia yet, I've used it with success with my patients.

It is also worth noting that adults with fibromyalgia have, on average 30 percent less somatomedin C—the crucial co-worker of growth hormone—than the norm. One study showed that growth hormone therapy significantly reduced (by 25 percent) the number of tender points and the patient's perception of pain.

DHEA can also bring relief to an inflammatory disease such as fibromyalgia, although it is rarely a complete cure.

Do you have carpal tunnel syndrome? The hallmark of carpal tunnel syndrome is an unpleasant pricking feeling in the fingers, which is caused by the compression of the median nerve in the carpal canal—the sheath surrounding the hand's tendons at the wrist. It occurs more often in patients with low levels of thyroid hormones than in the general population. Only certain patients with low thyroid function will develop it. Fortunately, it clears up when the hormonal deficiency is corrected.

Carpal tunnel syndrome might also improve with estrogen and progesterone therapy.

Do you have gout (arthritis in your thumbs and/or big toes)? Gout, which occurs more often in men than in women, attacks by coating the joints with irritating deposits of uric acid crystals, causing inflammation and severe pain. It usually affects joints in the foot, especially the big toe, though joints elsewhere, especially in the thumb, are often involved as well. High levels of uric acid, which greatly increases the risk of developing gout, are more common in people low in thyroid hormones. So you won't be surprised to learn that gout occurs more often in people with low thyroid function. The good news is, patients with gout have far fewer crises when they use appropriate thyroid hormone therapy.

Did your arthritis pain start with menopause? Patients taking estrogen at menopause have a lower incidence of arthritis.

Do you have lupus? Lupus is an inflammatory disease of the connective tissue that can have a variety of symptoms; joint pain similar to rheumatoid arthritis is a common one.

The many anti-inflammatory properties of cortisol (see more information under the question about rheumatoid arthritis, page 119) make it useful in treating lupus.

Lupus is usually accompanied by low levels of DHEA. Patients who take DHEA clearly improve, though a cure with DHEA alone is rare. The studies indicate a fairly high dose is required (200 mg per day)—too high, in my opinion. I do recommend DHEA to my patients with lupus, however, just at lower doses and in partnership with other deficient hormones. With the synergy that exists between hormones, the larger dose isn't necessary for effectiveness. For example, cortisol and DHEA work together to fight inflammation—and the two together, in physiologic doses, work better than either alone.

SUMMARY: ANTI-JOINT-PAIN HORMONES

Hormone Deficiency	Symptoms	See also pg.
Calcitonin	rheumatoid arthritis; acute pain such as from vertebral fractures or crushes	26
Cortisol	rheumatoid arthritis; fibromyalgia; lupus	26
DHEA	rheumatoid arthritis; osteoarthritis; lupus; fibromyalgia	27
Estrogen	rheumatoid arthritis; fibromyalgia; arthritis pain that started with menopause; carpal tunnel syndrome	28
Growth Hormone	osteoarthritis in your hips; rheumatoid arthritis; fibromyalgia; back pain	29
Melatonin	rheumatoid pain; fibromyalgia	30
Pregnenolone	rheumatoid arthritis	31
Progesterone	rheumatoid arthritis; carpal tunnel syndrome	32
Testosterone	rheumatoid arthritis, fibromyalgia, lupus, osteoarthritis	32
Thyroid	osteoarthritis; stiff or painful joints; rheumatoid arthritis; carpal tunnel syndrome; gout; fibromyalgia	33

CHAPTER EIGHT

RIGHT DOWN
TO THE BONE

As we age, our bones lose mass, protein, and minerals, becoming thinner and more porous. When this loss of bone density becomes rapid enough or severe enough, it shows up as the condition we know as osteoporosis. At minimum, this means an increased risk of fractures, especially in the vertebrae and hips, and difficulty healing when they occur. And you've seen some of the more extreme signs, like an elderly person permanently bent forward because of the curve of his or her spine as the vertebrae collapse into each other. In some cases, as when it leads to hip fracture, osteoporosis is life-threatening. Short of fatality, it is always a threat to quality of life.

For years medicine has shrugged all this off as an unavoidable part of aging. More recently, bone loss has been treated in women with standard hormone replacement therapy (estrogen, or estrogen and progesterone). And indeed, osteoporosis occurs more often and at younger ages in women than in men, and the menopausal drop in hormones is the major reason why. What we'll look at in this chapter, however, is just what a variety of hormones—well beyond estrogen and progesterone—are involved in making and keeping bones healthy, dense, and strong. With the appropriate hormones in the appropriate doses, osteoporosis is preventable and even reversible.

CARINE

When she was still in her twenties, Carine had a complete hysterectomy—removal of her uterus and (hormone producing!) ovaries—as a consequence of large uterine fibroids, ovarian cysts, and excessively heavy menstrual bleeding. Such a condition is often caused by an uncorrected progesterone deficiency, although that was never investigated in Carine's case—but I cringed to think of the simple solution that would have been open to her if it had.

Instead, Carine had had the drastic surgery, and for twenty years she had been living with its drastic consequences. Without ovaries, her body made practically no estrogen or progesterone, and as a result she now had severe osteoporosis, although she hadn't yet reached the age when most women go through menopause. Without these crucial hormones, her bone mineral density was not even half of what is considered optimal. That meant her bones would break easily, and she was at high risk of having vertebral fractures and the collapsing spine that results in loss of height, a hump back, and often severe bone pain.

Now Carine had tried hormone replacement therapy using estrogen and progesterone immediately after her hysterectomy, but she had tolerated it badly and quit. After nearly twenty years of living essentially without those hormones, she had recently begun a new regimen of estrogen and progesterone replacement, this time without the negative side effects she had experienced the first time around. She was using transdermal estrogen—a good idea, as this form has been shown to not only slow or stop decreases in bone density, but also to stimulate an increase in bone formation, which oral estrogen does not—and oral progesterone, but the doses weren't high enough to protect her deprived bones. So the first thing we did was move her to the top range of physiologic doses— gradually, to make sure her body would handle it. Her testosterone level was also low, so we added small doses of that, too.

Carine's history and exam revealed one possible explanation for why she did not tolerate medications, like the original hormone replacement therapy, easily: a cortisol deficiency. She had other hallmarks of the condition too, complaining of joint and muscle pain not only in the spine and back muscles, as is common with osteoporosis, but also in her limbs. In addition, her resistance to stress was low, as was her blood pressure, and she craved sugar and sweets.

She also had symptoms of thyroid deficiency, including excessive sensitivity to cold; a swollen, puffy face in the morning; waking up tired; and dry skin. Thyroid deficiency can also cause stiffness and joint pain such as what she was experiencing.

When lab tests confirmed both of these deficiencies, we added cortisol and thyroid hormone supplements to her daily regimen. Although these treatments have been blamed for *causing* osteoporosis, that is only in cases in which doses are inadequate, excessive, or imbalanced. In physiologic doses balanced with other hormones (like the male and female hormones Carine was taking), they do the opposite, protecting the bones and eliminating the conditions that lead to low bone density in the first place. Cortisol might improve the intestinal absorption of amino acids and other nutrients, building blocks for the bone, by calming down inflammation of the digestive tract. Thyroid hormones keep waste materials from accumulating between bone cells. For Carine, the full combination meant strengthening her bones and lowering her risk of fractures as well as clearing up her other annoying symptoms of deficiency. All that, and her bone density increased 12 percent over four years (6 percent the first year, and an average of 2 percent per year after that, according to annual bone density scans).

TESTING

Just in the way hormone deficiencies can be detected (and, for a lot of our history, *had* to be detected) via more or less subtle physical signs, osteoporosis has long been diagnosed only after it was so advanced that obvious symptoms (fracture prime among them, but also height loss, spinal curvatures, and sagging muscles) appeared. Fortunately, now there's an alternative. In addition to testing your hormone levels and nutritional status, when there's a question of the health of your bones, I recommend having your bone density tested. There are several methods of doing so, but the current front-runner is dual-energy X-ray absorptiometry (DEXA). It's painless, takes only ten to twenty minutes, and exposes you to less radiation than a chest X-ray or a full set of dental X-rays (or a year of just living in the world). The bad news is that it costs upward of $300. Fortunately, more and more health insurance plans are providing coverage.

NUTRITION

The most important nutritional step you can take to safeguard your bones is to moderate the amount of protein you get, especially animal protein. The digestive process for protein requires a lot of calcium, sapping the mineral that is crucial to bone strength. The more protein you

NUTRIENTS FOR STRONG BONES

VITAMINS

Vitamin C: 1,000–1,500 mg daily
Vitamin K: 9–10 mg daily
Vitamin D: 800 IU daily

MINERALS

Calcium: 1,500 mg daily for menopausal women not taking HRT
    1,000 mg daily for premenopausal women over
        thirty-five
    500–1,000 mg daily for everyone else

TRACE ELEMENTS

Silicon: 90 mcg daily

eat, the more calcium is excreted in your urine and the less calcium is available to your bones. But your bones definitely need the amino acids proteins provide, so you do need to get enough in your diet. What you need is a diet moderate in protein.

Menopausal women have a much higher rate of bone loss than anyone else because of the drop in hormones that occurs at menopause, so diet is particularly important for them. Several studies have shown that menopausal women who get moderate protein by eating vegetarian have significantly less bone loss than other menopausal women. You want to limit dairy products, however, for the reasons laid out in chapter 17, and also because some studies show an *increase* in bone loss in women who eat a lot of dairy products.

You also should limit high-fiber grains to some extent and keep your intake of carbohydrates in general moderate, too. It is also important to limit or, better yet, avoid caffeine and alcohol, both of which have been linked to bone loss and low bone density.

Beyond that, several vitamins and minerals help fight bone loss and osteoporosis, while deficiencies in these same nutrients can *cause* the problem. Front and center is calcium, which protects against fractures, especially in the spine and hip (the most vulnerable places). It is helpful for everyone, particularly women, who face a greater risk, and particularly menopausal women not taking standard hormone replacement therapy (estrogen, or estrogen and progesterone).

Vitamin D works so closely with calcium in supporting bone strength that most people should take them together. If you live where it is sunny and get sun exposure every day, your body might make all the vitamin D it needs. For everyone else—and even those sun-worshipers— a supplement is a good insurance policy. A lot of the studies of supplements and bones in fact use a combination of calcium and vitamin D, like those showing protection against fractures in the spine and hip.

Studies have shown that vitamin C tends to be low in menopausal women not using hormone therapy and whose bone density is low. Vitamin K, too, is important for bone density, as it assists with new bone formation and calcification. Finally, silicon is important in preventing bone loss.

DECODING YOUR DEFICIENCIES

Do you have idiopathic osteoporosis? People with osteoporosis from unknown causes have low levels of somatomedin C, an indicator that they are low in growth hormone. Growth hormone levels drop with age (as does somatomedin C)—in fact, it is one of the first to do so. Its importance in bone density is seen most dramatically in cases of severe deficiency. At puberty, young adults deficient in growth hormone (even if they use supplemental hormone) have bones that are less dense than other people their age. In fact, their bone density is proportional to their somatomedin C levels (and so their growth hormone levels). Adults who develop a deficiency later in life, through the loss or damage of the pituitary gland through injury, surgery, or stroke, also have low bone density.

On the other end of the spectrum, during the first six months a growth hormone deficient patient takes growth hormone supplements, bone metabolism accelerates. The normal process, called bone remodeling (where some cells are broken down and others built up) is continual but slows down as we get older. After six months of treatment, the increase in bone density becomes visible. After two and a half years of treatment (in young adults), bone density increases close to 8 percent in the vertebrae and as much as 10 percent in the forearm. In one study, the improvement in bone density over two years exceeded 20 percent!

We can also learn something from cases of acromegaly, a disease in which *too much* growth hormone is produced. Bone density increases in all parts of the skeleton. Unfortunately, it does so to the point of excess. This is tantamount to an overdose, however; at prudent doses, growth hormone allows for a substantial increase of bone density but won't verge into excess.

Have you lost bone density in the spine? (women) The drop in estrogen as you get older plays a large role in decreasing bone density; estrogen supplements can halt bone loss and even rebuild bone. At menopause, where the decline in estrogen is the steepest (though it starts a downhill slide many years earlier), women lose bone at the rate of about 2 percent a year, up from 0.2 percent. That's a huge difference.

That much is widely known. What is less well publicized is that estrogen works closely with growth hormone. Estrogen is necessary for maintaining sufficient levels of somatomedin C, which is necessary for maintaining sufficient levels of growth hormone, which is necessary for maintaining bone density. Studies of female monkeys with an artificial estrogen deficiency injected with growth hormone show they retain bone density.

Do you have vertebral fractures or crushes? Pain from vertebral fractures? Have you lost height? Do you have a forward curve in your upper back ("dowager's hump" or "hump back")? Have you been bedridden or immobilized for any significant length of time? Do you have Paget's disease? Calcitonin is one of the first treatments for osteoporosis, slows bone loss, and increases bone mass. It blocks the cells responsible for bone breakdown (the osteoclasts). It is especially effective when bone loss occurs because of paralysis, weak ovaries, menopause, and simply being over sixty.

Women treated with calcitonin have one-third the fractures of women of the same age taking calcium tablets only (but no hormones). The best part about this approach to osteoporosis is that calcitonin is an efficient remedy for relieving the pain—which can be intense—of vertebral fractures.

Paget's disease, a bone ailment occurring in the second half of life, also responds to calcitonin.

MARTHA

All her life, Martha had worked hard running her farm. Now she was in her eighties and had moved into an assisted-living facility. One morning when she woke up, she had a sharp pain in her back that didn't go away once she was up and moving around. On the contrary, the pain got so intense she had to call for the nurse, who in turn called in her doctor, a colleague of mine. A bone scan of her spine revealed she had several crushed vertebrae that had clearly been there for a long time—a not uncommon occurrence in patients with undiagnosed and untreated osteoporosis—as well as some newer ones that had caused the actual intense pain. Martha's bone density was very low and obviously already in the fracture zone.

Her doctor prescribed daily injections of calcitonin, which not only improves bone density and can help prevent fractures, but also provides pain relief from bone pain, particularly pain from fractured vertebrae. (Injections are cheaper and more efficient, but many doctors and patients prefer the more convenient nasal spray.) They started with a very low dose, just 25 mg a day, to make sure there were no side effects (nausea being the main concern), and gradually increased to 75 mg a day.

After two weeks, Martha's pain subsided 80 to 90 percent, she estimated—a very fast response—so this story has a reasonably happy ending. However, no doubt Martha would have preferred to avoid those painful fractures altogether, and earlier intervention with calcitonin could have done just that.

Have you lost muscle mass, tone, or strength? Are your muscles sagging? Are you constantly depressed or fatigued? Women: Have you lost bone density in your hip, wrist, or other extremity? Men: Do you have decreased sexual potency? Lack of testosterone is one of the principal causes of bone loss, in women as well as men. While the effects on the bones might be hidden until it is too late, you can use other clues to spot a testosterone deficiency: diminished muscle mass, tone, and strength, fatigue and depression prime among them. Other signs, though they can also indicate low estrogen or low growth hormone, are a sagging belly pushed downward by a more pronounced forward curve of the spine (lordosis), an asymmetrical spine, and thinning bones (especially in the jaw and fingers).

Men's testicles produce testosterone as well as a very small quantity of estrogen, and both hormones contribute in a significant way to maintaining bone mass—significant enough that you should make sure testosterone, too, is included in treatment of osteoporosis, though currently it is often overlooked.

You might be interested to know that most of the testosterone that permeates the bones is converted into estrogen in men as well as women. As this portends, women need this male hormone, in addition to the female hormones, to keep their bones solid. Women who have the densest bones also have the highest testosterone levels. Testosterone stimulates the production of cortical bone—the surface of the bones. The more testosterone a woman has, the more solid the outer part of her bones. A form of male hormone released by the ovaries stimulates trabecular, or interior, bone.

The best results of hormone replacement therapy against osteoporosis occur when testosterone is prescribed in addition to estrogen and progesterone. Results, in the hips and extremities especially, improve with the combination.

Of course, testosterone is important to men's bones as well. Elderly men with osteoporosis, for example, heal faster after fractures if they take testosterone supplements. We can learn a lot from an extreme example in men of any age: testosterone-deficient men with osteoporosis from hemochromatosis (a metabolic disorder that accumulates iron in the tissues). In one study, patients' bone density increased by 13 percent in their spines and 5 percent in their forearms after two years of testosterone treatment (one injection every three weeks), whereas men with the same disorder who didn't take testosterone because lab tests showed their hormone levels qualified as sufficient *lost* 3.5 percent of their spine bone mass over the same period. (Forearm bone density was stable.) This is a lesson in the power of testosterone to maintain and improve bone density as well as on just how insufficient "sufficient" levels of hormones can be.

*Do you take cortisol (cortisone) or other steroids? Do you
have low bone density or osteoporosis as a result of steroid
use?* Anyone taking cortisol, especially in massive doses, should balance
it with DHEA. In the process of producing energy, cortisol consumes
bone mass. DHEA maintains or builds bone mass, so it can counter any
negative effects of cortisol. (The problem with cortisol generally comes
with its traditional use, involving synthetic derivatives in doses several
times too high for our purposes; at the physiologic levels discussed in
this book, and in conjunction with a hormone that builds up bone, such
as DHEA, bone density isn't harmed.)

DHEA is not as powerful as growth hormone when it comes to bone
density, but it deserves our attention nonetheless as it is very useful in
its own right, particularly when prevention rather than treatment is the
aim. DHEA stimulates bone growth from the membrane of the inner
bone as well as from the outer membrane. In the leg, new bone growth
has been shown to be enhanced by 35 to 45 percent with DHEA treatment. DHEA stimulates bone density well at the joints, like the hip, but
also in the vertebrae. The bone density of the spine depends on the
DHEA level to a degree. The higher the DHEA level in the blood, the
denser are the vertebrae, according to a study of menopausal women.
Likewise, the bone density in the forearm increases as the DHEA blood
levels rise.

As you would predict, people with Addison's disease, a severe
adrenal gland deficiency that results in low cortisol and DHEA levels,
generally have low bone density.

Do you have scoliosis or an asymmetrical spine? Animal studies have linked melatonin deficiency and scoliosis (in chicks with no
pineal gland). Treatment with melatonin avoided the problem.

*Do you have (or have you had) bone cysts in your arms or
legs?* Although cortisol is often criticized as contributing to bone loss,
it nonetheless plays a positive role in the treatment of bone cysts in the
humerus, femur, and tibia (the long bones of the arms and legs). Just be
wary of synthetic derivatives and excessive doses, either or both of which
encourage bone loss by slowing calcium absorption and increasing the
level of a hormone from the parathyroid gland (called parathyroid hor-

mone) that extracts calcium from the bones. In rats, this bone loss can be countered by taking zinc, and although I think this works in humans as well, it probably doesn't to a sufficient degree to solve the problem. Physiological doses (1 to 4 mg a day) of cortisol derivatives like (methyl)prednisolone (which is five times more powerful than natural cortisol) has been shown *not* to cause bone loss. But doses of 5 mg or more create a problem.

Are you menopausal? Menopausal women who take testosterone in addition to estrogen and progesterone have the best bone density. The addition of the male hormone often gives better results than the female hormones alone, especially when it comes to bones.

Have you had PMS, breast cysts, or uterine fibroids for many years? These are signs of progesterone deficiency, and over many years another effect of low progesterone is a decrease in bone density. Dr. John Lee, a leading expert in natural progesterone use, claims excellent results in building bone density with progesterone creams applied to the skin. His patients have had increases of more than 10 percent in their bone mass. I am eager to see this reproduced by other doctors, and if the promise bears out, this will be an excellent new option for preventing or curing osteoporosis in women—and maybe in men, too, as their adrenal glands produce small amounts of the hormone as well. For now, I don't use progesterone alone to treat low bone density; I combine it with estrogen and testosterone. And when you are using estrogen, you need to make sure you get sufficient progesterone to temper its effects—and progesterone skin cream, Dr. Lee's preferred method, is not always strong enough for the job.

Are you taking thyroid hormones? In thyroid hormone deficiency, bones swell with an accumulation of mucus waste products between the cells (myxedema). Fortunately, supplying the missing hormones reestablishes healthy calcium content, at least partially, and strengthens the bone. But some studies have suggested that otherwise healthy post-menopausal women using thyroxin alone (the thyroid precursor hormone) experience a drop in bone density of up to 5 to 7 percent—but only in estrogen deficient women. (Fortunately, treatment with female hormones prevents such an adverse effect.) Other studies show no bone loss. Still, it is concerning. Work by Dr. C. Ribot and his colleagues has shown that any bone loss that occurs is temporary and transitional, as defective old bone is replaced by new bone. After the first year of thyroid hormone treatment, the creation of new high-quality bone at the very least stops the loss and very often outpaces it, thereby increasing bone density once again.

SUMMARY: BONE-DENSITY HORMONES

Hormone Deficiency	Symptoms	See also pg.
Calcitonin	vertebral fractures or crushes; pain from vertebral fractures; loss of height; forward curve in upper back ("dowager's hump" or "hump back"); bedridden or immobilized; Paget's disease	26
Cortisol	bone cysts in arms or legs	26
DHEA	cortisol, cortisone, or other steroid use; low bone density or osteoporosis as a result of excessive steroid use; bone density loss in spine or hip	27
Estrogen	in women: bone density loss in spine	28
Growth Hormone	idiopathic osteoporosis; osteoporosis from advanced age; bone density loss in spine, hip, hands, and feet	29
Melatonin	scoliosis; asymmetrical spine	30
Progesterone	long-standing PMS, breast tenderness, breast cysts, heavy periods, and/or uterine fibroids	32
Testosterone	loss of muscle mass, tone, or strength; sagging muscles; constant fatigue or depression; in women: bone density loss in spine, hip, wrist, or extremities	32
Thyroid	use of thyroid hormone for osteoporosis in estrogen deficient women; hypothyroidism	33

CHAPTER NINE

MATTERS OF
THE HEART

Heart disease is the number one cause of death in the United States. Twenty-one million new cases are reported each year, and nearly three-quarters of a million people die of it. Nearly three out of four people die of heart disease. Like so many other serious health conditions, heart disease is generally associated with aging. It doesn't always wait until you're "old" to break out, of course, but most of the time it does take many years to develop. By now I'm sure you can guess: Heart disease and its risk factors increase as hormone levels decrease, and that's no accident.

In the fight against disease—and heart disease, given its "popularity," always prime among them—science has revealed hormones to be at least palliative and often curative. Hormones play an enormous role in the circulation system, supplying blood to the organs, and the deterioration of the heart and arteries crucial to the process can be attributed to the lack of various hormones. Although this insight is typically given short shrift in the typical medical practice, study after study has shown the favorable effects of hormone therapy on heart disease and risk factors. The right balance of hormones keeps the cardiovascular system (the heart and blood vessels) strong and resilient, reducing heart disease and its risk factors.

WALLACE

Wallace is an excellent example of the power of hormones to heal the heart. Wallace was in his early fifties when I met him, and he was recovering from triple bypass surgery after a second heart attack. He'd had to retire, although he was only in his mid-forties. He was haunted by the fact that his father had died of a heart attack at fifty. Wallace feared for his own life, and he was right to do so.

Wallace had seen enough doctors to staff a small hospital. He'd changed his diet and exercised when he could, but his cholesterol stayed sky high (350 mg/dl), and, like any bypass patient, he faced reclogging of the arteries within five to eight years. None of his doctors could say he wasn't going to suffer another heart attack at any moment.

Wallace told me all about his heart and the surgery and the attacks and the hospitalizations and the various treatments and his family history. Way at the end of his saga, almost as an aside, he mentioned that his hands and feet were always cold, his skin was always dry, he had periods of intense fatigue and depression, and he had joint pains and was particularly stiff in the morning. He'd been diagnosed with Raynaud's syndrome: His fingers turned blue as soon as they touched anything cold, due to a lack of fresh oxygen supply from poor circulation. I could see his eyes were puffy, his lips were almost purple, and his hands and feet looked bluish. Tests showed his heartbeat was slow and weak, his temperature was very low in the morning (not quite 97°—with optimal being 98.6°), and his cholesterol high. All of this suggested a thyroid deficiency.

Because heart patients must gradually build up to the proper doses, Wallace started taking natural thyroid hormone slowly, working up to 120 mg and eventually 150 mg daily. This brought about big improvements in his quality of life. Within three months, his mood and energy improved, and he was able to exercise again, including his old favorite, biking long distances. But a year later, he still had bouts of fatigue and depression. With so many of his other symptoms cleared up, Wallace now noticed his muscles seemed weak, his sex drive was low, and he occasionally had hot flashes (a phenomenon common at midlife and not limited to menopausal women). On exam I found other signs of testosterone deficiency, including dry eyes and a "spare tire." I also confirmed his suspicion that his muscles were weakened. A lab test of Wallace's testosterone levels confirmed he was running low.

He started taking testosterone capsules, which helped, but he saw even more improvement when he switched to injections. Still, occasional depression and lack of energy plagued him, though definitely not as severely as before, so I checked other systems. Both his pituitary gland (maker of growth hormone) and adrenal glands (source of cortisol) were not up to par. The subtle signs of deficiency, including excessive emotionality, thick skin, and increased fat under the skin (growth hormone), and low blood pressure and low resistance to stress (cortisol) revealed themselves. Once he began small doses of growth hormone and hydrocortisone, Wallace finally found the right balance of hormones for his body. He felt strong and well and rated himself as having a very high quality of life. And so it remains ten years after beginning treatment, with no further heart problems. Without hormone treatment, I believe Wallace would be an invalid or perhaps dead by now. The right hormones keep him vibrantly, vigorously alive and healthy.

DIET AND LIFESTYLE

When it comes to keeping your heart and cardiovascular system healthy, nutrition is of paramount importance. Eating right might be enough to improve your hormone balance and protect your heart. If not, good nutrition is necessary to allow the hormone supplements to work most efficiently and effectively.

But before we get to the details of that, I want to cover a few other lifestyle points important for heart health. I don't think you'll find any of them to be big newsmakers. Get regular, moderate exercise. Lose any excess weight. Don't smoke or use any tobacco products. Control your cholesterol levels. Maintain a good blood pressure. If you have diabetes, manage it well. And here's one I hope will be most enjoyable: Get enough sleep and plenty of rest.

The nutritional strategies below, though most are designed to create hormone balance, will help you achieve several of those, including controlling weight, cholesterol, and high blood pressure, all of which are key factors in risk of heart disease.

First and foremost is eating a diet with moderate levels of fat that is rich in fruit and vegetables. Another across-the-board recommendation is avoiding caffeine—coffee being the most common culprit. Beyond that, diet strategies depend on the specifics of your condition. If your triglycerides are high or you have diabetes, eliminate sugars and simple carbohydrates, cold cuts, and dairy products. If you have high blood pressure, be sure to drink lots of water.

Drinking plenty of water might also be good for lowering choles-

NUTRIENTS FOR HEART HEALTH

Be sure to get at least these minimum doses daily.

VITAMINS

Folic acid: 15 mg
Riboflavin: 12 mg
Vitamin B_6: 15 mg
Vitamin C: 200 mg
Vitamin E: 400 mg

MINERALS

Zinc: 20 mg
Copper: 2 mg
Magnesium: 150 mg

TRACE ELEMENTS

Chromium: 0.5 mg
Manganese: 2 mg
Selenium: 100 mcg
Phosphatidylcholine: 50–100 mg

terol. People with high cholesterol should also make sure that most of the fat in their diet is unsaturated—that is, mainly nonanimal fats—but also has sufficient (not excessive!) amounts of saturated fats in order to be able to produce enough sex and adrenal hormones. The catch is that saturated fats and anything with cholesterol must not be cooked at high temperatures. If they are, structural changes from high heat can make them toxic.

And although you want a diet that is low in fat, you do *not* want a no-fat diet. Your body needs moderate amounts of healthful fats to stay healthy itself. If your LDL (bad) cholesterol is too high, you should avoid cooking your food in oil at high temperatures (including baking). Don't overcook your eggs, either, lest the high temperatures render them toxic, too.

SUPPLEMENTS

*E*ven with an excellent diet, nutritional supplements can be an important part of any program for heart health. **B-vitamin** deficiencies, particularly **folic acid, riboflavin,** and **vitamin B$_6$,** raise the blood level of homocysteine, which increases the risk of arteriosclerosis. Supplements lower homocysteine levels.

Vitamin C—particularly in combination with **vitamin E**—lowers blood pressure, raises HDL (good cholesterol), and lowers blood viscosity. Vitamin E also lowers LDL (bad cholesterol). Many studies have proven the correlation between lack of vitamin E and the development of cardiovascular disease.

Copper and **zinc** strengthen blood-vessel walls. **Chromium, manganese,** and **zinc** prevent plaques from building up in the arteries. **Selenium** lowers blood pressure and viscosity, and **magnesium** stabilizes cardiac rhythms. **Phosphatidylcholine** supplements lower cholesterol.

DECODING YOUR DEFICIENCIES

CHOLESTEROL

Cholesterol levels tend to rise with age, and it is much more than a coincidence that it happens as hormone levels drop with age. Several different hormones act on the fats in the blood, and deficits in one or more generate disturbances of fat metabolism—the major sign of which is rising cholesterol counts. Since risk of heart disease rises quickly in proportion to cholesterol levels, we simply cannot afford to keep overlooking this connection.

Seventy to eighty percent of the cholesterol in the body is not from what we eat, but rather is produced internally, by the body itself. That's why diets so often don't work to regulate cholesterol levels—and why hormones are much more important than we are generally led to believe. The pharmaceutical industry sells drugs that can reduce cholesterol 10 to 30 percent as the answer. But why not use natural substances the body already makes for this purpose rather than these artificial products, which are foreign to the body and associated with unpleasant side effects? The results are just as good—and often better.

Do you have high cholesterol? Taking thyroid hormones, for example, drops elevated cholesterol levels. An excessive rise of cholesterol is a characteristic sign of low thyroid hormone levels, and a cholesterol level that is too *low* is a sign of thyroid hormone excess. With appropriate treatment, cholesterol levels stabilize in the healthy range. The greater the dose of thyroid hormones a patient takes, the more the cholesterol will drop. The reduction is usually proportional to the blood level of T_3, the active thyroid hormone.

Testosterone is also important to maintaining desirable cholesterol levels in men. A study of male rabbits, for example, showed that castrated animals (so, animals deprived of most of their testosterone supply) have dangerously high cholesterol but that in those same animals, given supplemental testosterone, the cholesterol level drops.

DHEA can also diminish cholesterol levels, but the drop is fairly modest and requires a higher dose than I'd usually recommend. I recommend it to my patients in small doses aimed at preventing further increases in cholesterol levels.

Is your bad cholesterol (LDL) too high or your good cholesterol (HDL) too low? The risk of heart disease rises not only with total cholesterol levels, but also proportionally with the level of LDL cholesterol (low-density lipoprotein, the bad cholesterol) and inversely with the level of HDL cholesterol (high-density lipoprotein, the good cholesterol). Growth hormone lowers LDL and raises HDL—just the opposite of what happens as the body ages.

The sex hormones also act positively on cholesterol levels. Estrogen (in women) and testosterone (in men) also bring down the bad and bring up the good cholesterol. Women taking supplemental estrogen will see their HDL rise and their LDL fall. In men, the higher the level of testosterone and its derivatives in the blood, the higher the HDL level and the greater the level of protection for the heart. (A word of warning: Some doctors tell heart patients not to take testosterone for any reason. That's because taking some forms can provoke a drop in HDL. Note, however, that this drop comes when patients are taking the hormone orally and using a synthetic form. Natural testosterone via injection or from a gel applied on the skin has no such down side and is, in fact, protective.)

Do you have high cholesterol because of poor kidney function? EPO, which stimulates the production of red blood cells, also helps maintain a healthful cholesterol level in people with renal insufficiency. Poor kidney function often leads to low EPO levels.

Do you have arteriosclerosis? Men with arteriosclerosis generally have low testosterone levels. A German study compared sterile men with low levels of testosterone to men with arteriosclerosis and to normal men, and the group with arteriosclerosis had the lowest testosterone levels of all. All the men with low testosterone also had high blood levels of apoprotein B, a fat-protein complex harmful to the arteries. Though studies are sparse, the ones there are indicate that taking natural testosterone by injection or skin cream can help reverse arteriosclerosis.

Is your cholesterol high from a diet too rich in fat? Is it hereditary? Is your cholesterol high only now that you're older? Did medications you are taking increase your cholesterol level? Melatonin often lowers high cholesterol levels, particularly in cases of fatty diets, heredity, old age, or medications, according to studies of mice. Mice with low melatonin levels (having damaged pineal glands) have cholesterol levels 30 percent higher than normal. When elderly mice receive melatonin, they escape the progressive rise in cholesterol that mice undergo with aging.

Melatonin might work this way in humans, too, as it increases the conversion of precursor thyroid hormone T_4 into T_3 and this increases thyroid function and the thyroid-hormone-related drop in cholesterol.

Has your cholesterol risen excessively? Pregnenolone, a precursor of all the other adrenal hormones, fights an excessive rise in cholesterol.

DECODING YOUR DEFICIENCIES

HIGH BLOOD PRESSURE

Americans make more than thirty million visits to doctors' offices each year because of high blood pressure; that's because 23 percent of Americans between the ages of twenty and seventy-four have it at any given time. For the majority of us, sooner or later our blood pressure is going to get too high. The artery walls lose their flexibility and no longer dilate as well with each heartbeat; the rigidity of the walls increases the pressure within the arteries—increasing the blood pressure. High blood pressure accelerates the aging of the heart and blood vessels, causing atherosclerosis and increased risk of heart disease and heart attack, and prompting negative symptoms such as headaches and fatigue. The constant threat to a person with high blood pressure is suffering a stroke due to excessive pressure in the brain. The risk is much higher than for a person with healthy blood pressure.

Once again, here is a condition that increases gradually with age and, once again, the coordination with declining hormone levels is no coincidence. And here again, the drug companies have poured money and time into producing products that control high blood pressure. While I want to give them their due for their search for a cure, it is important to remember that these medicines aren't always effective, and they often bring with them undesirable side effects like fatigue, dizziness, headaches, and coughing that can easily be enough to make a patient stop treatment.

Fortunately, there are powerful (if often overlooked) alternatives. Deficiencies of several different hormones can lead to high blood pressure, and filling in those deficiencies often normalizes blood pressure. And since natural hormones are not alien substances to your body, they can be at least as effective as drug treatment without provoking negative reactions. (Not to mention the other problems they can solve, ostensibly not related to high blood pressure. Unlike much of what the drug companies market, hormones are not one-trick ponies.)

Is your blood pressure too high? Thyroid hormones keep the arterial wall flexible and blood pressure stable. Without sufficient thyroid hormones, waste accumulates between the cells of the arterial walls, slowing the entry of nutrients into the cells, thereby disturbing their proper functioning. A swelling forms around this waste pileup, swelling the arterial walls and limiting their flexibility. Blood pressure rises. Thyroid replacement therapy, fortunately, restores healthy blood pressure. Better still, taking thyroid hormones if you have a deficit can prevent high blood pressure from occurring. The best study in this regard followed more than one thousand patients using thyroid hormones for twenty years. Someone whose body doesn't make enough thyroid hormones has three times the risk of developing high blood pressure than a normal person over that kind of time frame. That is, three hundred out of one thousand patients with low thyroid, and not using thyroid hormone supplements, would get high blood pressure. But only five patients did. That's sixty times less than would otherwise be expected.

DHEA also plays a role in preventing high blood pressure. It dilates the arteries and, in addition, lowers blood pressure by taming excess levels of glucocorticosteroids—stress hormones. It fights, therefore, the stress-related components of high blood pressure. Patients with high blood pressure tend to have low DHEA levels.

Taking DHEA can help with high blood pressure in cases of excessive use of mineral corticosteroids causing high blood pressure. Mineral corticosteroids (including aldosterone) retain water and salt in the body.

Is your systolic blood pressure (the top number) high? People with high blood pressure have lower than average levels of melatonin. Melatonin also fights high blood pressure. One study shows a one-third drop in systolic pressure in patients taking melatonin compared to a control group treated with a placebo. The diastolic pressure dropped more than 20 percent. I must mention that the doses were given at bedtime, when the body has the maximum number of melatonin receptors.

Melatonin's importance is underlined by the fact that animals with very low melatonin thanks to damaged pineal glands have high blood pressure. This normalizes as soon as they are given supplemental melatonin.

Is your diastolic blood pressure (the bottom number) high? Are the diastolic and systolic too close together? Without enough thyroid hormones, blood pressure rises—especially the diastolic number, which is even more crucial to heart health than the systolic number. Systolic and diastolic readings are closer to each other than normal because the inflexible artery walls can't give clear pressure differences between the two. In patients with thyroid levels that are too high, on the other hand, systolic and diastolic pressures are abnormally far apart.

Do you have high blood pressure that started at menopause or, for men, at midlife, with high systolic and diastolic readings? The sex hormones, estrogen for women and testosterone for men, protect against developing high blood pressure, as long as you do not take them orally, which can *increase* blood pressure. So can the synthetic versions, so you must stick to natural preparations, molecularly identical to the hormone naturally present in the body, via skin cream, patch, or implant or, as an additional option for testosterone, via injection.

Natural estrogen taken through the skin has been proven to lower systolic and diastolic blood pressure, while synthetic derivatives taken orally induce a rise, especially in the diastolic number.

In men with high blood pressure, testosterone levels are 30 percent lower than normal and might normalize when given sufficient testosterone. Testosterone dilates the arteries, including the aorta and the coronary arteries of the heart, which lowers blood pressure.

Do you have high blood pressure due to poor kidney function? Growth hormone quickly improves kidney function by increasing the flow of blood to the kidneys and increasing the elasticity of arterial walls. Many people respond within weeks. This is important because kidneys in bad shape, worn down, and poorly irrigated increase blood pressure. Furthermore, the lower the blood level of somatomedin C, growth hormone's close working partner, the higher both the systolic and diastolic readings will be. Maintaining proper levels of somatomedin C, and thus of growth hormone, brings blood pressure into the healthful range.

DECODING YOUR DEFICIENCIES

LOW BLOOD PRESSURE

Significantly less common than high blood pressure, low blood pressure is nonetheless problematic to those who have it. It can occur in people over sixty-five, as the endocrine glands wear out. Symptoms include feeling woozy, low stress resistance, and feeling faint when standing.

Do you have low blood pressure? Cortisol, aldosterone, and vasopressin play major roles in maintaining sufficient pressure in the arteries. Vasopressin retains water in the body, especially at night, playing its part in maintaining blood pressure. Aldosterone slows the loss of salt and water from the kidneys, keeping these basic components of blood pressure regulation available for the body to use to raise blood pressure.

If your body is deprived of cortisol, you will die in a matter of days, in large part because your blood pressure drops, ultimately to zero. Cortisol helps maintain appropriate blood sugar levels to nourish the cells, not least of which are the smooth muscle cells of the artery walls, keeping them strong. It increases the sensitivity of the blood vessels to other hormones that raise blood pressure. Cortisol also retains water and salt in the body, preventing them from being unnecessarily excreted in the

ERICA

It was just about all Erica could do to get out of bed and keep her first appointment with me. For three years she had suffered from severe, disabling chronic fatigue syndrome. Although she was only in her mid-twenties, she had "retired" from her job a year before, simply unable to get up and go to it each day, she was so intensely tired. Financial stress compounded her problems. Worse, no one around her really understood what she was going through—or even believed her.

Along with her chronic fatigue, Erica had been diagnosed with low blood pressure. It hovered around 75/40. To normalize it she was taking two medications—at double doses, yet with only about half the expected effectiveness. Without the drugs she couldn't even get out of bed.

Her history and physical exam revealed multiple hormone deficiencies, which is usual in cases of longstanding, overwhelming fatigue. Her adrenal glands in particular weren't functioning well, which is known as adrenal burnout syndrome. Her cortisol level was especially low, which would affect blood pressure and create fatigue.

Even more telling was her relative lack of aldosterone, which is even more important for blood pressure. Its only major function is to keep salt in the body, keeping water at the same time, thereby ensuring good blood pressure along with a clear mind and good energy when on your feet. Without enough aldosterone, Erica always felt an urge to lie down. When she remained upright, she felt drowsy and confused. Since she wasn't retaining enough salt and water, she had to urinate often. She always voided lots of urine soon after drinking anything.

Erica was afraid of taking too many medications and distrusted hormone therapy. But having come to a low point in her life, she was more than ready to try just about anything promising. She agreed to try thyroid hormones and cortisol supplementation. She improved considerably within just two months. But she still felt exhausted in the upright position, and her blood pressure, while improved, was still low at 105/50 and she still needed her medications. The progress she had made already allowed her to trust me a bit more, and so she added aldosterone to the mix. She used a synthetic derivative commonly called fludrocortisone, 100 mcg a day.

Four months later, Erica was back in my office and couldn't stop smiling. The immense fatigue that had kept her in her bed or lying on the couch for most of the last few years was practically gone. In fact, she said she felt better almost immediately upon beginning the fludrocortisone. To check her results, she had halved the dose of her original low blood pressure medications, but she continued to feel better. She no longer had to go to the bathroom so often, and she rarely felt dizzy. Eventually she found she could discontinue that medication without feeling any less well, though she still took it in times of stress or hard physical or professional activities. She was back at work part time, and eight months later she was back full time. "I feel like the person I used to be!" Erica beamed.

Erica has been well for years now, with no real setbacks. She does notice some regression if she doesn't follow a healthful diet, but this is easily corrected by getting back on the good-nutrition bandwagon.

urine. This trio of functions come together to maintain proper blood pressure.

Small doses of cortisol (15 to 25 mg a day) increase systolic blood pressure by 15 percent and diastolic by 20 percent. Excessive cortisol, or synthetic versions thereof, on the other hand, create high blood pressure in many people.

DECODING YOUR DEFICIENCIES

PROTECTING THE HEART AND BLOOD VESSELS

Time and life bring minor deterioration and microscopic damage to everyone's tissues and organs, including the heart. Tissue-building anabolic hormones, despite their undeserved bad reputation thanks to abuse by overly ambitious athletes using industrial-strength derivatives of natural hormones, actually rectify and repair any tissue damage. They improve the condition of the heart, healing where necessary and protecting in any case.

Do you have heart muscles or arteries that are already damaged (including just by normal wear and tear as you age)?

Growth hormone is one of the most important hormones for the heart. It plays a large role in determining its volume and muscle tone and has a hand in setting the heart rate as well. To underline its importance, consider that a person who has always been deficient in growth hormone, like a midget, has a smaller than expected heart that beats weakly. Whether they know it or not, people who have growth hormone levels that are normal for most of their lives but decline as they age experience a slackening of all the structures in the body, including the heart, which becomes soft and less well supplied with blood. It beats more weakly, as the walls get thinner and contract less strongly, pushing less blood toward the organs with each beat. People with low growth hormone levels are more likely to die of cardiovascular disease than those with normal levels.

Supplemental growth hormone in adults with declining growth hormone secretion allows significant reversal of the aging process of the heart tissues. Growth hormone injections make the heart pump 15 to 20 percent more blood at rest and 45 percent more during exertion.

For full protection of the heart, patients most likely need growth hormone *as well as* the hormones listed below. The remaining ones won't be as powerful on their own as in combination with growth hormone.

Thyroid hormone deficiency can damage the heart. So can significant excess. So you must use care in reaping the full heart benefits without causing any harm. This has been enough to keep many doctors from recommending thyroid hormone to their cardiac patients, and that's been a loss. If you have a thyroid deficiency, there is no need to fear appropriate doses of a supplement, started low and slowly and progressively increased.

Thyroid hormones strongly influence the heartbeat. They build up the muscle cells in the heart. They increase the calcium level in cardiac cells, helping the muscle fibers to contract, and provide the cells with energy. People with different levels of active thyroid hormone (T_3) will have different heart rhythms at rest. Thyroid hormones help the heart move more blood, and to do it with greater velocity.

In men, treating any testosterone deficiency is a good preventative for heart conditions of all sorts. And all men develop a deficiency sooner or later as the tissues that produce testosterone wear away. Supplemental testosterone relieves even hearts and arteries that are already not up to par. The heart is supremely sensitive to testosterone. Testosterone accumulates in the heart twice as much as in normal muscle and five times as much as in the prostate, which is famously receptive to it.

In studies of rats treated with testosterone, their hearts stayed healthy even when their aortas were purposely narrowed. Narrowing of this principal artery overloads the heart and forces it to exert much greater effort just to push the blood through. Without enough testosterone, the heart simply can't do it. On the other hand, a heart with a plentiful testosterone supply remains oxygenated, strong, and tough.

Estrogen plays a similar protective role in women, through similar mechanisms. Estrogen dilates coronary arteries, increasing the blood supply to the heart. Then it increases the strength of the heart's contractions as well as boosts its capacity for relaxation, which also serves to increase the blood flow. Furthermore, estrogen calms the heart by lowering the heartbeat and decreasing noradrenaline discharge at times of mental stress.

More important than the reasons are the results. A woman taking estrogen at menopause not only has a better quality of life (eliminating annoying and disruptive menopausal symptoms such as hot flashes and mood swings), she also lives longer and develops heart disease much more slowly or not at all. She has close to two times less risk of dying from a heart attack than a woman of similar age not taking estrogen.

The natural form of progesterone protects the arteries against spasms. Many, many heart attacks in women occur when there is no real obstruction of the coronary artery. They are most likely due to spasms in the cardiac arteries that simply last too long. This type of heart attack typically happens after menopause, when the ovaries have quit producing most of their hormones, including progesterone. Replacement therapy remedies this kind of arterial problem.

Note well that some synthetic progesterone (progestin) can actually contribute to that type of spasm. Using only natural progesterone to protect your heart is crucial.

Do you have cardiovascular disease? Thyroid hormones can slow the development of cardiovascular diseases.

Do you have angina? Intermittent claudication? Arterioscle-
rosis? Leg ulcers? Gangrene? Testosterone, especially by injection,
reduces the intensity, duration, and frequency of angina (pain resulting
when the heart does not receive enough blood) and intermittent claudication (pains in the calves when walking due to arteriosclerosis). In high
doses it accelerates the healing of leg ulcers (which occur due to poor
blood supply) and even gangrenes for which surgery and amputation
were once considered the only solution left.

Melatonin also plays a role in angina. Men with angina typically
have a lower melatonin level—up to five times lower at night—than
other men their age. No study yet proves that taking melatonin reduces
angina, but it might well since it makes blood more fluid.

Is your red blood cell count low? With EPO therapy, the heart
functions more effectively. EPO increases the production of red blood
cells. EPO treatment increases the amount of oxygen carried in the
blood. Tissues all over the body, including in the heart and arteries,
experience better oxygenation as a result.

Do you have a weak heartbeat? Rapid heartbeat? Do either or
both happen to you when you are under stress or exerting
yourself? Do they happen more often when you are standing
up? As described above, both growth hormone and testosterone can
improve a weak and slow heartbeat. As for a weak and rapid heartbeat,
especially under the conditions in the question above, cortisol can be
helpful.

Cortisol is important for good cardiac functioning. It stimulates the
cardiac cells' sensitivity to adrenaline (the "fight" part of "fight or
flight"), allowing the heart to contract strongly. When it is released in
response to stress, cortisol increases the flow of blood, sending blood to
the parts of the body that need it most urgently by narrowing the arteries farthest from the heart. Without enough cortisol, the heart beats
weakly and too rapidly, especially when standing or in stressful situations, and isn't able to handle exertion or stress.

Cortisol is a catabolic hormone, meaning that it consumes tissue in
order to make energy. So it is appropriate for treating the heart only when
balanced with the tissue-building effects of an anabolic hormone like
DHEA or, as second choice, testosterone. Growth hormone, while not
anabolic, or its partner somatomedin C, can also play the supporting role.

Do you have atherosclerosis because of a fatty diet? Angina? Are you at increased risk of heart attack and/or heart disease? DHEA has impressive benefits for the heart, at least in men. I think it helps women, too, but few studies indicate that yet, as most of the work has been done on males. With my female patients I don't use it solely for prevention or cure of heart problems. Animal studies have shown that DHEA slows atherosclerosis due to an excessively fatty diet. For men with atherosclerosis in the coronary arteries, the lower their DHEA blood level, the greater their risk of strictures of their coronary arteries and the less well they feel.

Studies have shown that people with good DHEA levels are less likely to have a heart attack than are those whose DHEA levels are low. In addition, the chances of surviving a heart attack are greater in patients with higher DHEA levels. Compared to other men their age, men over fifty with low DHEA (under 140 mcg/dl, which is frequent in people over sixty) have up to three times the risk of dying from cardiovascular disease, twice the risk of dying whatever the cause, and three times the risk of developing angina or another condition of insufficient blood supply to the heart. On the other hand, with each 100 mcg/dl (1000 ng/ml) increase in DHEA blood level, the risk decreases by half.

Do you have diabetes? Insulin is another anabolic hormone that continually builds and restores cardiac tissue. It does this by stimulating the production of proteins essential to the survival of cardiac cells. When insulin is low, as in diabetes, the cells of the body, including the heart, become more and more resistant to its action and the heart ages more quickly. Furthermore, when the level of sugar in the blood and the tissues is high (as it is when insulin is low), a sugary "glue" slows the passage of oxygen to the arteries supplying the heart's cardiac cells. The cells are deprived of oxygen, which can lead to a heart attack. Among heart attack patients, 5 percent have diabetes, a rate much higher than in the general population.

DECODING YOUR DEFICIENCIES

STROKE

The success of hormones in the prevention and treatment of cardiovascular diseases is repeated in the arteries of the brain, lowering the risk of stroke and speeding recovery. The arteries that supply blood to the brain keep our neurons alive, allowing us our consciousness and all our movement. Tragedy strikes when they are blocked, as when a clot forms, generally in the heart or in an artery below the heart. The arteries can become blocked slowly, too, by the formation of plaque (thrombosis) and can burst and cause a cerebral hemorrhage or stroke. Paralysis, problems speaking, memory loss, and disorders of consciousness and impaired sense of touch can result. Fortunately, hormones can prevent them in the first place and help repair the damage if it's already been done.

Do you have a tendency to get blood clots? Melatonin acts as a nocturnal anticoagulant. It diminishes the ability of blood-clotting platelets to stick to the walls of blood vessels and keeps the blood fluid during the night, both of which act to prevent thrombosis, the clotting within a blood vessel that can lead to stroke.

The beneficial effects of melatonin on the blood vessels practically disappear upon getting up in the morning. That's a good thing because blood should be able to coagulate during the day, when humans are active and at risk of hurting themselves and bleeding. We wouldn't want melatonin to be unlimited this way, as we need platelets to avoid bleeding too easily in general and specifically to avoid having abnormal hemorrhages, including stroke.

Have you had cerebral hemorrhage? People with cerebral hemorrhage (loss of blood in brain tissue between the arteries of the brain) have low thyroid levels. Thyroid hormones are important in getting the brain the blood it needs. In people with unhealthy brain blood vessels, the level of active thyroid hormone (T_3) is generally low, while the less active forms (like T_4) increase.

Do you feel dizzy or drowsy? Cortisol and aldosterone help maintain proper pressure in the cerebral arteries.

Do you have arteriosclerosis? DHEA keeps the artery walls in good shape and lessens the degree to which blood-clotting platelets cling to each other, preventing thrombosis. It also helps prevent buildup of plaque in the arteries to the brain. Testosterone has an even stronger blood-clot-dissolving effect.

Do you have diabetes and atherosclerosis? Insulin protects the arteries in general and the cerebral arteries in particular against aging and atherosclerosis. People producing little or no insulin—people with diabetes—get the most benefit in this regard from treatment with insulin. It isn't something you'd use for protection against stroke unless you were diabetic.

Are you at increased risk of stroke? Using sex hormones, via injection or through the skin, is an important way to prevent stroke. Animal studies show that, in females, estrogen helps prevent strokes and limits the damage when they do occur. When necessary it can curb the excess flow of blood to the brain, which causes damage by compression.

In men, testosterone benefits the arteries of the brain by two principal mechanisms. First, it develops the muscle cells of the artery walls, keeping them flexible and preventing deterioration. Second, it has anticoagulant properties—but only when not taken orally. In fact, taking it orally can actually lead to unwanted thickening of the blood, although one study shows an oral testosterone with anticoagulant effects.

Are you at increased risk of stroke? Adults low in growth hormone are more likely to have a stroke than those with sufficient levels. If you do have a stroke, animal studies show that growth hormone precursor somatomedin C can limit the damage, particularly in areas of the brain responsible for memory and emotion.

Women: Do you have swelling from a brain injury? Progesterone reduces brain swelling from trauma. It keeps the neurons from degenerating and protects spatial memory, which keeps you oriented in space.

SUMMARY: HEART AND ARTERY HEALTH

Hormone Deficiency	Symptoms	See also pg.
Aldosterone	low blood pressure; dizziness or drowsiness; rapid heartbeat when standing up	26
Cortisol	low blood pressure; weak heartbeat; rapid heartbeat; weak and rapid heartbeat when under stress or exerting yourself or standing up; dizziness or drowsiness	26
DHEA	high blood pressure; high cholesterol; atherosclerosis because of a fatty diet; angina; increased risk of heart attack and/or heart disease; arteriosclerosis	27
EPO	low red blood cell count	28
Estrogen	high cholesterol with high LDL; low HDL; high blood pressure that started at midlife or menopause; damaged heart or arteries; increased risk of stroke	28
Growth Hormone	high LDL; low HDL; high blood pressure due to poor kidney function; damaged heart or arteries; weak heartbeat; slow heartbeat	29
Insulin	high cholesterol and diabetes; atherosclerosis and diabetes	30
Melatonin	high cholesterol from a fatty diet; hereditary high cholesterol; high cholesterol as a result of aging; high cholesterol due to medications; high systolic and diastolic blood pressure; angina; tendency to get blood clots	30
Progesterone	damaged heart or arteries; spasm of the coronary arteries; swelling from a brain injury	32
Testosterone (in men)	high LDL; low HDL; arteriosclerosis; high cholesterol; high blood pressure that started at midlife; damaged heart or arteries; angina; intermittent claudication; leg ulcers; gangrene; weak heartbeat; slow heartbeat; increased risk of stroke	33
Testosterone (in women)	high blood pressure that started at menopause	32

SUMMARY: HEART AND ARTERY HEALTH
(continued)

Hormone Deficiency	Symptoms	See also pg.
Thyroid	high cholesterol; damaged heart or arteries; cardiovascular disease; high blood pressure; high diastolic blood pressure; diastolic and systolic blood pressure readings too close together; diastolic and systolic blood pressure readings both too high; cerebral hemorrhage; slow and weak, almost inaudible, heartbeat	33
Vasopressin	low blood pressure	34

CHAPTER TEN

YOUR IMMUNE
SYSTEM

*J*ust to warn you, this chapter will be a little different than the others in Parts II and III. Here there is no specific condition that can be addressed with specific hormones. Instead, we're taking a more general approach. The main point is to help you understand the potential problems of hormone deficiencies, which can include a weakened immune system and so increased susceptibility to infections and cancers. You wouldn't take hormones specifically to fight an infection or cancer you already have, but balancing your hormones can help prevent them in the first place.

It is true, however, that the sicker a person gets, the more important it becomes for him to get the hormones he needs. Better still, of course, is to fill in any deficiencies you have sooner rather than later and perhaps avoiding getting sick at all. Timely hormone replacement therapy can help prevent infections and cancer. Once a disease is in place, the endocrine glands might be further weakened and hormone deficiencies aggravated. Correcting deficiencies can increase immunity. And some hormones, including thyroid hormones and melatonin, appear to have some anticancer properties. Finally, there are some cases in which hormones might be beneficial as part of actually treating cancer.

LISE

*L*ise was the very picture of what can go wrong when your immune system isn't up to snuff. She didn't have the big baddie, cancer, so it could always have been worse. But it was plenty miserable the way it was. Lise always had some kind of infection. It had been this way since childhood: No sooner did one cold dissipate than she got a sore throat. Or an earache. Or the flu. Or bronchitis. Or tuberculosis. After more than forty years, Lise was more than tired of this routine. But she didn't know what to do.

Thyroid deficiency brings major immunity problems in its wake, leaving the body sensitive to all sorts of infections, mild and severe. Tuberculosis is a possible sign of immune problems caused by thyroid deficiency. Children with thyroid deficiency—and Lise most probably had been one—might catch one thing after the next all winter long (and perhaps year round). There's usually little relief until the rise in sex hormones at puberty enhances immunity, usually enough to break the seemingly never-ending loop of infections. Lise had found some relief as she became an adolescent, but it turned out to be temporary. In recent years she had been once again plagued by a long chain of infections. Her current specialty was hard-to-control bladder infections.

Lab tests did indeed detect a thyroid deficiency, but they also revealed an estrogen deficiency. That probably explained the resurgence in infections, and bladder infections in particular. The urinary tract is dependent on a healthful balance in the female hormones. If estrogen levels are low, the mucous membranes (the inside layer) of the urinary tubes and the bladder are thin and weak and can't defend themselves well against bacteria and other microbes.

Lise began using supplemental thyroid hormones, an estrogen gel on her skin from the fifth to the twenty-fifth day of her menstrual cycle, and oral progesterone from the fifteenth to the twenty-fifth day. She was free of urinary tract infections within two months, as estrogen works more quickly than thyroid hormones, and after five months she felt fine, even though it was the middle of winter, her usual busy season from the germ perspective. (The female hormones she was taking, in the way she was taking them, did not interfere with ovulation, so she had to use some other method of contraception; birth-control pills were out of the question, as they would have disturbed her hormonal levels as we were trying to find their equilibrium.) With the thyroid deficiency corrected, as it was in Lise's case after four to five months, her infections were less severe and became less frequent. After ten months of treatment, she'd gone five months without any infection at all, not a single cold. It's now been years since she first consulted me, and Lise comes back in for regular checkups. But she rarely has more than one cold or flu a year and has had only a couple of mild bladder infections. Her immune system has been able to recover its strength and go back to doing its job—and doing it properly.

STIMULATING IMMUNITY

*I*t is possible to match specific hormones with specific immunity issues, and we'll get to that later in the chapter. Before we do, I want to look at a number of hormones and how they boost immunity in general. The first three (DHEA, melatonin, and thyroid hormones) are the most important, although there is a good list of second-string players, as you'll see.

DHEA

DHEA stimulates the immune system, reversing some of the immuno-logical changes that come with age, as various important immune system chemicals decline. For example, as we age, humans produce fewer and fewer antibodies to protect themselves from external invaders (germs) or internal aggressors (like cancer). DHEA therapy increases production of antibodies, including the kind that stick around after an infection is over with their capacity to recognize and attack that specific germ still in place and vigilant. These antibodies are known as G immunoglobu-lins. We have them to thank for getting chicken pox a maximum of once, for example. They are what make vaccinations work.

As we get older, we also make less and less interleukin 2, a chemi-cal that helps cells in the immune system communicate with each other. DHEA boosts the production of it. It also increases the amount made of a similar messenger, gamma interferon, which is produced by cells infected by a virus to alert healthy neighbors to the infection.

DHEA can also fight autoimmune diseases. With age the immune cells sometimes choose the wrong target and produce antibodies against the body's own tissues, as in some forms of rheumatoid arthritis and lupus. Animal studies have shown that DHEA slows the production of these "auto-antibodies."

For all these reasons, DHEA should improve resistance to infec-tions. It is best able to influence the immune system when taken via injection or gel applied on the skin, as the skin (like the brain) can trans-form DHEA into an even stronger immune booster, androstenetriol.

MELATONIN

Melatonin reinforces the actions of immune-system cells. For example, it increases levels of at least five types of infection-fighting white blood cells. It stimulates the bone marrow to make more of the type of white blood cells the body uses to fight bacterial infection. It boosts levels of another type—eosinophils—that the body uses to combat parasite-caused infections. Melatonin also increases the level of a third type of white blood cell used to make antibodies to control viral infections and makes them more sensitive and more active. It creates more of a fourth type known as "humoral" immune cells, which otherwise decrease with age. Levels of the fifth type, thymus lymph cells, known as T cells, jump as well. T cells work locally, going into specific tissues and working there when they are needed. Without enough melatonin, the making of T cells slows, weakening immunity.

The thymus is an essential immune gland in children, but it degenerates almost completely over the years. Supplemental melatonin can reactivate it, particularly when any other hormonal deficiencies are also filled in. The research on this point has been done mostly in mice. Just as in humans, as mice get older their melatonin levels drop and their thymus glands break down, so they make fewer T cells. Given melatonin supplements (or, thanks to the magic of microsurgical transplant techniques, a new pineal gland to make more melatonin), their thymuses recover and resume immune activity. The number of active thymus cells increases—some of them up to the level of young mice—and the thymus gland increases in size and weight.

The secret is apparently the way melatonin improves zinc absorption. Zinc boosts several immune functions itself, and you need healthful levels to keep your thymus in good working order.

Melatonin therapy also helps the spleen, another immune-system component, recover its youthful levels of activity in the face of the decline brought on by age.

It is important to note that for greatest effectiveness, melatonin must be taken at night, when the body has the most melatonin receptors ready and waiting. In the daytime, the number of melatonin receptors is much lower, and results won't be as outstanding.

THYROID HORMONES

Thyroid hormones stimulate immunity on all possible levels. For starters, with thyroid hormone deficiency, heat production is low, resulting in slow metabolic reactions as well as sluggish immune reactions. When the immune system reacts slowly, microbes have time to multiply and proliferate before the body gets it together to intervene.

Thyroid hormones also increase the size of the organs of the lymph system—and the larger they are, the stronger the immune response possible. In addition, thyroid hormones maintain a healthful ratio of two types of T cells. Studies on chickens show that thyroid deficiency upsets that ratio, compromising immune response.

ESTROGEN

Estrogen stimulates immunity and diminishes susceptibility to infections. It activates proliferation of monocytes (large white blood cells). It increases production of B lymph cells, which, in contrast to T cells, work from a distance, secreting antibodies into the blood. The benefits occur only in sexually mature animals—so, in humans, only after adolescence. Estrogen counters urinary infections. Studies in chickens demonstrated that estrogen fights certain viral infections.

TESTOSTERONE

Male hormones, in physiologic doses, stimulate immunity. Testosterone protects the thyroid gland from autoimmune inflammation, which 10 to 15 percent of women over forty have. The most common form is known as Hashimoto's disease. In some parasitic infections, you'll find low testosterone levels. Low testosterone levels might encourage the tissue damage done by viral infections, including AIDS.

GROWTH HORMONE

Growth hormone enhances cellular immunity. It increases the number of cells in the thymus, and its volume, and reactivates the gland and the production of the thymus hormones, increasing cellular immunity and local immunity in each part of the body. It can up the number of beneficial CD4 immune cells and stimulate phagocytosis, again stimulating local immunity. Then, if something happens in a tissue, there are already immune cells there to combat it. Growth hormone increases production of B lymph cells and the level of immunoglobulins. It might help fight the damage done by viral infections and bacterial infections like salmonella. Studies of patients with severe burns show growth hormone helps reduce infections. In fact, there's a list of studies showing benefits. Unfortunately, there are also some that show unfavorable effects. Fortunately, it is clear that filling in a known growth hormone deficiency with physiologic doses is a good thing. For now, no one else should use it just on the promise of immune-system benefits.

CORTISOL

At excessive doses, cortisol and its derivatives tend to lower immunity, but in physiologic doses, they increase it. Cortisol stimulates the production of and protects T cells and beneficial CD4+ cells, stimulates communication and interaction between immune system cells, and raises the level of white granulocytes to improve local immunity. Cortisol increases the level of the antibodies known as M, G, and A immunoglobulins, though excessive doses bring them down. It has been proven to counter a range of viral infections, including the flu, measles, and mononucleosis/Epstein-Barr virus. The list of bacterial infections it is good for is even longer and includes bacterial pneumonia, Legionnaire's, typhoid fever, tuberculosis, bacterial meningitis, bacteremic shock, bacterial infection of the cornea (via local application), and bacterial superinfections in AIDS patients. It does not, on the other hand, seem to help with parasitic or yeast infections—or at least no benefit has yet been proven.

PROGESTERONE

Progesterone benefits the immune system. It supports the thymus.

CANCER

More than half a million Americans die of cancer every year—and that's only a fraction of those who suffer with the disease in one of its myriad forms. Over the years, medicine has accumulated more and more efficient weapons in the arsenal against cancer, all of which either directly attack the cancer cells, as in chemotherapy, or stimulate immunity—the body's own defense systems against cancer. Total effectiveness of these treatments is still much more rare than we'd wish, and the ideal would obviously be to avoid cancer altogether. A strong immune system is the key to that plan, and balanced hormone levels are key to a healthy immune system. Hormones, with a few rare exceptions, don't kill malignant cells directly; they accomplish the same goal indirectly, however, by stimulating the immune system.

If immune defenses drop, the risk of developing cancer increases. When some hormone levels drop, immune defenses drop. Hormones, appropriately used, can reduce the risk of cancer, although they cannot banish it completely or permanently. What preventive treatment might actually do is delay, perhaps greatly, the day cancer will eventually strike. If and when cancer does occur, the hormones will have made the body more resistant to malignant tumors, increasing the chances of a cure. (I'm talking only about hormone therapy supporting medically proven anti-cancer treatments. Hormones alone are never a treatment for cancer.)

We'll look here at several specific hormones and their effects on cancer risk.

ESTROGEN AND CANCER

Estrogen has gotten a bad rap as a cause of cancer. Excessive doses of some synthetic forms have been associated with increased risk, but the appropriate forms in the appropriate doses might actually be protective against cancer. A number of studies show estrogen's anticancer properties. The overall cancer risk—the risk of having any sort of cancer—is lower in women taking estrogen. For example, estriol, and in some circumstances estradiol, might offer protection against breast cancer. The studies showing the most positive results are of breast cancer caused by chemicals in animals. Estrogen also seems to slow the spread of cancer throughout the rest of the body. That might be one reason women with higher estrogen levels thanks to taking the hormone prior to the appearance of breast cancer live longer after the disease has appeared than women with lower estrogen levels. Caution is still in order, as there is a 10 to 20 percent increase in breast cancer incidence in women taking estrogen even though mortality from all forms of cancer is reduced.

TESTOSTERONE AND CANCER

Testosterone might be protective against cancer, even prostate cancer. For advanced or terminal prostate cancer patients, testosterone therapy might improve the length of survival after cancer, according to two studies. Men from families predisposed to prostate cancer generally have lower testosterone levels in the blood than other men of similar ages. This suggests that men with higher levels of testosterone have less risk of prostate cancer than those with low levels.

GROWTH HORMONE AND CANCER

Various studies have shown growth hormone (and somatomedin C) to be beneficial in cases of breast cancer (in rats), liver cancer (caused by carcinogens), prostate cancer, and endometrial cancer. Growth hormone supplements inhibited metastases of prostate cancer in rats. Patients with endometrial cancer and liver cancer usually have low levels of growth hormone. With liver cancer, it is still uncertain if the low growth-hormone levels contribute to the cancer or are a consequence of it. All this raises the important question: Would correcting the deficiency combat the cancer? Unfortunately, no study has yet answered this question, although at least one physician in the United States is using growth hormone supplements in deficient terminal cancer patients with success in improving quality of life and prolonging survival, and tumor growth seems to be contained.

Growth hormone should be useful as a palliative in terminal cancer, helping to maintain body weight and muscle tone to improve quality of life and duration of survival.

Despite its promise, I think it wise to restrict growth hormone for cancer to the rare cases of symptomatic and proven severe deficiency, when everything else has been tried unsuccessfully, and only in physiologic doses designed to just fill the deficiency. Not enough is established about growth hormone and cancer to recommend its wider use.

CORTISOL AND CANCER

Cortisol might be useful as a component of cancer treatment, as it can lessen inflammation, eliminate fever, relieve pain, stimulate the appetite, and produce feelings of well-being. It is especially useful in treating leukemia and lymphoma, especially in children, and might have some benefits in ancillary treatment of myeloma and metastatic brain cancer. It can be used to reduce the swelling of breast cancer metastases in the brain and spine, lessening compression and pain. Cortisol can lower excessive calcium levels from bone metastases eating away bone and letting calcium escape into the blood. We need calcium, of course, and low levels are problematic, too, but we need it mostly in the bones, not the blood, and high levels bring their own problems, including cardiac arrhythmias.

Cortisol and its synthetic derivatives are often used in combination with other anticancer drugs to help tolerate their side effects. They are part of a reliable cure for leukemias and lymphomas and work against multiple myeloma and prostate cancer, too.

THYROID AND CANCER

Thyroid hormones apparently help prevent cancer and improve survival in those who do get cancer. It might slow the growth of cancer cells. For people with thyroid hormone deficits, correcting those deficits can significantly diminish their risk of cancer.

One study of hypothyroid (low thyroid) patients showed that only 3 percent of those treated with 130 mg or more of dried animal thyroid gland powder developed cancer, while 74 percent of those receiving 65 mg or less (insufficient amounts to correct a deficiency) did. The most common cancers in that group were colon and rectal cancer, followed by uterine cancer, then lung cancer, and Hodgkin's disease. And all this although patients in the well-treated group were followed for longer than the thyroid-deficient group, on average (fifteen years versus ten years).

Another study followed three thousand patients treated at a clinic specializing in thyroid disorders. They were divided into three groups: patients with thyroid hormone deficiency (7 percent), patients with an overactive thyroid (38 percent), and patients with normal thyroid levels (55 percent). The average age of each group was comparable, forty-seven to fifty years old. Seven percent of the deficient patients developed malignant tumors. Only half as many (3.5 percent) did in the normal group, and only 2 percent in those with excess thyroid hormone.

All the patients in this study were women, and breast cancer was the most frequently detected cancer in the group. Patients with higher levels of thyroid hormone showed a clearly higher survival rate. Of the eight women in this category who developed breast cancer, only one died within eight years after diagnosis, and one more when that time frame was stretched to twenty years. The situation was far gloomier for the three women in the deficient thyroid group who developed breast cancer: All died within sixteen months after diagnosis. The study fails to mention the mortality rate of women with normal thyroid levels.

Another study confirms this pattern. One hundred eighty-four breast-cancer patients proved to have a thyroid gland significantly larger than average, indicating some abnormality of the thyroid gland and a tendency toward insufficiency. The thyroid gland increases in size to capture more iodine from the blood in order to make more thyroid hormone, so an enlarged thyroid gland reveals a need for more thyroid hormones. Forty percent of women with breast cancer have abnormally enlarged thyroid glands, compared to just under 9 percent of healthy control women.

While we're on the breast cancer–thyroid connection, I want to take a minute to note that breast-cancer mortality rates are highest in the regions of the world where goiter is most frequent. Goiter, the swelling of the thyroid gland to the point where it is easily visible, is a disease of iodine deficiency. And iodine is key in making thyroid hormones. Geographically speaking, areas without much iodine overlap with the areas of greatest frequency of thyroid insufficiency. Breast-cancer mortality, on the other hand, is lower in iodine-rich regions.

DHEA AND CANCER

DHEA helps prevent cancer. Several studies have shown how this hormone stimulates immunity, offering protection from several specific kinds of cancer, including breast, prostate, testicular, liver, thyroid, and colon cancers.

For example, in several studies, women with breast cancer and men with prostate cancer have lower than normal levels of DHEA in their blood. Breast-cancer patients have fewer than normal DHEA metabolites in their urine, too (the metabolites being substances derived from DHEA after its use; their presence indicates the body has in fact been able to use DHEA).

In animal studies (on rats), DHEA has been shown to slow or prevent the appearance of prostate cancer caused by chemicals, testicular tumors, and malignant breast tumors.

DHEA also protects the liver from tumors. It prevents a fearsome carcinogen produced by fungi (aflatoxin B-1) from making liver cells cancerous in the laboratory. In another study, other carcinogens (nitrosamines) caused almost no liver tumors in rats eating food laced with DHEA. Nitrosamines can also cause thyroid cancer in animals, though animals treated with DHEA are resistant to the tumors.

Two experiments on mice indicate that DHEA is also protective against colon cancer. A known toxin (1,2-dimethylhydrazine, if you must know) induces malignant tumors in the large intestines of the mice, but DHEA therapy significantly reduces the appearance of these tumors, making them smaller and having them show up less frequently than would otherwise be expected in animals exposed to the toxin.

Keep in mind that it isn't necessarily DHEA on its own that is responsible for these excellent results—or the lack of it that creates danger. The body converts DHEA into several other hormones, particularly testosterone and estrogen. These, as we've seen, have anticancer properties of their own. Those same hormones are also suspected, however, of favoring prostate and breast cancers, respectively. Nevertheless, no studies contradict the hypothesis that male hormones derived from DHEA (in physiologic doses) do not seem to have negative effects on the prostate. DHEA-derived estrogens, however, probably can have the same risk-increasing effect of any other estrogen on breast cancer—but that's only when it is excessive compared to progesterone and testosterone.

SERGE

Two of Serge's brothers had had prostate cancer, and one had died of it. The men in his family seemed prone to it, and there were enough other cases that Serge knew he should be grateful when he got prostate cancer in his mid-sixties because it was a well-differentiated, nonaggressive type. He had surgery to remove his prostate.

With surgery behind him, however, Serge came in to see his regular doctor—my father, as it happens—complaining about fatigue, irritability, anxiety, and little tolerance for physical exertion. Plus, he felt as if his muscles were melting off his body. The diagnosis was soon made: Serge had a deficiency of male hormones.

Because of his history of prostate cancer, Serge's urologist had told him it wasn't safe to take testosterone, which has been suspected of encouraging growth of prostate cancer. He didn't object to small doses of DHEA, however, on the condition that Serge be closely monitored.

Lab tests had shown a low level of DHEA and its metabolites, and a PSA (prostate specific antigen) test, a marker of prostate inflammation and cancer, was so low as to be undetectable, so Serge went ahead and started taking 25 mg a day of DHEA. Happily, it was enough to curb most of his negative symptoms. Even better, none of the regular PSA tests he took ever showed any increase. Serge increased his dose to 35 mg, which resolved the last of the symptoms, and still showed no change on the PSA. It is now almost a decade since Serge started daily DHEA therapy, and he's had no cancer recurrence.

DHEA therapy won't be right for every cancer patient, prostate or otherwise, but when used carefully and properly, Serge would be the first to tell you, it can be a powerful weapon. If nothing else, it relieved many of the health complaints that were nagging at him. But it might well have played an important role in making him a cancer survivor rather than a cancer victim.

MELATONIN AND CANCER

A variety of studies show that people diagnosed with cancer have low melatonin levels in their blood. The more severe the cancer, the lower the melatonin level usually is. A high level of melatonin seems to provide some protection against cancer.

Hormone replacement therapy is generally not used as a treatment for cancer, with rare exceptions. One of those might be melatonin, which blocks the multiplication of certain fast-growing breast cancer cells (in lab cultures). Unlike most available cancer treatment, it is not toxic for healthy cells.

On another tack altogether, melatonin is helpful in the wake of anti-cancer radiation therapy, which releases lots of free radicals in the body. Melatonin, a powerful antioxidant, helps neutralize those potentially damaging molecules, reducing the negative consequences of radiation therapy.

PROGESTERONE AND CANCER

Natural progesterone is considered protective against cancer in general, and specifically against breast, endometrial, and ovarian cancer. (The more common synthetic derivatives don't have nearly as clear an effect.) Physiologic doses of natural progesterone, combined with estrogen, work on T cell and B cell immunity. In rats, natural progesterone by itself can prevent the significant age-related reduction of thymus volume and activity, preserving the ability to produce plentiful T cells.

If you take excessive doses of progesterone when you have an estrogen deficiency, you can actually lower immunity, so it is especially wise to use a physiologic dose and to combine it with estrogen (particularly if you have low levels). Progesterone should always be added to estrogen therapy to protect the breast.

CALCITONIN AND CANCER

Here the use is very specific. Calcitonin relieves the pain of spinal fractures due to cancer metastasized to the bone.

INFECTIONS

THYROID HORMONES AND INFECTIONS

Thyroid hormones stimulate immunological defenses against infectious germs. Well-adjusted doses in deficient patients significantly diminish the risk of infections and can even treat infections. They counter viruses, bacteria, and parasites. They defend against common offenders including colds, sore throats, earaches, and bladder infections as well as more serious threats like pneumonia, parasites, bone infections (osteomyelitis), and opportunistic diseases that prey on people with compromised immune systems (such as with AIDS).

In infection, thyroid hormone levels are generally low. Is this the cause or the consequence of the infection? Well, . . . yes. The stress of the infection itself leads the body to consume more hormones, including thyroid hormones. Infection also weakens the conversion in the liver of precursor thyroid hormone (T_4—thyroxine) into active (T_3) hormone. Infections caused by viruses, bacteria, and parasites lower the level of thyroid hormones in the blood and can even damage the thyroid gland. A weakened thyroid gland creates a vicious cycle, with lowered hormone levels, lowered immunity, more infections, more thyroid damage, and so on. But it is also clear that low levels of thyroid hormones encourage the infection process.

Some infections can even be treated with thyroid hormones. Several experiments show positive results. For example, patients with hepatitis A, a viral liver infection, and low thyroid hormone levels, recovered faster than expected when they were given thyroid hormones. Another study demonstrated that rabbits with tuberculosis treated with thyroid hormone had fewer lesions and quicker recovery. Additionally, more of the treated rabbits survived the infection. In yet another study, this one of men only, thyroid treatment accelerated healing of mycosis, a parasitic disease provoked by fungi that was resistant to all traditional treatments.

CORTISOL AND INFECTIONS

Cortisol stimulates immune cells to help in fighting off viral, bacterial, and (more rarely) parasitic infections—but only in small, safe, physiologic doses. At excessive doses, cortisol and its derivative are known to depress the immune system.

DHEA AND INFECTIONS

DHEA protects against viruses, bacteria, and parasites. For example, a study of mice showed that elderly mice did not create significant antibodies in response to a vaccine against a bacteria that causes pneumonia. (Mouse immune systems decline with age, just like humans', one key measure being the ability to produce antibodies.) Given DHEA, however, their immune systems were reactivated, reaching a level comparable to that of much younger mice in the antibody-making department.

Parasitic infections are less common but more often serious, so it is fortunate DHEA can be an effective defense against them. One study showed that in hamsters inoculated with cryptococcidiosis, the germs overwhelmingly invade the small intestine and then cross over into the rest of the body, causing generalized infection. Hamsters given DHEA when infected, however, are able to fight off the invaders, and the parasites are for the most part unable to colonize the intestine. Those that do are unable to cross the intestinal barrier to reach the rest of the body.

DHEA can also protect against chronic viral infection. To take just one example, in the lab, DHEA partially blocks the replication of the most common form of HIV. People with HIV have less DHEA sulfate in their blood than noninfected people. As the disease progresses and immunity drops, DHEA sulfate levels decrease. A study of HIV-positive people who feel well and haven't developed signs of the disease showed their DHEA was 28 percent lower than normal. In people who had developed symptoms, DHEA levels were down 50 percent. Another study, over seven years, of 108 HIV-positive men showed that DHEA sulfate levels that go below 18 mcg/dl in those who are still in good health is a good predictor of the first appearance of symptoms.

PROGESTERONE AND INFECTIONS

According to studies of AIDS patients—and viral bronchitis in chickens!—progesterone might be helpful against viral infections.

GROWTH HORMONE AND INFECTIONS

Growth hormone is effective against viral and bacterial infections. How it works in AIDS cases provides a good example of the positive synergy between two hormones. Separate treatment with growth hormone or insulin does not get much in the way of positive response; neither allows a patient to regain appropriate weight. But if patients receive daily injections of both, they regain weight where and how they should (gaining muscle and organ volume) and regain their strength as well. Each hormone stimulates the effects of the other.

TESTOSTERONE AND INFECTIONS

Testosterone fights the physical consequences of viral infections, including AIDS.

ESTROGEN AND INFECTIONS

Estrogen has shown benefits in cases of viral and bacterial infections.

NUTRITION

*E*ating specifically to boost general immunity has not been extensively studied. Most work focuses on specific conditions. But, clearly, being well nourished is key. Take, for example, a recent study exploring whether the often observed decline in immune function with age is inevitable. Researchers looked at well-nourished older women in good health and found they showed no decline in immune function compared to a similar group of younger women. Women over sixty were screened to make sure they were getting enough protein, iron, vitamin B_{12}, and folic acid. Those who were were the equals, when it comes to immunity, of women twenty to forty years old.

So my eat-for-immunity recommendation would be to follow the diet that's most healthful for you given your particular hormone levels and health conditions, as outlined in other chapters.

There *has* been a lot of research, however—and a lot of publicity—about diet strategies to avoid cancer specifically, presumably in part through fortifying the immune system. In summary, the findings point toward increasing your intake of vegetables and, to a lesser degree, fruit, and cutting down on fats and, to a lesser degree, animal protein. When you do have animal protein, fish is the most healthful source, so make that a regular part of your diet. Whatever meat you choose, be sure not to burn it by cooking it at high temperatures in butter or oil. At high temperatures, carcinogens might be formed from the overheated fats.

Just a few other guidelines give you most of what you need to know to have a healthy foundation for your immune system to work from. Avoid alcohol (just two glasses of beer a day can increase the risk of

---

NUTRIENTS FOR
BOOSTING IMMUNITY

Be sure to get at least these minimum doses daily.

VITAMINS

Vitamin A: 2.5 mg (2,500 IU)
Beta-carotene: 18 mg
Riboflavin: 5 mg
Vitamin B_{12}: 250 mcg
Vitamin C: 100 mg
Vitamin D: 20 mcg
Vitamin E: 20 mg

MINERALS

Calcium: 500 mg

COENZYMES

CoQ10: 30 mg

---

breast cancer in women, for example). Avoid environmental pollution as much as you possibly can and—although I'm sure I don't have to tell you this—don't smoke!

Vitamins seem to help prevent cancer only when they come from a well-rounded diet and not when they are taken in separate supplements. A few studies show promising results in *treating* cancer with very high doses of several vitamins, though they'll need to be validated by larger-scale scientific studies before being declared of definite value.

For our purposes now, I just want to review what work has been done linking specific nutrients with benefits in cases of specific cancers.

Vitamin A and its precursor **beta-carotene** can play a protective role against lung cancer. A diet poor in either increases the risk of cancer of the cervix, esophagus, stomach, breast, bladder, intestine, larynx, and ear/nose/throat. Vitamin A is effective in the treatment of certain lesions of the mouth and esophagus that can be cancerous. Carrots, melons, spinach, greens, and apricots are particularly rich in vitamin A and/or beta-carotene. A form of vitamin A, retinoic acid, has been proven effective against skin cancer.

Studies done in China show a greater risk of esophageal cancer with **riboflavin** (vitamin B_2) deficiency. A **vitamin B_{12}** deficiency is found in leukemia and cancer of all the organs covered by otorhinolaryngologists (ear, nose, throat, mouth, and related structures in the head and neck).

A diet poor in **vitamin C** increases the occurrence of stomach, esophageal, mouth, pharynx, and breast cancers. An epidemiological study has shown that the risk of mortality from colon or rectal cancer goes down as the supply of **vitamin D** and **calcium** go up.

A low blood level of **vitamin E** has been found in patients with lesions in the stomach and lungs that could prove cancerous. Researchers are in the process of measuring the efficacy of preventive treatment with vitamin E in several kinds of cancer.

Coenzyme CoQ10 (or simply CoQ10) stimulates immunity. Some studies have shown benefits in treating advanced cancers in part with high doses, which appear to significantly lengthen remissions.

DECODING YOUR DEFICIENCIES

- Are you having or have you had radiation therapy?
  Read more about . . .
  melatonin
- Do you have or are you at increased risk of cancer?
  Read more about . . .
  growth hormone
  cortisol
  thyroid hormones
  DHEA
  melatonin
  progesterone
- Women: Do you have or are you at increased risk of breast, endometrial, or ovarian cancer?
  Read more about . . .
  thyroid hormones
  DHEA
  melatonin
  progesterone

    growth hormone

    cortisol

- Do you have metastases in the bones?

    Read more about . . .

    calcitonin

- Are you at risk of being exposed to a parasite, virus, or bacteria?

    Read more about . . .

    melatonin

    thyroid hormones

    DHEA

    growth hormone

    cortisol

    estrogen

- Do you have a viral infection (including AIDS)?

    Read more about . . .

    melatonin

    growth hormone

    thyroid hormones

    DHEA

    cortisol

    estrogen

    testosterone

- Do you have a low ratio of CD4+ to CD8+ (a high ratio is an indicator of immune strength)?

    Read more about . . .

    thyroid hormone

    growth hormone

    DHEA

- Have you been diagnosed with any condition of the thymus or spleen?

    Read more about . . .

    melatonin

    thyroid hormones

    growth hormone

    DHEA

    progesterone

- Men: Do you have or are you at increased risk of prostate cancer?

    Read more about . . .

    DHEA

    testosterone

- Do you have fever, pain, inflammation, or lack of appetite from cancer treatment?
  Read more about . . .
  cortisol
- Do you have leukemia, lymphoma, or myeloma?
  Read more about . . .
  cortisol
- Do you catch one cold after another? Do you have frequent sore throats or earaches?
  Read more about . . .
  thyroid hormones
- Do you take a long time to recover from an infection?
  Read more about . . .
  cortisol
  growth hormone
- Do you have a compromised immune system, as with AIDS?
  Read more about . . .
  thyroid hormones
  DHEA
  cortisol
  melatonin
  growth hormone

SUMMARY: IMMUNE-SYSTEM HORMONES

Hormone Deficiency	Symptoms	See also pp.
Calcitonin	cancer metastases to the bones	26, 169
Cortisol	susceptibility to negative physical side effects of cancer or cancer treatment; leukemia, lymphoma, or myeloma, especially in children; risk of exposure to parasite, virus, or bacteria; viral infection (including AIDS); fever, pain, inflammation, or lack of appetite from cancer treatment	26, 163, 165, 170
DHEA	cancer; increased risk of cancer; risk of exposure to parasite, virus, or bacteria; viral infection (including AIDS); in men: possible increased risk of prostate cancer	27, 160, 167, 171
Estrogen	cancer; increased risk of cancer (except breast and endometrial cancer); in women: increased risk of ovarian cancer; risk of exposure to parasite, virus, or bacteria; viral infection (including AIDS)	28, 162, 164, 172
Growth Hormone	cancer; increased risk of cancer (though this is controversial); risk of exposure to parasite, virus, or bacteria; viral infection (including AIDS); low ratio of CD4+ to CD8+; diagnosis of any atrophy of the thymus	29, 162, 165, 171
Melatonin	radiation therapy; cancer; increased risk of cancer; in women: breast cancer or increased risk of same; viral infection (including AIDS); diagnosis of any condition of the thymus or spleen	30, 161, 169
Progesterone	cancer; increased risk of cancer; in women: breast, endometrial, or ovarian cancer or increased risk of same; viral infection (including AIDS)	32, 163, 169, 171
Testosterone	viral infection (including AIDS)	32, 162, 164, 172
Thyroid	cancer; increased risk of cancer; in women: breast cancer or increased risk of same; risk of exposure to parasite, virus, or bacteria; viral infection (including AIDS); low ratio of CD4+ to CD8+; frequent colds, sore throats, earaches, or other infections	33, 162, 166, 170

PART III

MIND

CHAPTER ELEVEN

SUPER SEX (NO VIAGRA NECESSARY)

Sexuality is perhaps the most widely known area controlled by hormones. Hormones (together with neurotransmitters) are at the root of our amorous desires. They enable us to behave erotically and maintain sexual relationships. Hormones are love's messengers; they incite us to love those who give us the most pleasure, whether sexual or platonic. That's one reason we are emotionally touched by those we love physically.

If our hormones aren't up to snuff, desire is dulled. Our sexual potential fades. That's more than common with age. Fortunately, we can maintain—or regain—our full sexuality with properly tailored hormone treatments. With them, we can rekindle sexual desire and boost performance.

Later in this chapter we'll go over each of several hormones and the specific aspects of our sex lives they affect. But first I'm going to give you an overview of the various stages of sexual arousal, intercourse, and recovery controlled by hormones so you can understand exactly how intrinsic they are to the whole process. The whole rhythm is set by the ebb and flow of various hormones. Of course, there are as many ways to feel and express sexual desire as there are people, and hormones would be behind each and every one, perhaps in slightly different patterns. The following simply traces a typical course. As you'll see, there's quite a lot going on underneath the surface when we're simply "doing what comes naturally."

HORMONES, FROM FOREPLAY
TO AFTERGLOW

*I*t all starts with physical attraction. All sorts of desires appear at this time, and they might include hunger or thirst, for example, alongside sexual longing, thanks to the catecholamines dopamine and noradrenaline and other neurotransmitters (which in some circumstances are considered hormones).

The next hormone that comes directly into play actually affects other people more than it does you. During foreplay, hormones known as pheromones communicate to your partner through subtle sexual fragrances, arousing sexual desire. Your partner actually inhales the pheromones (often unconsciously), which are secreted by sweat glands in the armpits and pubic area.

Once desire is aroused, estrogen not only allows for good vaginal lubrication, it also enhances the sense of mutual attraction by stimulating certain neurons in the brain and prompting release of more pheromones. Studies have shown that women with higher than average estrogen levels report feeling more attracted to images of individuals than are women with low or average levels. Studies in monkeys, which have yet to be repeated in humans, indicate that estrogen works in similar ways in males as well as females.

Sexual desire gently increases as DHEA and especially testosterone stimulate sexual odor and sweat (in both men and women, though DHEA has a stronger effect in women than in men). Meanwhile, two pituitary hormones, LH and FSH (luteinizing hormone and follicle-stimulating hormone), compel production of more sex hormones, secreted in greater amounts. They also stimulate sexual desire in the brain, the most powerful sex organ of all.

Once sexual desire is aroused, testosterone stirs things up even more by stimulating fantasies. During passionate kissing, hugging, and other physical contact, more pheromones, derived from DHEA and estrogens, secreted through the skin and saliva, arouse desire and enhance pleasure. More and more cortisol is secreted, supplying energy and enthusiasm and generally getting both partners highly excited.

Vasopressin levels also increase, helping blood accumulate in the penis and clitoris to allow erection, assisted by the neurotransmitter acetylcholine (another sometime-hormone), which dilates the blood vessels and makes blood flow into the penis and clitoris. Testosterone brings on a man's erection (and eventually ejaculation). Meanwhile, neuro-transmitters like serotonin (which can act as a hormone) activate various areas of the brain to provoke erections of the nipples, clitoris, and penis.

As both partners hug and caress, giving themselves over to love play, growth hormone provides physical endurance. It also encourages a firmer and prolonged erection of both the penis and clitoris.

As excitation peaks, the nerves and adrenal glands secrete noradren-aline (a hormone) that allows quick reactions to the unexpected, sexually speaking. Orgasm and ejaculation occur with a sudden discharge of adrenaline (another sometime-hormone). During orgasm, the hormone oxytocin provokes the contraction of the uterus and the muscles of the vagina. (Oxytocin is also the hormone that signals for the release of milk in nursing mothers, explaining both the similar effect orgasm can have and the pleasant feeling that can occur during breastfeeding.)

After orgasm, progesterone intervenes to subdue sexual desire, bringing on a state of serenity, relaxation, and a feeling of fullness as well as a certain passivity and drowsiness. This effect is stronger in women than in men, as women make much more progesterone. Prolactin is also secreted profusely, encouraging drowsiness and reducing sexual desire, in men and women, although women might secrete more of it. (Pro-lactin is the hormone that enables milk production, so it, too, plays a role in milk discharge during and after lovemaking in women who are nursing a baby.) Prolactin is reinforced by melatonin, which encourages deep sleep after sex. Endorphins (a type of neurotransmitter) are also released, and while they are famous for their ability to fight pain, here their role is to inhibit sexual desire and make you feel drowsy but good.

And that certain sadness that can take hold of you after all is said and done? That's thanks to the severe post-orgasm drop in aphrodisiac neurotransmitters and hormones.

NUTRITION

A closer look at individual hormones is up next, but the first step to super sex should always be excellent nutrition, so I'll cover strategies for that now.

Protein and (healthful) fats increase sex hormones, fortifying libido and erections. Spicy and salty foods increase the effects of adrenal hor-mones, including testosterone, DHEA, and cortisol.

A diet designed to increase energy and vitality is the next best thing

```
┌─────────────────────────────────────────────────────┐
│                                                       │
│         NUTRIENTS FOR SUPER SEX                       │
│                                                       │
├───────────────────────────────────────────────────────┤
│                                                       │
│   VITAMINS                                            │
│   Vitamin A: 10 mg daily                              │
│   Vitamin E: 400–800 mg daily                         │
│                                                       │
│   MINERALS                                            │
│   Zinc: 10–20 mg daily                                │
│                                                       │
└───────────────────────────────────────────────────────┘
```

for your sex life. That would entail plenty of animal protein and fruit. Meat increases adrenal hormones and the levels and/or efficiency of sex hormones. Fruit increases your level of thyroid hormones and along with it your vivacity, intelligence, and quickness of reaction. Fruit is good for helping you be seductive.

Vitamins A and E and zinc increase sex hormone levels and/or sex-gland functioning. You should take enough vitamin A to correct any detected deficiency. Often, 50 mg a day for two to four months is sufficient.

DECODING YOUR DEFICIENCIES

Do you lack sexual desire? Are you unable to fantasize? Do you have problems feeling aroused? Or turning desire into action? Make sure you are getting enough testosterone. It arouses desire, promotes sexual fantasies, and makes you feel more in love—in both men and women.

DHEA can also be an effective treatment. A recent study helped women with loss of libido, low motivation, and fatigue (most of whom were in menopause or had had their ovaries removed) regain a satisfying sense of their sexuality after six to twelve months taking 50 mg of DHEA a day. And although DHEA has a more potent effect in women, recent studies show that it also increases potency in men with erectile dysfunction.

Estrogen arouses sexual desire. It might surprise you, but the effect may be even more powerful in men than in women—and even more powerful than testosterone in men. A study of male monkeys, for example, revealed that sexual desire increased more in male monkeys given estrogen than in those given testosterone.

Once you've gotten the ball rolling, cortisol provides energy and enthusiasm during sexual activity.

Do your sex organs seem insensitive? Testosterone (and in particular dihydrotestosterone) increases the sensitivity of the glans of the penis and the clitoris. Estrogen moistens and lubricates the vaginal mucous membranes, sensitizing the nerve endings in the vagina.

Do you have a problem developing or keeping an erection, or are your erections not firm enough or too brief? Do you have a problem ejaculating? Is your clitoris hard to stimulate? Testosterone gives men greater sexual capacity, enabling ejaculation and erections. DHEA has similar effects, although more moderate. Cortisol peaks excitement during sex, maintaining erection longer and providing energy to the muscles, including the heart, for endurance.

During intercourse, growth hormone encourages a firmer and more prolonged erection of the penis and clitoris. It provides significant endurance for sexual efforts in both male and female bodies and enables good tone and volume of the penis. Increasing growth hormone's partner, somatomedin C, boosts recovery capacity and helps tissue in the genital areas retain water and volume.

Vasopressin helps retain water in the body and blood in the arteries, so it contributes to the accumulation of blood in the penis that enables erection. It does the same for the clitoris.

Has your sexual odor changed or decreased? Have you lost body hair? DHEA and testosterone increase sexual odor and sweat. They also develop hair in the pubic area and under the arms.

Do you have a hard time calming down and relaxing after sex? Do you no longer fall into a deep sleep after making love? Melatonin helps you relax, makes you drowsy, and causes you to fall into a deep sleep after lovemaking. Progesterone calms sexual desire and brings on feelings of fullness, serenity, passivity, relaxation, and calmness.

CHRIS

Chris, nearly fifty, was a successful businessman despite nearly ten years of struggle with severe fatigue, lack of concentration, memory problems, and ever-increasing weight. Things had gotten so bad that he and his wife divorced, and now being apart from his children was an added stress. When he was thirty, he told me, everyone called him "the marathon man" because of his seemingly never-ending energy and his participation in so many sports. Now it took him a good long time to recover from any physical exertion whatsoever.

It wasn't until his third visit to my office that he revealed his main complaint, however: Like forty million men in the United States alone, he suffered from erectile dysfunction, or what used to be known as impotence. His penis wouldn't get fully erect anymore, making sexual intercourse difficult or impossible.

Further details on history and exam revealed that what Chris actually had was Peyronie's disease, in which dense strands of fibrous tissue form in the penis, causing a deforming curvature, painful erections, and mechanical difficulties with intercourse. It is generally considered irreversible.

In addition to this central finding, I saw many signs that suggested hormonal deficiencies. In addition to the constant fatigue and difficulty achieving full erections, Chris also had hot flashes and bouts of excessive emotionality, all of which can indicate testosterone deficiency. There were signs of thyroid deficiency as well, including low body temperature, morning fatigue, fatigue at rest, drowsiness, constipation, hair loss, dry skin (especially on the face), episodes of dizziness, and memory and concentration problems. I suspected low growth hormone, too, given his low-back pain (enough to stop him from playing any sports), flabby belly, and difficulty recovering from physical exertion.

Lab tests confirmed this trio of deficiencies, so Chris took supplemental hormones to correct them. Before long, he was no longer exhausted all the time, his concentration and memory improved greatly, and his flabby belly clearly decreased. He started

exercising extensively and playing sports again. And happily—
although I admit it wasn't a result I felt we could count on—
within a year and a half the Peyronie's vanished, thanks to
testosterone injections administered every two weeks, a testosterone gel (dihydrotestosterone) applied daily directly to the penis,
and 2 g daily of vitamin E (which makes tissues more supple, flexible, and elastic). Chris is happy in a new romantic relationship—
and his ex-wife, persuaded by his excellent results, is now a patient
of mine, too, and doing very well.

Do you have a problem with vaginal lubrication? Estrogen helps
maintain moist membranes and keeps the vagina lubricated.

Have you lost the feeling of attraction to your partner? Estrogen and testosterone enhance feelings of sexual attractiveness and make
you feel more in love.

Wish you had more endurance? Growth hormone can prolong erections of penis and clitoris and enhance endurance for any physical activity, including sex.

SUMMARY: SUPER SEX

Hormone Deficiency	Symptoms	See also pg.
Cortisol	not initiating sex with a partner	26
DHEA	lack of sexual desire; problem feeling aroused; problem turning desire into action; problem getting or keeping an erection; weak or short-lasting erections; problem ejaculating; hard-to-stimulate clitoris; decreased sexual odor; loss of body hair (note: effects are significant, but less than testosterone and estrogen)	27
Estrogen	lack of sexual desire; problem feeling aroused; problem turning desire into action; lack of vaginal lubrication; loss of feeling of attraction to partner	28
Growth Hormone	problem developing or keeping an erection; weak or short-lasting erections; lack of endurance	29
Melatonin	hard time relaxing after sex; not falling into a deep sleep after making love	30
Progesterone	hard time calming down and relaxing after sex	32
Testosterone	problem getting or keeping an erection; weak or short-lasting erections; lack of orgasm; lack of sensitivity of the penis; clitoris hard to stimulate; sex organs seeming insensitive; lack of sexual desire; inability to fantasize; problem feeling aroused; problem turning desire into action; decreased sexual odor; loss of body hair; loss of feeling of attraction toward partner	32
Vasopressin	problem getting or keeping an erection; penis or clitoris difficult to bring to full erection	34

CHAPTER TWELVE

SLEEPING
BEAUTIFULLY

Sophie hadn't slept in ten years. Not literally, of course, but almost. She couldn't seem to fall asleep most nights. She didn't sleep deeply, woke up frequently, didn't dream. She was, not surprisingly, tired all the time. The worst fatigue hit her in the morning and in the week before her period. (She also had trouble with PMS.) This had been going on since her early thirties.

At a glance, I was ready to put my money down on lack of melatonin as the root of Sophie's problems. Melatonin is the major hormone that promotes good sleep. And women with PMS often have lower melatonin levels in their blood during the night. Sure enough, as soon as she started taking melatonin, she slept much better.

When a case like this comes up—with a simple solution available that no one has thought of for ten years—I feel bad the patient has had to wait so long to resolve his or her problem. Of course sometimes it's taken ten years because it is a truly tough nut to crack. But not always. Not for Sophie.

Even once she was sleeping better, Sophie still had occasional trouble, and she showed signs of other deficiencies, too. She was in her early forties, so her estrogen, progesterone, and testosterone levels were low, and in addition to PMS she had droopy breasts, painful periods, easy bruising, obesity around her belly and hips, muscle loss, dry eyes, smaller than normal breasts, and cystic breasts.

Lab tests confirmed the trio of deficiencies, so Sophie started taking estrogen and progesterone balanced with a little testosterone. That did away with her sleep problems once and for all, and the rest of her symptoms cleared up, too. Most impressively, she no longer needed the antidepressant she'd been taking for years. It's a wonder what a good night's sleep can do.

SLEEP WELL

Getting to sleep. Staying asleep. Waking up rested. These are simple things most of us pay absolutely no attention to until we are deprived of them. Sleep is easy to take for granted, but once it is gone you deeply appreciate how much good it contributes to your life.

Sleeping well means feeling rested and restored and ready to face the day when you get up in the morning. Sleeping well improves your mood and lets you get done whatever you need to with enthusiasm, ease, and pleasure.

But as we age, the quality of our sleep declines. The deep and easy sleep we had as children is replaced by a lighter, more agitated sleep. We start to have trouble falling asleep or getting back to sleep when we wake up during the night. We just lie there, drowsy, with too-short periods of real sleep breaking in now and then. We "wake up" in the morning more tired than we were the night before. Too many of us too often turn to tranquilizers and other sleeping aids, but they offer only the illusion of help: When they "work," all they do is induce poor-quality sleep anyway. (And some can even impair memory.)

GOOD NIGHT

Fortunately, there is a better way. For most people, correcting hormonal deficiencies can restore the days of sound, refreshing sleep. This chapter covers them all. But first, let's look more closely at just what goes on during a single night's sleep. The process of falling asleep and the different phases that make up sleep are variously affected by hormones.

Sleep is a five-stage cycle repeated three to five times a night. Each cycle lasts one and a half to two hours, and there are a few minutes of downtime between each cycle.

When you go to bed, as soon as you close your eyes, brain waves in the characteristic low-and-short beta pattern change into alpha waves, which are higher and longer. You remain awake, but your muscles relax.

Progressively, sleep sets in. You slip, at first, into light sleep, now with larger, irregular theta waves. This is stage one.

You doze off, overwhelmed by an agreeable sleepiness and exhibiting different large, irregular brain waves called single-complex K waves. After brief states of consciousness during light sleep, your heart begins to beat more slowly and your blood pressure and temperature drop (stage two).

The duration of stages one and two lengthens over time. When you are forty-five, they take about forty minutes combined. By the time you are sixty-five, they average seventy-three minutes.

Next, you gently enter into deep sleep. This heavier sleep features large, slow delta brain waves, which induce a pleasant state of well-being (stages three and four). Stage four features slower wavelengths on the electroencephalogram (EEG) than stage three. These stages together last close to three and a half hours a night in young adults, declining to less than two hours in people over sixty-five.

You now enter into the REM (rapid eye movement) phase, or dream sleep (stage five). Short and fast waves cross the brain, a sign of intense activity. This is sometimes called paradoxical sleep because it brings together a state of deep sleep in which almost all the muscles relax and the limbs go soft with a state of hyperactivity in the brain and the eyes. This dream phase, repeated many times during the night, is very important. It lets you recover from exertion and assimilate the day's happenings into your memory. The longer your REM phase, the better your memory will be. At twenty, it will last almost three hours a night, but that is gradually reduced over time to little more than an hour and a half in people over sixty-five.

GOOD NUTRITION

Before you start taking any hormones, or to allow the hormones you do take to work most efficiently, some simple diet and nutrition strategies can improve your sleep habits. The main thing is to restrict what you eat in the evenings for three to four hours before bedtime. Keep dinner—and everything you eat for the rest of the day—light, avoiding protein-dense, fatty, and raw foods, including fruit. Avoid caffeine in the afternoon and evenings and, if that doesn't work, anytime after breakfast. You should avoid alcohol as well in the afternoon and evenings.

NUTRIENTS FOR SLEEP

VITAMINS
Vitamin B_6: 50–125 mg at bedtime

MINERALS
Calcium: 100–1,000 mg at bedtime

You might also try taking 1,000 mg of calcium at bedtime, which will help calm you. Vitamin B_6 taken at bedtime is also calming. Experiment with doses between 50 and 125 mg to find what works for you.

DECODING YOUR DEFICIENCIES

Do you have trouble falling asleep? Melatonin speeds up the getting-to-sleep process, widening the spectrum of brain waves when sleep sets in. It slows down the heartbeat and lowers blood pressure. It can shorten the total time it takes to cycle through stages one and two, to the point where it can help people over sixty-five match twenty- to twenty-five-year-olds who, on average, spend almost half as much time in these stages.

Progesterone can help, too. Taken orally, natural progesterone can bring on extreme sleepiness. As it passes through the liver, progesterone is metabolized into a variety of substances that reduce anxiety and pain and make you drowsy. Anyone who takes this form for any reason should therefore take it only at night, just before going to bed.

Do you wake up unrefreshed, even if you've slept through the night? Melatonin, which your body releases mostly at night, lets you sleep longer and deeper—or, rather, sleep deeper for longer. In fact, melatonin improves sleep at all stages. Its benefits are most impressive in older people, who generally have lowered levels of melatonin produced by their own bodies. The market for chemical sleep aids has shrunk in this country since over-the-counter sales of melatonin began. And no wonder. Standard sleeping pills don't produce high-quality sleep. Most lengthen the duration of the less useful light sleep (stages one and two) and diminish the duration of good, deep sleep (three through five).

Like melatonin, more growth hormone is released during the night than during the day, and it is beneficial to sleep. Without enough growth hormone, you sleep longer but not as well. You'll get more stage one and two sleep but less of stages three through five. With growth hormone supplements, you'll sleep less when you go by hours on the clock, but it will be better, deeper sleep, mainly in the later stages. For many people, this is the best of all benefits from growth hormone.

Thyroid hormones also improve sleep quality, which is a bit surprising given their energizing nature. These are the hormones, after all, that so often snap apathetic, lethargic individuals right out of their sluggishness and sleepiness. But the explanation is simple: People low in thyroid hormones doze for longer, lingering in stages one and two but sleep less deeply (stages three and four). When they take supplemental thyroid hormones, the restorative deep sleep lasts longer and the superficial sleep is shorter.

Cortisol also, surprisingly, lends a hand here. It's a "wake-up" hormone in the morning, when it is secreted most abundantly. But in certain circumstances it has a beneficial influence on deep sleep as well. People who enjoy more energy during the day, thanks to cortisol, are more active and generally sleep better at night.

Still, don't take cortisol or a derivative before going to bed or you'll risk insomnia. Better to take it in the morning, upon arising, and again at noon and during the afternoon. Whenever you take it, be careful to avoid excessive doses, particularly in the second half of the day and definitely at bedtime. Moderate doses have been shown *not* to interfere with brain waves during sleep.

Progesterone encourages good sleep in men and women both. Estrogen improves the overall quality of the sleep women get, as does testosterone in men. The more testosterone a man has, the deeper his sleep. Sleep-deprivation, on the other hand, causes testosterone levels to drop. This starts off an infernal spiral: Less testosterone means more insomnia, which means less testosterone. More than 60 percent of testosterone-deficient men complain of sleep problems.

Do you wake up frequently? Thyroid hormones often help people who snore or have sleep apnea. The obstruction of the airways that causes snoring might be due in part to a swelling in the airway created by the accumulation of sticky waste materials between the cells. With thyroid treatment in those who are deficient, the swelling goes down, so they snore much less and wake up less often during the night. Therefore they sleep better. But avoid taking too much thyroid hormone or you might find yourself waking up in the middle of the night with your heart beating fast.

DHEA can also be useful. One woman I treated slept terribly for years, waking frequently because of sleep apnea and its severe snoring. She experienced major improvement—almost complete disappearance of her symptoms, in fact—with DHEA.

Are you not dreaming as much as you used to? In the dream phase, the information you've taken in is integrated into your brain. If you don't dream enough, you brain won't work as efficiently as it should.

Melatonin lengthens the REM phase of sleep, encouraging dreaming and allowing more time for dreaming. So does estrogen. In men, the higher the testosterone level, the more numerous the dreams. Finally, DHEA lengthens the REM, or dreaming, phase and increases its intensity, though to get this effect usually requires large doses, about 500 mg a day. That's too large, in my opinion. I generally recommend doses between 10 and 50 mg, depending on the person. So I don't use DHEA specifically to address lack of dreaming. I'm mentioning it here, however, to let you know that if you are taking DHEA in physiological doses for other reasons, you might experience some improvements in this area, too. People low in growth hormone dream less—and when they take supplements, their sleep becomes richer in dreams. When people low in thyroid hormones take supplements, the length of their REM sleep increases significantly.

Does jet lag hit you hard or do you have a hard time recovering from jet lag? This is the condition melatonin is most famous for, and rightly so. Taking melatonin just before going to bed upon arrival in a new time zone resets the physiological cycles of hormone secretion. When you are jet lagged, your rather mixed up biological clock tells your body to release energizing hormones during the night rather than during the day. Melatonin suppresses the nighttime release, shifting it to daytime and catching your body clock up to your actual time zone.

SUMMARY: SLEEP HORMONES

Hormone Deficiency	Symptoms	See also pg.
Cortisol	waking unrefreshed, even if you've slept through the night	26
DHEA	not dreaming as much as you used to	27
Estrogen	waking unrefreshed, even if you've slept through the night; superficial sleep; not dreaming as much as you used to	28
Growth Hormone	waking unrefreshed, and eventually exhausted, even if you've slept through the night; sleeping superficially, waking up frequently; anxious sleep; not dreaming as much as you used to; needing more than 9 hours of sleep per 24 hours	29
Melatonin	trouble falling asleep, and falling back asleep when you wake up during the night; waking unrefreshed, even if you've slept through the night; superficial sleep; anxious or agitated sleep; not dreaming as much as you used to; jet lag; impression of having no dreams	30
Progesterone	trouble falling asleep; waking unrefreshed, even if you've slept through the night	32
Testosterone	waking unrefreshed, even if you've slept through the night; superficial sleep; not dreaming as much as you used to	32
Thyroid Hormones	waking unrefreshed, with swollen face and puffy eyelids, even if you've slept through the night; waking up frequently; disruptive snoring; not dreaming as much as you used to	33

CHAPTER THIRTEEN

REMEMBERING
NOT TO FORGET

"It's the same thing that happened to what's-his-name . . .

"You know, he had that . . . that . . . what do you call it?

"Yes, and his doctors had him taking that stuff, I forget what he said it was . . .

"Now when was that? Let me see . . ."

Okay, raise your hand if you've ever had a conversation like this. If you're over forty-five, I'm betting yours is up there waving. Memory deterioration is one of the most frequent complaints people express as they get older. Some people, especially those who have had painful experiences with parents or loved ones with Alzheimer's, fear that these little gaps are just the first symptoms of that dreaded condition. Others find the lapses just as they are horrifying enough. We might cover it up with jokes about losing our minds, but this is a fear that strikes deep—and not without reason. According to a recent study done in Sweden, close to 30 percent of people eighty-five and older suffer from Alzheimer's.

Beyond that, the number of people with garden-variety memory deterioration is staggering. Almost everyone experiences it in some shape or form eventually. It happens to most of us sooner rather than later. It certainly isn't a phenomenon limited to the over-eighty-five crowd. It is so common, in fact, that we believe it is inevitable, just part and parcel of getting older.

Like most things we all "know," there's a degree of truth in that. As we get older, cognitive function, with memory as its hallmark, progressively declines as specific areas of the brain deteriorate. The brain actually gets smaller. The number of brain cells (neurons) shrinks, too. So do the number of connections between neurons, which limits the flow of information-exchange. The supplies of enzymes and neurotransmitters the brain needs to function diminish. The brain does not receive enough blood. It doesn't work as quickly or smoothly as it once did. Memory problems is what most people notice first and most often.

But, for most of us, all this is *not* inevitable. Hormones play a large role in the brain, as they do everywhere in the body, and so a decline in their levels can cause a decline in memory and other brain functions. The good news is, maintaining and even improving memory is often only a matter of achieving correct hormonal balance.

KEN

Ken is a case in point. Over the last couple of years before he reached fifty, his memory and concentration started to go. His main complaint was that after a half-hour of reading he'd get distracted and forget what he'd just read, whereas he used to read for hours on end and retain what he'd read. It was especially bad in the morning, and his thinking seemed foggy then, too, he told me, though the memory lapses and loss of focus could happen anytime.

The more I asked, the more nagging problems it turned out Ken had: coldness, weight gain, lack of energy, puffy eyes and face in the morning, cold feet and muscle cramps at night. On exam, I could see he also had a slow Achilles tendon reflex, high diastolic blood pressure, and a slow and weak heartbeat. All of this suggested a thyroid deficiency.

Since he was a man over forty, I guessed his sex hormones were declining. Many of his symptoms pointed toward lack of testosterone—the memory loss, occasional excessive sweating, small wrinkles, decreased libido, decreased frequency and firmness of erections, reduced muscle strength, back pain, and enlarged prostate, lax testicles, and that telling spare tire.

I picked up several other signs pointing toward low growth hormone, including fatigue, low resistance to stress, slow recovery from any kind of exertion, easy exhaustion if he stayed up late or exercised, excessive emotionality, pale face, thin hair, poor muscle tone, and the tendency to isolate himself (probably because of the fatigue and low stress resistance).

His terrible sugar cravings, especially under stress, clued me in to

Ken's cortisol deficiency. (Low cortisol can lead to low blood sugar, especially under stress.)

In short, Ken was prematurely aging, both physically and mentally.

Lab tests confirmed all four deficiencies, so I prescribed thyroid hormones, testosterone, DHEA, hydrocortisone (cortisol), and growth hormone in physiologic doses for Ken. I also gave him an antiyeast medication because of his bloated belly and coated tongue. He cut back on sugars and sweets, breads and cereals, dairy products and wine.

Before long, he was like a new man. He even *looked* younger and healthier. He was no longer fatigued all the time. His memory was back to normal. His thinking cleared and his concentration returned. And that was what mattered most to him.

NUTRITION

Ken is a good role model not only for balancing your hormones, but also for understanding the importance of good nutrition. To maintain your memory, and even boost its capabilities, you must eat right. Good nutrition keeps you and your brain healthy and gives your hormones everything they need to do their jobs unimpeded.

To support your memory, get plenty of fruits and vegetables, plenty of complex carbohydrates, and sufficient healthful fats. You should avoid dairy products but otherwise maintain a diet rich in protein from meat, poultry, and eggs. Eat lightly and eat light foods. Don't eat anything or in any way that causes you to bloat. Bloating is one sign of fermentation or rotting of food in the digestive tract, food that is "eaten" by bacteria and yeasts for energy rather than by the body. That process produces gases (and bloating) as well as toxins. It is those toxins that make you drowsy and cloud your thinking after a meal, making it difficult to commit anything to memory or retrieve anything from memory after a meal. That's a good chunk of each day, if you think about it.

There are some exceptions.

If your thyroid hormones are low, moderate the amount of animal proteins and fats you get.

If your estrogen level is low, regulate—but don't eliminate—the amount of whole grains you eat, as large amounts of fiber can bind to estrogen and carry it out of the body.

You might also want to consider supplements of the antioxidant vitamins A, C, and E, which delay cerebral aging at the cellular level by

NUTRIENTS FOR MEMORY

Be sure to get at least these minimum doses daily.

VITAMINS

Vitamin A: 5 mg
Vitamin C: 200 mg
Vitamin E: 20 mg

MINERALS

Magnesium: 100 mg
Phosphorus: 60 mg
Manganese: 2 mg

TRACE ELEMENTS

Selenium: 50 mcg

preventing the accumulation of free radicals. Selenium is also an antioxidant, and it does the same. Magnesium, phosphorus, and manganese also play significant roles in improving memory.

DECODING YOUR DEFICIENCIES

Is your thinking slower than it used to be? You should check for a thyroid hormone deficiency. The age-related changes in the brain, and so your thought processes and memory, are caused or worsened at least in part by hormonal deficiencies, thyroid hormones prime among them. In the brain's gray matter, where thinking takes place, the blood begins to flow more slowly as thyroid levels decline. As a result, less oxygen and fewer nutrients reach the brain cells, the brain becomes malnourished, and the brain's owner thinks and moves less. In the extremely rare case in which a person is totally deprived of thyroid hormones, intelligence, memory, and emotions just disappear. Unless the person is treated in time, the absence of thyroid hormones provokes rapid aging of the brain's blood vessels, causing severe arteriosclerosis. Without enough thyroid hormones, the number of connections (dendrites and synapses) between the brain cells decreases, weakening the brain cells. All this causes you to think and move slowly and to have problems concentrating and remembering, particularly upon rising in the morning and when you are at rest.

Thyroid hormones are, in short, essential for good memory. Taking thyroid hormones can reverse premature aging of the arteries and accelerate blood flow throughout the brain. After correcting a deficiency, the neurons that had been deprived of sufficient oxygen can once again nourish themselves properly. Gradually, you'll start thinking more clearly and acting faster.

Thyroid hormones are essential for intelligence from the beginning of life. During the first months in the womb, the fetus needs thyroid hormones for the proper development of its brain. If the mother is deficient during pregnancy, the IQ of the child will be affected. If the baby is born with hypothyroidism, corrective treatment is essential immediately. In untreated children, the volume of the brain, the number of neurons, and the thickness of the coating protecting the nerve endings are reduced. Fifty to 70 percent of children who have not had enough thyroid hormone before birth have neuropsychic disturbances including attention deficit, difficulty orienting in space, slow thought processes, and poor physical performance. A study of adolescents has even shown that long-term memory (which allows recalling past events) and spatial memory (which allows, for example, the memory of a sequence of movements) depend on thyroid hormone levels in the mother's blood during pregnancy. The higher the thyroid hormone level in the mother, the better the adolescent's memory will be. Every woman planning a pregnancy should have her thyroid hormone levels checked.

Are you unable to trust your memory in general? Male hormones, including testosterone, fortify not just the muscles, but also the brain and nerves. (Testosterone is useful for women's memory, too, but it is more powerful in men, and in women estrogen is more powerful than testosterone.) They provide a steady and determined state of mind and reinforce memory. Without enough of them, a man's blood coagulates too easily, increasing the risk of thrombosis (the same effect occurs in women) and decreasing the level of good HDL cholesterol. The arteries of the brain weaken, growing too soft in some places (increasing the risk of blood clots and stroke) and too stiff in others (increasing the risk of high blood pressure and cerebral hemorrhage)—none of which is good for the memory! When the arteries of the brain wear out, blood can no longer properly circulate there or to any other organ. When the resulting lack of oxygen and nutrients to the brain is chronic, memory weakens.

Year after year, this degeneration proceeds—unless hormone supplements come to the rescue. Hormone therapy can save your memory and even restore it to what it once was. Scientific experiments confirm that testosterone can increase the size and number of connections between neurons, although it does not seem to be able to increase the number of brain cells. It also thickens and fortifies the protective sheath (myelin) around nerves, allowing transmission of information to proceed uninterrupted from one brain cell to the next.

Research with mice has shown that supplemental testosterone allows elderly animals to regain their earlier capacity to learn difficult tasks with the same effectiveness as they did when they were young. In humans, testosterone has been shown to influence several components of memory. Men and women who have better spatial memory (which allows precise movements in space, such as handling tools or dancing) have higher levels of testosterone than their peers. Women who excel in mathematics have also been found to have high testosterone levels. It is interesting to note that transsexual women (that is, women undergoing treatment to become men) perform spatial tasks better once they begin testosterone treatments—while, on the other hand, their inclination to talk declines.

Estrogen is similarly powerful. Ask enough women in menopause, and you'll soon enough hear about how memory problems arise as estrogen levels decline. Estrogen therapy improves memory in women, particularly those whose ovaries have been removed or blocked by medication or who have serious problems with their central nervous systems, such as multiple sclerosis. It is important for men, too. One study showed that men recall images better as the dose of estrogen they are given goes up.

Do you have losses of memory? Studies have shown DHEA can significantly promote memory, although some studies do not show a benefit at physiologic doses on the order of 50 mg per day. Most studies cover periods that are too short, however. They look at about two weeks, when significant improvement in memory would take months.

A series of studies on mice and rats demonstrates what power

DHEA has over memory. Mice given drugs that cause amnesia keep their memories when they also receive DHEA, which seems to nullify the memory blockage. This requires, however, very precise dosages; neither too much nor too little will work.

It is when DHEA is given in larger doses for prolonged periods of time (months) that memory is improved. I don't recommend doses of that size, as they are no longer physiological (what your body would make on its own). So I don't use DHEA solely for memory, though you might see benefits here if you take it for other reasons. Still, some results are tantalizing. For example, Dr. Kenneth A. Bonnet of New York used DHEA when he treated a young woman with terrible memory losses— and a very low level of DHEA in her blood. An EEG showed abnormal functioning in the left hemisphere of the brain, which is active in various memory processes. It was normalized with DHEA treatment, and her memory was completely restored.

Do you want to improve your memory? Pregnenolone works in the brain as a neurotransmitter, stimulating thought processes. Pregnenolone is present in very high concentrations in the brain—two to four times more than DHEA, the next most abundant hormone in the brain. That is especially true in the hippocampus, the main memory center.

Many patients taking pregnenolone say it does improve their memories. This might be one of the reasons the brain produces large quantities of pregnenolone, as high levels are found in the cranial nerves and many regions of the brain, particularly areas associated with memory.

Research in mice has shown that pregnenolone works at least as well as DHEA (the second best) when it comes to stimulating memory—in doses 100 times lower. It takes five hundred times as much testosterone to get the same effect on memory as pregnenolone. Other studies, also in mice, showed remarkable improvement in performance on memory-related tasks in animals given pregnenolone.

Do you have trouble concentrating? ACTH, which stimulates the adrenal glands and, in particular, the secretion of cortisol, acts like a neurotransmitter in your brain, so it has a significant role in memory. Animal research shows that ACTH treatments increase motivation, vigilance, attention spans, the capacity for learning, the ability to perform tasks well, and memory for what you see (as opposed to what you hear

SHEILA

Sheila was the kind of woman who always remembered everyone's birthdays and anniversaries. She could reel off the phone numbers (home, office, and cell) of all her family members and close friends. She remembered the addresses of and directions to just about every place she'd ever been. If she cooked a dish once, she never had to look up the recipe again. She didn't bother with a date book; she kept everything in her head. She never missed an appointment. She never forgot a name.

Imagine her distress, then, when she got home from a trip to the grocery store and realized she'd forgotten the steak she needed for dinner that night. And the shampoo, with not a drop left in the current bottle. She had to go back.

This happened again and again. For the first time in her life, Sheila had to go shopping with a list. She'd noticed a few other lapses as she got closer and closer to fifty, but she had attributed these to inattention and overwork. She had to admit, though, that her memory was getting worse, and she had to write down more and more things to avoid the embarrassment of missed lunch dates, forgotten addresses, and calling someone she'd met several times by the wrong name.

Needing a shopping list was the last straw, and Sheila finally mentioned her memory complaints to me. She had already begun using hormone replacement therapy composed of thyroid hormones, estrogen, progesterone, testosterone, and growth hormone. Since she'd started, her memory hadn't worsened any further, but it hadn't gotten better either.

Researching her options on her own, Sheila "discovered" pregnenolone and added it to her regimen. Although the mechanisms haven't been pinned down yet, it has been proven to be a safe hormone, and animal studies showed spectacular results on memory. Sheila liked what the other hormones she was taking had done for her, and she decided to give one more a try. She took 100 mg a day.

After about a month, Sheila felt her thoughts were less con-

fused, and she even had the impression that her eyesight, when
reading, was improved. After another month, she realized she no
longer needed to write so many things down lest she forget them.
Whole days went by, and then weeks, without her ever having the
awful realization that she'd forgotten something important. But
Sheila didn't get really excited about her results until she com-
pleted a whole supermarket trip without needing to consult the
list she'd taken with her. The next time, she didn't even take a list.
Or the next time, or the next. Now Sheila felt sure that it wasn't
a fluke. Her memory was back. She had pregnenolone to thank.

or read or feel). When the part of the pituitary gland that produces
ACTH is destroyed in rats, they learn more slowly and less well and dis-
play poor behavior and poor memory.

ACTH stimulates the formation of ideas and thoughts. In humans,
ACTH therapy accelerates the recall of memories and improves visual
memory.

Melatonin protects our brains as well. In addition to making us
sleep well, wearing its antioxidant cap, it defends our neurons against
attack by free radicals. The brain is very vulnerable to free-radical damage because it generates more toxins than any other organ. Most of these
toxins are free radicals, and if these highly reactive molecules aren't stabilized, they will destroy brain cells. Melatonin is, in fact, one of the
most powerful antioxidants the body makes to neutralize free radicals.

Just melatonin's ability to improve sleep and dreaming is a tremendous boon to memory. Being well rested helps. In addition, dreaming
helps us consolidate our memories.

Still, if you use melatonin, moderate the dose. Too much will make
you feel muddled and distracted in the morning, which will do
absolutely nothing good for your memory.

Do you feel confused? Are you easily distracted? One sign of a
cortisol deficiency is confusion. A person low in cortisol is also easily distracted. Taking supplemental cortisol clarifies thoughts, sharpens ideas,
allows efficient memorization, and prevents memory gaps.

Mice low in cortisol have difficulties finding solutions to stressful
situations. They recognize the situation poorly and don't know how to

face it effectively. On the flip side of the coin, when mice receive corticosterone, the rodent version of cortisol, they better remember stressful situations and are better able to handle moderate stress. Other animals studies, on chickens, rats, and more, confirm the beneficial effect of cortisol and its derivatives on memory, particularly for tasks in which the animals have to learn to avoid a stressful situation.

You must be careful about dosing with cortisol, however, as excess can *impair* overall memory.

Do you have poor recall? Do you have memory problems after moderate physical trauma? Vasopressin can stimulate memory. Many studies, focusing on volunteers between fifty and sixty-five years old, show that vasopressin improves visual memory recall and the speed with which people react to information—as well as how *well* they react. People born with a severe lack of vasopressin complain of short- and long-term memory problems and difficulty concentrating. Taking vasopressin supplements brings significant improvements.

Vasopressin works best in healthy people, in people who are having memory problems due to moderate cerebral trauma like a concussion or surgery on the area around the pituitary gland, and in people over sixty-five with moderate memory loss due to aging. It works less well in patients with memory problems from other causes. Patients with severe brain damage are not good candidates for vasopressin therapy.

Animal studies underline its promise. In rats, for example, vasopressin has been shown to improve recall of information. In fact, it is so powerful that rats with amnesia due to toxins, electric shocks, or chemical blockers regain their memory with vasopressin treatment.

Vasopressin, administered by nasal spray, works incredibly fast, improving memory within four hours. The gains last at least forty-eight hours. But the best results on memory with vasopressin are obtained with the natural form, identical to what the body makes. Pharmacies generally sell only the synthetic derivatives, which are good for keeping fluid in the body, another of vasopressin's duties, but less efficient when it comes to memory.

SUMMARY: MEMORY HORMONES

Hormone Deficiency	Symptoms	See also pg.
ACTH	trouble concentrating	25
Aldosterone	poor memory or poor concentration when standing up	26
Cortisol	confusion; easily distracted	26
DHEA	losses of memory	27
Estrogen	inability to trust your memory in general	28
Melatonin	trouble concentrating	30
Pregnenolone	memory needs improvement	31
Testosterone	inability to trust your memory in general	32
Thyroid	thinking is slower than it used to be; memory loss	33
Vasopressin	poor recall; memory problems after moderate physical trauma	34

CHAPTER FOURTEEN

IN THE RIGHT MOOD

Since her early twenties, Pamela has been plagued with depression and anxiety, not to mention feeling constantly stressed out and irritable. She had family and social problems, and psychotherapy didn't seem to be helping. Seven years into it, to hear her tell it, she had so many problems she didn't know where to start. And she wasn't kidding. It was hard to get a straight story out of her. Clearly, her symptoms were overwhelming to her.

You couldn't blame her. I've rarely seen so many symptoms of hormone deficiency in any one person, among them fatigue, memory loss, poor concentration, severe PMS, and low resistance to stress. By the time I noted all the signs, the list of suspects included thyroid hormones, estrogen, progesterone, testosterone, and cortisol. Lab tests confirmed these deficiencies.

Pamela's deficiencies in estrogen and progesterone existed even though she was taking oral contraceptives made up of those two hormones. That's not uncommon. Even though they were doing the trick as far as her reproductive system was concerned, the dose was too low to meet her entire body's needs. She was taking synthetic thyroid hormones also, since her psychiatrist had noticed that deficiency. Pamela's personal pharmacy included prescription antidepressants already, too, but none had the desired effect. (That's a familiar story when it comes to chemical antidepressants, but the explanation, almost always overlooked, is simple: The "chemical imbalance" they fix often isn't the one that is out of whack; powerful as they are, they can't provide missing hormones.)

All this, and Pamela was *still* depressed and anxious, and she was annoyed by dozens of uncomfortable physical symptoms.

The first thing we did was switch her to a natural preparation of thyroid hormone. She stayed on the Pill for its contraceptive effects but added additional natural estrogen, progesterone, and testosterone to eliminate the effects of hormone deficiency that the synthetic versions couldn't. All those hormones increase cortisol production, but not enough to correct her deficiency, so Pamela started on small doses of cortisol as well. She also used melatonin to improve her sleep.

With the combination in place, Pamela finally made major improvements. She still had ups and downs, but they grew progressively less severe, and she felt better and better. Finally, her depression disappeared, her anxiety greatly diminished, and her energy came back in a major way. She felt less stressed and no longer had sugar cravings or felt dizzy. As a bonus—not that she wasn't already pleased with her results—as Pamela's physical and mental health improved so dramatically, so did her appearance. It was if the light inside her had come back on and now was shining through for everyone to see.

Pamela is just one of the thirty-two million Americans who suffer from mental disorders of one kind or another each year. Like just about every other bodily system, hormones play a part in mental health, too. This chapter looks at the two most common types of disorders, anxiety and depression, and the hormones that are most important for stabilizing mood.

ANXIETY

Roughly 10 percent of the U.S. population will experience serious or long-term anxiety at some point in their lives. The world seems to become more demanding and life more complicated each day. We all have our moments of irrational fears, and many of us have more permanent anxiety. It doesn't require a life of obvious or constant severe stress to be burdened with anxiety. The least worry can cause anxiety, which doesn't always have a clear reason behind it anyway. I estimate the frequency with which my patients say anxiety is their main complaint during their first visit to my office has doubled in the last five years. I'm not surprised that tranquilizers are high on the list of most commonly prescribed drugs.

Feelings of anxiety increase with age for most people. We (thankfully) grow beyond the invincible, invulnerable attitude of youth, leaving the most outrageous risk-taking behind us. Unfortunately, our carefree attitudes go right out the window with it. Still, all that would be well and good if it weren't for the encroachment of hesitation, worry, and brooding that is so common. Life is unexpected, if nothing else, so if we worry about everything or worry disproportionately, it can be paralyzing. Happily, to the extent that hormonal and nutritional deficiencies contribute to that tendency, we can calm even the most deep-seated anxieties quite simply.

DEPRESSION

More than one in five Americans will experience depression in their lifetimes—almost twice as many of them women as men. I'm not talking about "reactive" stress or depression, which is the result of a trauma or loss (such as major illness or the death of a loved one) or bad moods that are quickly overcome. Clinical depression lasts, and often can't be pinpointed to any particular cause. It can make you feel like your life has no meaning or that you can't feel happy and satisfied no matter how many good things you have in your life. It might show up as irritation at the least little thing, withdrawing into yourself, or a constant bad mood. And it can be devastating, even at this "mild" stage, wreaking havoc on relationships and careers. It ranges from here to the quite serious, including suicide. This sort of depression is often brought on by lack of hormones (accounting, no doubt, for most if not all of the different rates of occurrence in men and women). It is one of the most common complaints general practitioners hear from their patients. The only complaint I hear more frequently is fatigue.

NUTRITION

Nutritional as well as hormonal deficiencies can cause or exacerbate anxiety and depression. Good nutrition also supports the work of any hormone supplements you use. What you eat is as important as anything else you do to maintain your health, including your mental health.

NUTRITION AND ANXIETY

The rules for anxiety are much the same. Magnesium, vitamin B_{12}, and calcium are even more important here than in depression. They all have

NUTRIENTS FOR
ANXIETY AND DEPRESSION

Be sure to get at least these minimum doses daily.

VITAMINS

Vitamin B_6: 50 mg
Riboflavin: 15 mg
Thiamin: 30 mg
Folic Acid: 1 mg
Vitamin B_{12}: 2 mg
Vitamin C: 1 g (1,000 mg)

MINERALS

Calcium: 500 mg
Magnesium: 600 mg
Copper: 2 mg
Zinc: 30 mg
Iron: 100 mg
Potassium: 1 g (1,000 mg)

a calming effect. Other than that, the focus on fruits and vegetables, which calm you down, still stands, though you want to watch how much meat you get, as that can increase anxiety and nervousness. Sugar can provoke anxiety and even panic attacks, even in small quantities an hour or two after you have it, because of the resulting sudden drop of blood sugar levels (hypoglycemia), so you want to avoid it.

NUTRITION AND DEPRESSION

To fend off—preventatively or curatively—depression, the main idea is to get plenty of fruits and vegetables and small amounts of protein from fish, eggs, and poultry (you need only five to six ounces a day). The fruit boosts thyroid hormone levels, and the protein will increase adrenal and sex hormones, all of which improve your resistance to stress and help prevent a slide into depression . . . or assist a climb out of it. If you tend to be depressed in the morning, indicating low thyroid levels, the focus on increasing fruits and vegetables and decreasing dairy products is most important, as that will increase thyroid function. If your depression is more constant, meaning low sex hormones, or stress-related, meaning low cortisol, then increasing your animal protein intake (meat, poultry, fish, and eggs) is most important to boost the relevant hormones.

You might want to consider some supplements as well. For example, the liver makes **vitamin B$_6$** into a coenzyme that activates the metabolism of amino acids, including the making of tryptophan into serotonin (the lack of which can cause depression). Depression is also associated with low levels of **riboflavin, thiamin, folic acid,** vitamin B$_{12}$, and **vitamin C.** (Folic acid deficiency is especially common among women taking birth-control pills, alcoholics, smokers, and people over sixty-five.)

Scurvy, the disease defined by lack of vitamin C, has among its symptoms irritability and chronic depression, which often appear as the very first sign anything is wrong. Getting enough vitamin C clears up the symptoms.

Both too much and too little **calcium** can cause depression. Same thing for **magnesium.** These mineral deficiencies can cause excessive nervousness and muscular tension that fades away with adequate supplementation. Depression can also result from a lack of **copper, zinc, iron,** and/or **potassium** (this last being especially common in patients using diuretics).

DECODING YOUR DEFICIENCIES

ANXIETY

Are you anxious when you wake up in the morning but not while active? Thyroid hormones give us energy to face problems. If you are thyroid deficient, you might lack energy and the ability to quickly understand a situation, especially at rest, and that might make you anxious. In the morning, in bed, you might feel anxious about getting up, wondering what unpleasant events the day will bring. Later on, in the course of the day, if you remain quiet a little too long, you feel your fears return. At rest, blood circulates slowly in the brain and muscles if you are low in thyroid hormones. This disturbs the nervous and muscular cell activity, arousing the fear of not being able to face whatever life demands. Fortunately, the fears vanish as soon as you get active again and the blood circulates better. Although they are generally considered stimulants, taking thyroid hormone supplements to treat thyroid deficiency will calm you down.

This effect of thyroid deficiency is often overlooked even within the medical profession. There are a few studies, however, that underline the point. More than 60 percent of German refugees from the former German Democratic Republic who were treated for anxiety mixed with depression, for instance, had low levels of thyroid hormone. Another study showed that people with major depression are more likely to fear and avoid certain situations if their thyroid levels are low.

Too much thyroid hormone, on the other hand, can bring on anxiety and even panic attacks.

Men: Are you nervous and irritable? Easily excitable? Are you often ill at ease? Afraid? Worried? When male hormone levels are low, a man's body goes soft, his muscles shrink, and he becomes—sometimes literally, but often in his mind—less virile. He might, of course, keep right on with the macho behavior. But that would only be a front to hide an ever more insistent anxiety. He might start to look solemn and overburdened but be quick to attribute his irritability to simple overwork. These are also masks for his fear of not being able to cope. Emotional outbursts are staged to hide feelings of helplessness and the loss of ability to face any difficulty serenely.

Ninety percent of men diagnosed with low testosterone levels experience nervousness, and 80 percent of them irritability. Fifty-six percent report feeling ill at ease, 50 percent excessive excitability, 40 percent fear, and 25 percent useless worries.

All the above ailments die down or disappear when men take testosterone and/or DHEA therapy. DHEA enables you to better bear life's ups and downs and stay reasonable and peaceful. One study showed that a 50 mg dose of DHEA made men, averaging fifty-four years old, more relaxed and more able to react to stress. Experiments on mice subjected to excessive noise show that those given DHEA bear the racket much more easily. Finally, patients who take DHEA for other reasons report an increased sense of well-being and inner calm while they are using the therapy and nervousness, anxiety, and low stress resistance when they accidentally forget to take the hormone for a day or two.

Where DHEA generally makes a man gentler and more serene,

testosterone tends to encourage determination and even combativeness. It can reduce anxiety by making you feel fearless.

If your anxiety doesn't respond, or doesn't completely respond, to male hormones, it might be that you are experiencing purely psychological anxiety and should seek appropriate treatment. The other possibility, and the one I see most often, however, is that you have other hormones out of balance, particularly growth hormone (see below).

Women: Are you nervous? Are you irrational and irritable during the second half of your menstrual cycle? Do you worry about trivialities? Are you aggressive for no reason? Many women find DHEA calming, too, and testosterone even more so. In fact, women seem to be particularly sensitive to that effect of these hormones. But the hallmark of anxiety in women, particularly when it is synchronized with the menstrual cycle, is lack of progesterone. With an abundance of this hormone—as there should be in the second half of the menstrual cycle and during pregnancy—a woman feels serene, tranquil, gentle, contemplative, and receptive, as if nothing could ever disturb her. Progesterone is essential for good physical and mental balance.

Without enough progesterone, it is another story altogether. Deficiency of progesterone leaves the stimulating action of estrogen and some other hormones unopposed, making a woman irritable, nervous, and feeling on edge. She'll worry obsessively over unimportant matters, act overly aggressive for no apparent reason, and be quarrelsome and caustic . . . until a week or two later, when all that vanishes as if by magic.

If lab tests confirm a progesterone deficiency, natural progesterone will have significant tranquilizing effects. The body breaks it down into various derivatives that reduce pain and induce sleep—and can even block epileptic convulsions—as well as relieve anxiety. The effects are proportional to the levels of certain derivatives (allopregnenolone and pregnenolone) found in the blood rather than in the level of progesterone itself. But take note: The calming effect is not a part of the package—or at least not as significant a part—with the majority of synthetic derivative forms of progesterone (progestins).

Are you extremely anxious, to the point that it interferes with your ability to get or keep a job or relationship? Do you lack self-confidence? Do you isolate yourself from others? People of any age with a clear-cut deficit of growth hormone (or its partner, somatomedin C) often experience anxiety. They want to remain isolated, tucked away in their own little shells—and that alone, before you even factor in the underlying anxiety, can be extreme enough to cost them jobs or relationships. Not to mention the never-ending string of seemingly senseless worries, constant procrastination, endless reviewing of pointless details, and the lack of self-confidence.

Fortunately, taking growth hormone significantly lowers anxiety, inducing a state of calm and a feeling of inner peace. The reversal of the described symptoms of deficiency can transform someone's whole life, so dramatic is the shift to serenity.

Are you anxious at the end of the day and in stressful situations? Do small things set you off? Do you feel unable to confront or escape a situation? Cortisol helps you withstand stress, and escape the most unpleasant effect of stress: anxiety. Cortisol provides the additional energy your body needs to face unexpected situations. If the event is minor and lasts only a matter of seconds, no problem! Adrenaline triggers the release of the necessary energy to fight or flee, and that's that. Should the incident last longer—minutes or even hours—and require even more energy, your body needs cortisol, a lot of cortisol, fast. The adrenal glands can't always answer the demand. When they don't, anxiety sets in. You don't have energy to face whatever it is, and you know it. As these stressful situations recur, you'll fall victim to perpetual anxiety. Each unexpected event quickly piles up until one becomes the straw that breaks the camel's back.

Do you have nighttime anxiety? Sleep problems? If you don't have enough melatonin, anxiety might be the result. Anxiety from lack of melatonin happens at night and usually prevents its victims from sleeping well. Fortunately, this late anxiety dissipates with doses of melatonin before going to bed. The melatonin calms you down, makes you feel tranquil, and brings on a pleasant sleepiness and carefree yawning. It seems to dissolve minor worries that can significantly disturb sleep. One study shows that even patients with advanced cancer relax with melatonin.

Melatonin appears to have sedative properties separate from its soporific effects. That is, it would calm you down even if it wasn't putting you to sleep. Melatonin can relax involuntary (smooth) muscles like those of the artery walls and reinforce the part of the nervous system responsible for calming the body. It can also give orders to relax the voluntary (skeletal) muscles.

DEPRESSION

Do you feel depressed in the morning, when you wake up? Or when you are at rest (but not when you are active)? As with anxiety, this is the telltale pattern of a thyroid hormone deficiency. In this case, we're talking about the person who gets up on the wrong side of the bed—every day. The grouch proclaiming "I'm *not* a morning person." Or the person famous for always being active and never at rest— who probably doesn't stop moving during the day for fear of feeling bad—tired and blue. These are examples of morning depression and "rest-induced" depression, respectively, which are common when thyroid hormone levels are low.

These types of depression are quickly cured in most deficient people by taking thyroid hormones. They usually disappear within one to four months of treatment.

Some psychiatrists take advantage of thyroid hormones as antidepressants by prescribing a combination of traditional antidepressant drugs and a thyroid preparation, which often yields better results than prescribing the antidepressants alone. A Japanese study revealed that the patients with the lowest level of thyroid hormones at the outset responded best to this double therapy.

Men: Are you constantly depressed? More than three-quarters of men who are low in male hormones experience depression. So if any of my male patients complain of unrelenting depression, I make sure to check their testosterone levels. A study of men hospitalized for major depression showed they all had testosterone levels lower than nondepressed men of comparable age. And as the men gradually came out of their depression with psychotherapy and antidepressants, their testosterone levels progressively increased.

The inverse is also true—happiness can increase testosterone levels—which serves to underline the point. One study found that male college-student volunteers given a one-time injection of testosterone felt more optimistic. Men doping themselves with anabolic steroids— testosterone derivatives—report feeling enthusiastic, which is no doubt part of the appeal of this dangerous game. The same study also tested what happened to the young men's testosterone levels when they were told they had won a small monetary reward. It increased. This is a two-way street: Other researchers showed that bad news (being told you failed an exam) makes testosterone levels fall.

In almost every case, depression in male patients who are deficient in testosterone disappears after they begin using supplemental testosterone.

Women: Are you constantly depressed? Testosterone is also a powerful antidepressant in women. Part of its impact comes, no doubt, from the fact that the brain turns most testosterone into estrogen, in men as well as women, though females' brains might do it to a greater extent. We'll get to estrogen's effects next, but first I want to note that some testosterone remains vital for stabilizing mood in women. Women who are low in sex hormones who take natural estrogens have better results when they also take testosterone. Estrogen incites happiness and optimism, as we'll see, but testosterone adds self-confidence, tenacity, authority, boldness, and good resistance to stress. And it increases desire, including sexual desire, but also the burning desire for life itself and all that it holds.

Nearly half of women with sex hormone deficiency—including menopausal women—show signs of depression, such as sadness, loss of interest in regular activities, social withdrawal, and low self-esteem. Simply taking supplemental estrogen makes those signs disappear.

A study in France reveals that more than half of women who had attempted suicide had low estrogen levels (below 50 pg/ml). Very few had adequate levels (above 100 pg/ml). And consider this: Nearly half of suicide attempts in women take place during the first seven days of the menstrual cycle, when estrogen is at its lowest point.

Estrogen prevents or reverses depression in two basic ways. First, like some prescription antidepressants, it blocks monoamine oxidase, a brain enzyme that eliminates mood-stimulating neurotransmitters. With the enzyme blocked, the neurotransmitters can act longer and more strongly. Secondly, estrogen itself is used to make several neurotransmitters called catecholestrogens, which are mental stimulants.

Is your sex drive as depressed as you are? In addition to testosterone, sex drive is improved by DHEA. The effect is clearest in women, though it works on some men as well. Beyond that, DHEA is a general antidepressant, though its effects in that regard are not as powerful as testosterone and estrogen, at least at physiologic doses. Some people taking DHEA—for whatever reason—report feeling bad, sad, and sullen when they forget one or more doses. And they report regaining a good mood just as soon as they start up again.

Research backs this up. Studies show that low DHEA levels are associated with a rise in depressive feelings. A study in Canada revealed that patients' DHEA levels rise when they come out of depression, and they do so in proportion to how much the depression abates. Another study showed that people suffering from severe multiple sclerosis *and* depression feel better with DHEA. Yet another study compared two groups of businessmen and found significantly lower DHEA levels in those who were cynical and hostile and could not find pleasure in leisure activities than in their more optimistic counterparts.

Another study showed that in depressed patients, DHEA did not rise in the morning and lower in the evening, as it normally does. They had lost their natural circadian rhythm. That DHEA cycle is often decreased or absent in people over sixty-five as well, perhaps contributing to the increase in depression with age.

To obtain the antidepressant effect, women need to be on DHEA for at least four weeks (and generally three to four months) and men for at least six weeks.

Can even the littlest thing make you feel pessimistic and defeated? Are you excessively sensitive to stress? Are you confused? Distracted? Do you have trouble organizing your thoughts? Would you rather flee than fight, no matter what? When a situation demands additional energy, large amounts of cortisol are discharged into the blood in order to provide it. If you don't have enough of this stress-fighting hormone, you're likely to feel depressed, confused, and distracted and have difficulty organizing your ideas. Even the smallest stress can make you feel pessimistic and defeated. You'll prefer running away from difficult situations—literally or metaphorically—to facing them directly.

Depressed people generally adapt poorly to new situations. One of the reasons might be that cortisol secretion does not vary in depressed patients. It remains at a constant level, but it should increase under stress and diminish in periods of calm. Not enough cortisol during the day and during unexpected situations might make you unable to handle stress effectively, and too much at night can keep you awake, both of which contribute to depression.

Too *much* cortisol, on the other hand, comes with its own problems. People with too much cortisol seem to thrive on stress. They are somewhat energized and invigorated by the continuous flood of cortisol that stress produces. But if the cortisol-producing adrenal glands are too active or efficient, this can translate into excessive activity or euphoria or even disabling mania. The overabundance of joy and self-assurance makes all problems seem small, so they are handled only superficially, thereby allowing them to dig in and fester. When they finally surface, they might be worse than they originally were.

With appropriate amounts of cortisol, however, stress won't depress you; you'll have the wherewithal to face up to whatever it is. I do want to emphasize, however, that there can be big differences in the effects of natural cortisol and its synthetic derivatives, and nowhere does that show up more than when it comes to depression. Natural cortisol is much more psychologically active.

Here's an anecdotal warning for you, published in the medical literature: A woman had her adrenal glands (which make cortisol) removed then started on prednisone, a synthetic derivative of cortisol. Soon thereafter she became psychotic and didn't respond to any of the standard pharmaceutical treatments. When her doctors switched the prednisone to natural cortisol weeks later, however, she returned to normal within a few days! Of course, the synthetics are most likely *not* going to drive you crazy, but they do not have all the good mental effects that natural cortisol does. It is good to know what they each are capable of and to remember how different their effects can be.

Do you feel better lying down than standing up? Aldosterone improves your mood and increases your feeling of well-being when you are in a vertical position.

Have you lost your sense of well-being? Your physical endurance? EPO improves the feeling of well-being and stimulates endurance for long-distance or long-term physical efforts, in patients who need it—patients undergoing dialysis, for instance, or those with severe anemia because of kidney problems. It also increases endurance in athletes such as long-distance runners.

Do you have frequent, recurrent bouts of depression? Are you excessively vulnerable to stress? Do you feel fragile? Depressed people often have low levels of growth hormone, according to many studies. This is true especially when the depression is severe, with real mental breakdown possible. It is true regardless of age. Depressed adolescents diagnosed with suicidal tendencies, for example, secrete less growth hormone than is average for their age.

Depression resulting from the lack of growth hormone usually comes with a profoundly fragile mental state and excessive vulnerability to even the least stress. When significant emotional stress occurs, then, it is enormously difficult to overcome. Completing the circle, even a minor event can throw a person without enough growth hormone into depression, where they will be still more vulnerable to stress and so depression, and so on.

Taking growth hormone can restore your stress resistance, serenity, and self-confidence, improving your quality of life overall and leaving no room for depression.

SUMMARY: MOOD HORMONES

Hormone Deficiency	Symptoms	See also pg.
Aldosterone	feeling better lying down than standing up	26
Cortisol	anxiety at the end of the day; feeling provoked by small things; feeling unable to confront or escape from a situation; feeling pessimistic and defeated; excessive sensitivity to stress; feeling confused or distracted; having trouble organizing thoughts; would always rather flee than fight; becoming paralyzed by stress; outbursts of anxiety or anger during stress and feeling exhausted thereafter; suffering more than others from stress; suicidal thoughts at night	26
DHEA	nervousness; depressed sex drive; in men: irritability; feeling worried; in women: irritability; worrying about trivialities; anxiety	27
EPO	loss of physical endurance and/or sense of well-being	28
Estrogen	in women: constant depression	28
Growth Hormone	anxiety that interferes with job and/or relationship; lack of self-confidence; social withdrawal; frequent, recurrent bouts of intense, deep depression; excessive vulnerability to stress, with collapses possible from even minor stress; feelings of fragility	29
Melatonin	nighttime anxiety and/or depressive thoughts; sleep problems; suicidal thoughts at night	30
Progesterone	in women: nervousness, irrationality, and irritability during second half of menstrual cycle; worrying about trivialities; unprovoked aggression or anxiety	32
Testosterone	Constant depression; depressed sex drive; in men: nervousness, irritability, excitability; feeling ill at ease or afraid; worry; in women: irritability; worrying about trivialities; anxiety	32
Thyroid	anxiety and/or depression upon waking up in the morning or at rest, but not while active	33

CHAPTER FIFTEEN

STRESSING HEALTH

Some stress is good. It is energizing. It keeps you alert to danger. It keeps you safe. It keeps you ready to protect or defend yourself. It can help you perform at your peak or even better than you knew you could.

But lots of stress is bad. We all know it can make you feel awful. It can sap all your strength. Exhaust you. Make you sick and put you at high risk for getting sicker. It can paralyze you, so you no longer know how to face (or even flee from) whatever is making you stressed. One huge stress is bad enough, but chronic stress, even if each one is little on its own, is even worse.

Whether good or bad—and they coexist—prolonged, repeated, and excessive stress makes you age faster. Stress, and especially chronic stress, reduces hormone levels almost across the board—hitting the anabolic (tissue-building) hormones particularly hard—similar to the way getting older does. Too much stress makes you age too fast. The symptoms stress causes—from gray hair, wrinkles, and memory problems to fatigue, anxiety, and high blood pressure—could also be a catalog of the complaints of aging. The premature aging caused by stress is really the result of the decrease stress causes in hormone levels. You don't have to get older to get "old." You can stress yourself into it.

Fortunately, hormone replacement therapy in the correct doses addressing the hormone levels decreased by stress can prevent this premature aging. Beyond that, combating the stress and its symptoms will help keep you healthy—and young. There are shelves of books devoted to various stress-reduction techniques, and while that information might well be useful, it is beyond the scope of this book. Our focus will stay, no surprise, on the ways hormones either reinforce or undermine your resistance to stress.

Intense, short-lived stress provokes an influx of all sorts of fast-acting hormones into our blood. These chemical messengers open the floodgates of energy reserves to give the body the resources it needs to face up to the stress, whatever it is. These hormones, which work quickly and stimulate the nerves and the brain to produce energy by consuming body tissue, are known as catabolic hormones.

Anabolic hormones, on the other hand, build new tissue. They are produced more slowly, and act more slowly as well—and their levels in the blood drop significantly under stress. The resulting imbalance between catabolic and anabolic hormones can lead to overconsumption of body tissue. That might be an acceptable trade-off over short periods of time, but if it persists, the consequences can be severe.

When the stress lasts several hours, the level of other hormones, including thyroid hormones and insulin, also drops significantly due to simultaneously increased demand and decreased production. The reserves stored in the glands get used up gradually, while the production of new hormones progressively deteriorates. The glands just can't compensate for the overuse.

If the stress lasts even longer—days, weeks, years—then all the hormone reserves get used up. The endocrine glands—in fact, the whole body—get worn out. Minor tissue damage shows up, a feeling of fatigue sets in, and a deep-seated anxiety takes root. If something doesn't give, there will be irreparable harm. Interestingly, the hormones that drop during this kind of prolonged stress, regardless of age, are similar to the hormonal breakdown that weakens people over sixty-five. You could lose your hormones through simple wear and tear and the passage of time, or you could end up at the same place much earlier by living under constant stress. Either way, correcting any hormonal deficiencies you have or develop will help you bear up under unavoidable stress.

BERNARD

That's what happened with Bernard. Not yet thirty, Bernard was worried his fast-track career was stalled and feared it would be totally derailed. On paper, he was an excellent lawyer. He worked for a prominent law firm, specializing in international affairs, representing major clients in international courts in Europe. So far, so good. However, this required him to speak several different languages in court, and to speak them well and smoothly enough to convince the judges of the rightness of his case. This should not have been a particular problem, as Bernard had, indeed, mastered three languages. But during trials, the intense stress caused him to mix up the words of different languages, so that he became tongue-tied and unable to fully express the merits of his case. This, of course, only increased the pressure he felt.

Bernard had all the refined insights he needed to get to the heart of his cases, and all the legal knowledge and intuition, and in his own mind he could outargue any and all comers. Too often, though, his brilliance failed him when he was on his feet in the courtroom. He'd suffer from 20/20 hindsight. The exact right thing to say would occur to him . . . moments after he finished speaking. He had everything he needed to convince any judge, but too often he couldn't get it across effectively. As his win-loss record started to skew toward the loss column, Bernard started to think he simply wasn't up to the task.

Bernard finally made his way to my office, desperate for any solution. I listened to him describe his courtroom failings. It sounded to me like low resistance to stress was at the heart of the matter. He was obviously smart and capable, but he choked under pressure. If he could handle the stress in more productive ways, I thought he'd find his voice without a problem.

Hormone deficiency can weaken your stress resistance, and he had a few other nagging health problems that suggested the same thing: fatigue, especially in the morning; dry skin; slow reactions; and a slight tendency to obesity, particularly around his waist. Other than that, he considered himself very healthy.

Lab tests showed that Bernard was low in thyroid hormones, testosterone, and cortisol. He responded very quickly to treatment. Most of his symptoms soon abated when he started taking thyroid hormones and testosterone, and when he began very small doses (10 to 15 mg) of cortisol, he won his very next court case—a high-profile one at that—with a resounding victory. Even when the pressure was turned to the max in court, and even in a higher court than he was used to, Bernard kept a clear head. He felt sure of himself and his abilities. He spoke easily no matter what language he called upon, and he was able to hone precise and persuasive arguments on the spot as necessary. The best part for Bernard was hearing about how furious the opposing lawyers were to have been beaten by a young and relatively unknown lawyer on a case they had expected to win easily.

NUTRITION

As always, proper nutrition is key to successfully balancing your hormones—with or without additional hormone therapy.

When it comes to susceptibility to stress, poor nutrition in general often plays a part. A well-rounded, nutritious diet based around whole foods with very limited refined foods will do wonders. Or tailor your diet to the recommendations elsewhere in this book, depending on your other conditions or deficiencies. Think particularly about your intake of animal protein, especially meat, which will stimulate you and make you more aggressive—a welcome effect if you are too passive under stress, but not exactly desirable if you are irritable or excessively aggressive under stress. Also keep in mind that fresh fruits and vegetables are calming.

If you are being overwhelmed by stress, you should avoid or at least strictly limit caffeine and alcohol. Sugar is another culprit, and you probably have more of it in your diet than you realize if you eat prepared

NUTRIENTS FOR STRESS

Be sure to get at least these minimum doses daily.

VITAMINS
Vitamin B$_6$: 50 mg
Calcium: 500 mg

MINERALS
Magnesium: 350 mg daily (To get 350 mg of elemental magnesium, you'll need to take two to three grams of a magnesium complex. Read labels carefully to see how much elemental magnesium lurks within whatever complex you are taking.)

foods or are always eating on the run. Read labels, and fix your own meals when you can.

Magnesium helps you handle stress, and deficiencies are common.

DECODING YOUR DEFICIENCIES

You will notice that the signs of stress on this list could also be a list of the signs of aging—premature aging. They often appear between forty-five and fifty, not exactly a coincidence with the time of life during which hormone levels wane. Repairing your hormone levels will not only restore your ability to effectively manage stress (for no one's life is without it for long), it will also make you look and feel younger in general. But it is also true that stress ages your body—mainly by over-consumption and underproduction of hormones—which should give you an incentive to learn to manage it well, regardless of your hormone levels.

Do you have gray hair? This can indicate a lack of testosterone, especially in men. Men, especially younger men with gray hair and testosterone deficiency, might prevent the progression of gray or even noticeably decrease the number of gray hairs on their heads by taking testosterone, which stimulates production of the hair and skin pigment melanin.

Do you have wrinkles and tiny lines? They flourish after years of insufficient growth hormone, and sex hormone deficiencies including testosterone and estrogen. These hormones thicken and strengthen the outer layer of the skin, hydrate the skin, maintain the skin's elasticity, and strengthen the small muscle fibers in the skin.

Are you tired all the time? Check the levels of your sex hormones. Testosterone (for men and women) can be an underlying cause, especially when the fatigue worsens with physical activity. For women, progesterone and especially estrogen might also be low.

For young adults, particularly those about eighteen to thirty years old, chronic fatigue syndrome often develops after a long period of stress and hyperactivity followed by a major infection that stops them dramatically in their tracks for at least a while. Worn out after the infection, they can remain very tired indefinitely. (Some would say for the rest of their lives.) Their bodies show the signs of premature aging—the signs of stress—we are discussing here. When properly investigated, a multitude of minor (yet still potentially incapacitating) hormonal deficiencies are often found. Small doses of the hormones they lack can bring a veritable resurrection. In my experience, about 50 to 90 percent of cases of chronic fatigue will improve considerably with proper hormone treatment, even where no other treatment has worked.

Similar results are obtained in older and more stressed—but less severely tired—people.

Are you tired and slow to react to stress in the mornings or when you are at rest? This is a familiar sign of thyroid hormone deficiency, which causes slow blood circulation and thus an inadequate supply of nutrients and oxygen to the brain cells.

Do you feel easily confused or fatigued when under stress? A lack of cortisol might well be the cause. The confusion is due to a lack of blood sugar supply to the brain cells—hypoglycemia.

Do you feel dizzy when you are under stress? Do you need to urinate often and in large quantities? Suspect a lack of aldosterone.

Do you have little in the way of endurance? Do you have a hard time recovering from any kind of exertion? Suspect a lack of growth hormone.

Do you feel drained? This might signal a lack of sugar in the nerve and muscle cells, which happens with a drop in thyroid hormones, growth hormone, cortisol, and insulin, all of which help maintain proper blood-sugar levels.

Do you have digestive problems under stress? Check your cortisol and insulin levels.

Do you get headaches from stress? Are you paralyzed by stress? Are you irritable when you are stressed or have angry outbursts and feel exhausted afterward? Do you have digestive troubles or allergies or asthma that appear or worsen with stress? Check your level of cortisol.

Are you anxious? That's often the case when testosterone, growth hormone, and progesterone are lacking.

Do you sleep poorly? Light or interrupted sleep appears with low levels of melatonin, growth hormone, testosterone, and, in women, estrogen and progesterone. Without enough melatonin, you'll lie awake at night, thinking about stressful situations. Low progesterone will make you tense, nervous, and irritable enough to interfere with a good night's sleep.

Do you have memory problems? A lot of hormone deficiencies might be at work here, including thyroid hormone, testosterone, DHEA, pregnenolone, vasopressin, and ACTH.

Do you have low blood pressure? Low blood pressure can cause low resistance to stress. People with clearly low blood pressure are generally low in cortisol and aldosterone and tend to be paralyzed by stress. They become passive in the face of it, when they need to be active. A lack of vasopressin might also underlie low blood pressure.

Do you have high blood pressure? That's often the sign of lack of thyroid hormones, estrogen, and/or testosterone, all of which dilate the arteries and can naturally lower blood pressure or keep it healthfully low.

SUMMARY: STRESS-FIGHTING HORMONES

Hormone Deficiency	Symptoms	See also pg.
ACTH	feeling paralyzed by stress; memory problems	25
Aldosterone	low blood pressure; dizzy under stress or standing up; frequent urination and in large quantities, especially during the day, under stress	26
Cortisol	fatigue and/or confusion under stress; feeling drained; low blood pressure; headaches under stress; paralyzed by stress; irritable or angry under stress; digestive troubles, allergies, or asthma under stress	26
DHEA	memory problems; lack of calmness; low resistance to noise	27
Estrogen	wrinkles and tiny lines; tired all the time; poor sleep; high blood pressure	28
Growth Hormone	wrinkles and tiny lines; low endurance and poor recovery from exertion; feeling drained; exhaustion; anxiety; poor sleep	29
Insulin	feeling drained; digestive trouble under stress	30
Melatonin	poor sleep; nighttime anxiety and agitation	30
Pregnenolone	memory problems	31
Progesterone	anxiety, especially premenstrually; poor sleep; wrinkles and tiny lines; nervousness and irritability	32
Testosterone	gray hair; wrinkles and tiny lines; feeling tired all the time; anxiety; poor sleep; memory problems; high blood pressure	32
Thyroid	feeling tired or drained or slow to react to stress in the morning or when at rest; feeling drained; memory problems; high blood pressure	33
Vasopressin	memory problems; low blood pressure; urinating a lot (frequently and in large quantities), especially during the night	34

CHAPTER SIXTEEN

A MORE ENERGETIC YOU

"I'm tired all day long."

"I never feel fully rested."

"I'm twenty-eight, but I feel like a little old lady."

"The least little thing wears me out completely."

"I start yawning, or even fall asleep, at the drop of a hat."

"I just don't have the energy for exercise anymore."

I hear these and many more variations just about every day. Fatigue is often the main reason a patient comes to see me. It's often gone on for a long time, even years. A lot of the time, patients can no longer really remember exactly when they started feeling so tired. This kind of long-lasting fatigue can be brought on by hormonal deficiency.

GINA

Take Gina, for instance. She had chronic fatigue syndrome. This is a poorly understood and underrecognized condition, characterized by major, disabling fatigue lasting more than six months with spikes of fever, muscle and joint pain, low-blood-pressure problems, depression, and anxiety. It often starts after a difficult recovery from a serious infection.

Gina, not yet thirty, had had it for years. She was exhausted most of the time, and by this point she was almost completely inactive. She had quit her job long ago. She secretly hoped to paint or write poems, but even holding a pencil was too much for her and she'd have to rest after a matter of minutes. Like most people with this disease, Gina's friends and family, and even her doctor, couldn't really understand what she was going through. She felt they didn't believe she had a physical problem but was rather lazy or lacking in willpower or a hypochondriac—although she'd always been overactive, if anything, before her sudden collapse into exhaustion. It was as if she had simply used up all her energy.

There is no official cure for chronic fatigue syndrome. Gina had tried every commonly proposed treatment: vitamins, diet, meditation, a change of apartment, a new boyfriend. Nothing helped. Her doctor recommended psychotherapy. Now, psychotherapy is good for many things and might help patients learn to live with chronic fatigue, accepting it as their fate. But it would never restore Gina's energy. It couldn't get her back to normal professional work or a normal romantic relationship.

The cause or causes of chronic fatigue syndrome remain murky, but in my experience patients like Gina have burned out their endocrine glands, whether by infection, overwork, pollution, or poor genes. The result is multiple hormone deficiencies. The only treatment that will truly work, then, is correcting those deficiencies.

And, indeed, when Gina came to my office, blood and urine tests, our interview, and her answers to my standard questionnaire revealed several deficiencies. Although none of the lab results were outside the normal range provided by the lab, all were borderline low. Her levels were average—for a seventy-year-old woman! And her symptoms showed the grave impact of these low levels. She had clear signs of deficiency in thyroid hormones, testosterone, DHEA, estrogen, aldosterone, and cortisol. Situations like Gina's are why neither lab tests nor symptoms lists alone give you the full story when it comes to hormones. If I had to choose just one, though, I would go for the messages the body is putting out.

Gina took thyroid hormones, estrogen, DHEA, testosterone, aldosterone, and cortisol, though we started with just a couple and built up slowly and carefully to get everything calibrated correctly. Her muscle strength increased and her body firmed up (testosterone and DHEA). Her menstrual cycles normalized. Her skin colored up again, losing its paleness, and her breasts became more firm (estrogen). Her dry hair and skin and cold feet improved (thyroid). Her blood pressure stabilized and her dizziness and absentmindedness disappeared (aldosterone). Her eyes were no longer red, nor her muscles sore (cortisol).

Most important of all, her fatigue lifted, and it was gone completely six months after she started her hormone regimen. Gina resumed her normal life, going back to work and decorating a new house with enthusiasm. And though it surely mattered less to Gina, I was happy to see that further lab tests showed she now had average hormone levels for her young age. The supplemental hormones served only to correct the deficiencies, as they were supposed to, without pushing into overdose. It had taken quite a bit of adjustment, but we had found the right doses and combinations.

FATIGUE, FATIGUE, OR FATIGUE?

*E*ach hormone creates its own type of energy and, in the event of a deficiency, a different kind of fatigue. Paying attention to the timing and pattern of your fatigue is key to figuring out which hormone levels you should be concerned about, particularly if, like Gina, your lab results still put you in the "reference" range for the lab.

With thyroid hormone deficiency, you are tired when you wake up and when you are resting; the feeling of fatigue disappears as the morning goes on and you get active. Estrogen deficiency makes you tired all day long and so does testosterone deficiency, but with more extreme feelings of fatigue when you are physically active. With cortisol deficiency, you are profoundly tired in the evening, and during the day you feel exhausted whenever you are under stress. Growth hormone deficiency makes you mildly fatigued all day and exhausted in the late evening. You cannot stay awake after midnight and, if you do manage that, then you have a hard time recovering the next day. Finally, aldosterone deficiency makes you feel tired when you stand up.

NUTRITION

*N*o matter what pattern you identify with, you'll create a more energetic you by avoiding bread and anything else made with yeast, grains (unless they are sprouted), dairy products, and sugar. (A bread made with sprouted grains and no yeast that fits within this diet is Essene bread, which you can find at health-food stores.) Sugar provides quick energy, it is true, but a dramatic drop always follows, and it lasts longer than the boost ever did. It also promotes the growth of yeast in your body, which consumes a lot of blood sugar and hormones, including cortisol, sapping your energy. The fatigue caused by overgrowth of yeast in the body is characterized by ups and downs.

If you're having digestive trouble along with fatigue, spend several days eating only steamed, boiled, or pressure-cooked vegetables, fish, and meat.

Beyond that, those with low thyroid hormone fatigue (see below) should eat a more vegetarian diet, increasing their intake of fruits and vegetables and getting their protein from small amounts of fish, eggs, and poultry. Too much protein can decrease conversion of T_4 into the active thyroid hormone T_3. Avoid dairy products, as the milk protein casein can decrease thyroid hormone levels. Grains can improve thyroid function, but because they increase the growth of yeast can also cause fatigue, so they are best avoided. If your fatigue is related to low adrenal hormones—the sex hormones and growth hormone—you should eat more animal protein from meat, fish, and poultry. Avoid dairy products, however, as they decrease DHEA and other hormones and can cause digestive-tract problems besides. In either case, as long as you have low or normal blood pressure, do *not* follow a low-salt diet. Salt keeps blood pressure from dropping low enough to cause fatigue, and it increases energy. That's not to say you necessarily need to add salt to your diet; Americans generally get plenty of salt in their diets, especially if they eat any prepared foods at all. Too much salt is harmful. But as you transition to a healthful diet made up of whole, natural foods, you may not get enough salt unless you add it yourself—so you might in fact want to sprinkle some in, particularly if you live in a hot climate and perspire a lot (losing salt in the process).

Some supplements fight fatigue as well.

Vitamin B_{12} provides continuous energy. It helps create red blood cells. Without it the cells could not reach maturity and might not be able to survive. If they did they would not be able to properly oxygenate the body. The oxygen the red blood cells carry is vital to burning fuels for the body, like glucose. B_{12} is also important in building good myelin sheaths around the nerves. These are a kind of shield that protects nerve cells and improves communication between them. If you don't get enough B_{12}, you will be chronically tired and frequently breathless, particularly when you are making strong physical efforts.

Iron provides the energy necessary to make it through the day. Iron is used in many energy-producing metabolic reactions and is an essen-

NUTRIENTS FOR FATIGUE

VITAMINS

Vitamin B_{12}: 3,000 mcg orally for two to four months or four to eight weekly injections to correct deficiency

MINERALS

Magnesium: 350 mg elemental magnesium daily
Iron: 10 mg elemental iron daily or 80 mg in case of deficiency

ENZYMES

CoQ10: at least 50 mg daily

tial part of hemoglobin, the protein that transports oxygen in the blood. A severe oxygen deficiency can asphyxiate the cells of the body. People who are short on iron tire very quickly.

Magnesium also has an important role in many energy-producing metabolic reactions, serving mostly to speed them up. With low magnesium levels, your muscles become tense and tired. This increases under stress and will, in turn, aggravate that stress and make you nervous.

Coenzyme Q10 (CoQ10) facilitates activities requiring stamina, particularly affecting your heart. It also enhances the functioning of your heart (a muscle, after all), sometimes quite dramatically. One study showed that in healthy young adults, 50 mg daily of CoQ10 increased blood flow through the heart by 20 percent with no extra effort. That means the heart is able to pump 20 percent more blood at a time, and therefore more nutrients and energy reach all body tissues, resulting in more energy and endurance.

DECODING YOUR DEFICIENCIES

Do you have a hard time getting up in the morning? When you take a break during the day, do you seem to end up feeling even more tired? Thyroid hormones fight fatigue by providing the cells with the fuel they need by maintaining a constant sugar level in the body and speeding up energy and heat reactions inside the cells.

If you don't have enough thyroid hormone, you'll feel like staying in bed in hopes of recuperating just a little bit more. Then, thanks to loads of willpower, you'll get out of bed—and feel slow and dull. Thanks to what is really early-morning fatigue—often expressed as a bad mood—you'll be known far and wide as definitely not a morning person. You'll feel much better, though, by mid- or late morning, as you get more active. Your thoughts will be clearer and quicker as the blood circulates faster, providing vital oxygen and nutrients to the nerve and muscle cells. Your circulation slows down again when you sit or lie down, and your fatigue will be back. This cycle makes some people, especially very strong personalities, choose constant motion as their way of coping—anything to avoid that sluggish feeling at rest. In my experience, low thyroid hormone levels account for a lot of what is labeled as hyperactivity or attention deficit disorder, especially in adults.

Are you constantly tired? Do your usual activities exhaust you? The sex hormones—estrogen in women and testosterone and, secondarily, DHEA in both men and women—attenuate or relieve fatigue. Without enough of them, you'll be tired all day. And though you'll probably be determined to remain as active as you ever were, you'll have more and more difficulty keeping up the pace, at work and at home. You'll probably ignore that and claim to be full of energy, but your pale and weary face will give you away.

Does the least amount of stress wipe you out? When you are in good health, your adrenal glands contain large reserves of cortisol, which is released into the blood as soon as you need a burst of energy. Cortisol releases sugar from the body's stockpiles to provide the brain and muscle cells the fuel they need at strategic moments when the need for energy increases, like during physical exertion or in reaction to mental stress. Without enough cortisol, your blood pressure will be low under stress, which will make you feel too tired to face up to whatever problem is creating that stress. When you lie down, and your blood circulates better, particularly to the brain, you'll feel better—if only temporarily. Otherwise, you'll seek a sheltered life. You'll do everything you can to avoid stress, such as choosing relaxed work and low-key leisure activities. No candy, chocolate, sugar, or soda will be safe in your presence. You'll pounce on them in an attempt to compensate for your lack of energy. The more you fight this, facing up to everyday problems, the more persistent will be your fatigue at the end of the day, as you deplete the last of your body's cortisol reserves.

Do you feel light-headed and shaky while standing? Have your blood pressure and your aldosterone levels checked. Lack of aldosterone can cause excessively low blood pressure and that woozy feeling when standing or even sitting for a long time. This kind of fatigue fades or disappears when you're lying down. That's because aldosterone ensures the maintenance of appropriate blood pressure by retaining salt and water in the body, which affects blood volume and pressure in the arteries. It is thanks to aldosterone that sufficient blood reaches the head, despite the effects of gravity, when one is standing.

Patients bothered by low blood pressure are often prescribed medication to boost it, but simply correcting an aldosterone deficiency would bring the same results naturally.

Do you avoid brief physical effort because it leaves you breathless and tired and it takes a while to recover? Testosterone plays a large role in enabling you to carry out physical activity, insofar as, with other androgens, it largely determines health, muscle tone, and (in men) the size of muscles and blood vessels. Without enough of these "male" hormones (though that's a misnomer, because women have them, too, albeit about twenty times less), stamina decreases and constant fatigue sets in. Fatigue that seriously increases during physical effort—and particularly during sex—points toward a testosterone deficiency. DHEA is similarly, if secondarily, effective.

Do you avoid sustained physical effort for fear of being unable to finish? EPO reinforces the capacity to accomplish sustained physical efforts, which consume large quantities of oxygen, because it stimulates the bones to produce red blood cells, which carry oxygen to body tissues. (Some athletes have learned this lesson well and abuse the hormone by injecting large quantities to artificially enhance their endurance.) When an EPO deficiency sets in, the number of red blood cells and the level of hemoglobin (the part of the red blood cell that actually carries the oxygen) diminish. If this happens to you, you'll become pale and anemic. You'll also find that any physical activity requiring stamina, like running or even just climbing several flights of stairs, leaves you breathless and wears you out.

In just one example of how EPO is used, consider chemotherapy patients given EPO when their bone marrow, where red blood cells are created, is seriously damaged. With a series of EPO injections, a treatment starting to become more common in hospitals, the red blood cell level rises again, sometimes spectacularly, and patients report feeling better in general and being less tired in particular.

I almost never use EPO, however, and never to address fatigue alone, preferring to address anemia and fatigue with nutrients and other hormones.

Are you constantly fatigued and slow to recover after exertion or stress? Growth hormone releases a great deal of sugar into the blood in order to provide energy, particularly when there is an increased demand for fuel. It also pushes the body to produce the most active thyroid hormone and augments muscle mass and tone, making them stronger and more resistant to physical strain. Fatigue is a symptom of potassium deficiency, and growth hormone increases potassium (the main salt found inside cells) in the body and improves the functioning of cells in those deficient in potassium (as most people over sixty-five are). Without enough growth hormone, you'll be almost constantly fatigued and unable to recover your strength after exertion or significant stress. The way growth hormone creates difficulty in recovering from stress or unforeseen activity (to the point that it can be quite serious, even incapacitating) compounds the fatigue.

For people who are tired all the time, with tests showing growth hormone deficiency, two to four months of growth hormone treatment can restore a level of vigor and endurance equal to what you experienced in your thirties. You'll be able to stay out past midnight again without being exhausted the whole following week.

Numerous rigorous scientific studies, including meta-analyses, which combine the results of many studies, have confirmed the benefits of growth hormone on quality of life, and fatigue in particular.

If you are diabetic, do you lack energy for tiring work? Do you tire quickly or at the least effort? People with type I diabetes get breathless and tire quickly and often feel drowsy because the body can't properly use the main fuel for cellular activity: sugar. Furthermore,

SVEN

Severe chronic fatigue syndrome is often due to multiple hormone deficiencies. Sven could be a poster boy for the phenomenon. He was a flight attendant but hadn't been able to work for years, debilitated by constant and crushing fatigue. On his first visit to my office, he brought pictures of himself to show me the athlete he had once been. He was only in his mid-thirties, but you wouldn't have recognized him from those photos. He was now fat, with lax muscles and a puffy face.

The lab tests I ran revealed deficiencies in thyroid hormones, testosterone, cortisol, DHEA, and growth hormone as well as several vitamins and trace elements. Treatment got off to a rocky start until we got all the hormones in proper balance (and so eliminated some side effects). Sven also made some major dietary changes, increasing his intake of fruits, vegetables, animal protein, and water, and decreasing or eliminating dairy products, grains, sugars, and caffeine. The combination improved his energy levels enough for him to go back to work, albeit half-time. His body also firmed up again, giving him the literal strength to get through the day—as well as a much nicer appearance.

But there was still a problem: Sven was getting up three to five times a night to urinate large quantities. Losing that much fluid at night was not normal for a young man, and the interrupted sleep was keeping him fatigued, even though he was better than before. Poor sleep was also leaving him with memory and concentration problems.

Another test revealed a low vasopressin level. Taking vasopressin, using a nose spray, brought rapid improvement. Sven still had to get up to urinate at night, but only once, sometimes twice, and with much less volume. As his sleep improved, so did memory and concentration—and his energy itself.

sugar is plentiful in the blood and tissues, and particularly in the space outside the cells, and this unused abundance creates a sticky substance that partially prevents other nutrients from permeating the cells.

With insulin in small doses, diabetics' energy levels improve rapidly. Insulin transfers excess sugar from outside to within nerve, muscle, and heart cells, taking nutrients and energy levels back where they should be.

Note that patients with type II diabetes have too much insulin in their blood already and cannot use insulin effectively. This surplus drives sugar into the fat cells, where it is converted into fat (and not energy)—the reason diabetics get fat so quickly and why they get fatigued at the least effort. If you have type II diabetes, slimming down is your best bet for regaining your energy—and your health—and you should talk to your doctor about other treatments.

Do you lack energy and willpower? ACTH boosts this kind of drive by stimulating the secretion of hormones that release energy, including cortisol, DHEA, pregnenolone, aldosterone, and some thirty others. The increased level of cortisol, in particular, makes ACTH a fatigue-fighter.

For ACTH to work this way, the adrenal glands must be in good working order—they have to carry out the release of the other hormones. One drawback: ACTH must be given by intramuscular injection and is somewhat less predictable than the use of the adrenal hormones like DHEA, cortisol, and aldosterone, taken orally. It can be difficult to find the right dose.

Do you lack energy and enthusiasm for your regular activities? A pregnenolone deficiency causes periods of fatigue during the day because it is a precursor of all the other adrenal hormones. The body converts it into cortisol, DHEA, aldosterone, testosterone, estrogen, and progesterone—and a shortage of the precursor means a shortage of these products as well. Fortunately, any negative effects of the deficiency can be erased with supplements. Taking supplements provides additional energy, though its effects are not as dramatic as those of testosterone, thyroid hormones, and growth hormone.

Do you have a hard time getting going in the morning? If your melatonin level is low, you will sleep poorly and superficially, and so you won't get the rest you need to be refreshed and ready to face another day come morning. You'll be perpetually tired and poorly rested. Melatonin, in proper amounts, allows you to recharge your batteries at night. It reduces the amount of energy you lose during the night by slowing the secretion of catabolic (energy-producing but tissue-consuming) hormones like cortisol, which are useful during the day but should be decreased at night. Melatonin also increases or maintains the release of muscle-building anabolic hormones like growth hormone, which increase energy storage.

Furthermore, melatonin increases thyroid activity. It ups the production of the active thyroid hormone, T_3, which is why melatonin enables you to wake up in the morning ready and raring to go.

SUMMARY: STRESS HORMONES

Hormone Deficiency	Symptoms	See also pg.
ACTH	lack of energy and willpower	25
Aldosterone	feeling light-headed and shaky while standing	26
Cortisol	small amount of stress wipes you out	26
DHEA	constant tiredness; tired by usual activities	27
EPO	avoiding long-lasting physical effort for fear of being unable to finish	28
Estrogen	constantly tired; tired by usual activities	28
Growth Hormone	exhaustion; feeling unable or slow to recover after exertion or stress	29
Insulin	diabetics: lack of energy for tiring work	30
Melatonin	hard time getting going in the morning	30
Pregnenolone	lack of energy and enthusiasm for regular activities	31
Testosterone	constant tiredness; tired by usual physical activities; tendency to avoid physical efforts (even brief ones) because they leave you breathless and tired and take a long time to recover from	32
Thyroid	difficulty waking up and getting up in the morning; feeling tired at rest	33
Vasopressin	feeling of losing your energy; low blood pressure; excessive urine loss at night (getting up frequently to urinate)	34

PART IV

THE HORMONE SOLUTION

CHAPTER SEVENTEEN

THE HORMONE SOLUTION DIET

When it comes to "natural" ways to balance your hormones, you can't do better than eating right. You'll have to learn about just what eating right means as far as your hormones are concerned. (I'll give you a hint: It doesn't look at all like the famous Food Pyramid *or* the much-ballyhooed extremely low-fat diets.) But that turns out to be a simple matter. And once you do learn to eat right, you might be able to restore hormonal health without doing another thing. If you do still require hormonal supplements, the proper diet will ensure that those supplements can work most effectively and efficiently in your body, minimizing doses and maximizing results.

There is no one diet plan that can optimize hormonal levels for every single person. Even if we all had matching hormone levels, every body would still react uniquely, depending on a host of other factors. And, of course, we *don't* have identical hormone levels, and our choices of foods must address our own unique situation.

What I'll give you here, then, is an outline of the best way to eat to support your hormones—foods to eat, foods to avoid, the rhyme and reason behind it all, and the exceptions to the rules. We'll also look at the guidelines that apply to specific hormonal deficiencies and to specific health conditions—with information on how to work those into the overall Hormone Solution Diet. Finally, I'll give you sample menus you can use to make sure you're getting the best nutrition for your body and your hormones.

THE HORMONE SOLUTION DIET

*I*n the rest of the chapter, I'll get into the specifics, but to get you started, here's a summary of the Hormone Solution Diet: moderate to high protein (of the right type), moderate (but healthful) fats, limits on some types of carbohydrates, plenty of fruits and vegetables, and lots of water—all of it fresh and organic as much as possible. I'll give you guidelines about what types of foods you can mix and which should be eaten on their own, which foods to avoid altogether, and which foods are good for you only at the right time of day.

This is not a diet designed to make you lose weight, but most people find that eating this way will help them shed unwanted pounds. In any event, balancing your hormones is one of the best ways to stabilize your weight at a healthful level, whether or not weight is a major issue for you.

This is also not a diet bent on limiting the quantity of food you eat. As long as you are choosing foods that are good for you and are eating them within reason, you'll be getting what your hormones need. You'll have plenty of delicious choices, so feeling hungry or deprived just shouldn't be an issue on this plan.

And since nobody's perfect, and expecting perfection will only set you up for failure, I've built in a little escape hatch to make sure too much pressure never builds up, tempting you to give up on eating right for your hormones. Follow this program every day, but allow yourself one day a week to indulge in foods that are less than ideal. Just a little bit of cheating every day can undermine your results, but if your detours are limited to one day every now and then, you won't do much harm. So have that hot fudge sundae or those waffles or that wedge of Brie, even have them *all* if you must—but do it all on one day, then pick up where you left off with healthful choices the next day.

Most of my patients find that the better they eat, the less tempted they are on that free day anyway. As your body gets accustomed to only the highest quality food, the desire for junk food decreases. Part of that is physical—correcting hormone deficiencies makes a lot of your unhealthful cravings disappear. Part is experiential—you get used to how good you feel on healthful food and begin to notice just how bad you feel when you overdo it on exceptions. Once you've been there, you don't really want to go back.

Now, on to the specifics. We'll start with what you *should* eat.

FRUITS, VEGETABLES, AND MEAT

We're discussing evolving how you eat, and what it really involves is eating how you evolved. It takes tens of thousands or even *hundreds* of thousands of years for an animal species to evolve and adapt itself to new ways of eating. For millions of years, since the earliest days of humans stepping up from apes, we ate fruits and vegetables and, to a lesser degree, meat, poultry, fish, and eggs. With the invention of agriculture roughly six thousand years ago—a mere blip on the timeline of human evolution—we added in grains and eventually dairy products. But the genes of the cells of our digestive systems have not yet had time to fully adapt to these new food groups. So very often, they don't agree with us.

Hormone levels are optimized by the foods our bodies are designed to run on, because these are the foods that provide us with the most nutrition. For us that means the foods we've been eating since ancient times, since prehistory—vegetables and fruit, with a backup of animal protein.

FRESH ORGANIC FOODS

Get the most nutrients and the fewest additives and preservatives by buying fresh organic food whenever possible, for meat and eggs as well as produce. Processed foods might be contaminated with antibiotics, pesticides, and synthetic hormones that can worsen whatever imbalances you have. Vitamins and minerals break down over time, so the longer a good has sat around, the less of a nutritional punch it will pack. The fresher, the better.

HEALTHFUL FATS

I'm swimming against the tide of low-fat diets and anticholesterol hysteria, I know, but we need fats in our diets, including (gasp!) saturated fats. We *need* some cholesterol! What we *don't* need is superheated, cooked, or burnt fats or oils. Some fats from properly prepared meat, poultry, and eggs fit well in a healthful diet. So does a small amount of butter. Cold-pressed oils, like virgin olive oil, are good for you, and so are fish oils. Without enough fat in your diet, your body won't make enough cortisol, DHEA, estrogen, or testosterone.

WATER

Be sure to drink two quarts a day of pure, plain water.

Of course, there are also foods you must limit or avoid for hormonal health.

GRAINS

Humans are best adapted to foods that are generally easy to digest raw. Besides being a relatively new addition to the menu, grains are not edible raw. Thus they are second-rate food for us. Even cooked, grains are more difficult to digest than produce and meat. Some people seem to digest them better than others (perhaps they are our evolutionary leaders), but in my experience, few people really tolerate them well. It is a problem that often goes unrecognized, and the unpleasant symptoms—everything from bloating and flatulence to abdominal pain and drowsiness—remain unconnected to what we eat so commonly.

While I don't recommend eliminating grains from your diet, in most cases you should cut back on them drastically. Sprouting grains also makes them easier for your body to handle, so I recommend, for example, bread made entirely from sprouted grains. Certain proteins found in grains—gluten prime among them—are especially hard on the human digestive tract and should be avoided. Gluten is found in wheat, rye, barley, and oats. Rice is better, as it has little or no gluten. Corn is a common allergen, but if it doesn't bother you, you may have it in moderation.

LEGUMES AND NUTS

Beans and nuts are touted as sources of protein, and nuts are especially lauded as a source of healthful oils. But beans and nuts are difficult to digest raw and contain substances that inhibit enzymes and metabolism. (It's why they don't sprout without water, which no doubt is in the best interest of the plant, but imagine how it could mess up your body.) Sprouting them by soaking them makes them more digestible, and boiling beans helps, too, but still this isn't food you should be eating daily. Keep them to two servings a week at the maximum.

DAIRY PRODUCTS

We're not built to handle dairy products, either. Cheese is especially difficult. No other animal species consumes milk once it is past infancy. And none drink the milk of other species, as humans do. Coming from a different species makes it even harder to digest. It is designed for calves, after all, not with our interests in mind. As adults, we no longer have many of the enzymes required to digest dairy products. Some portion of all the dairy products we take in remains undigested by intestinal cells, just as with grains.

These undigested foods remain in the intestines two or three days before they are finally assimilated. A normal, healthy human intestine has a certain population of helpful bacteria, but as they feed on this undigested material, they multiply rapidly and easily get out of control. Yeasts in our bodies also thrive on the stuff and quickly come together and create large structures—what we recognize as fungus, also known as mycoses. The bread and milk literally get moldy inside you. Worse yet, the mycoses' waste products are toxins, poisonous to the human body.

SUGAR

Sugar, including honey, which is only marginally better for you, contributes to the overgrowth of yeasts and bacteria in our bodies, throwing our hormones off kilter.

YEAST AND FUNGUS

Any food containing yeast—the prime sources being breads and baked goods as well as cheese—obviously contributes to yeast overgrowth as well. It can provoke low-grade but tenacious fungal infections in our digestive tracts. From there they can spread into the blood and hence to tissue all over the body.

The problem starts with the simple fact that our bodies are not set up to properly digest these other foods. Bread is made out of grains, of course, which as we've already mentioned are hard on human intestines. The addition of yeast, itself a kind of fungus, puts it right over the top.

Repetitive fungal infections can profoundly disturb blood sugar and hormone levels. The mycoses extract the energy they need from the blood by eating up the sugar and consuming our hormones, and they do it in an irregular manner, causing alternating highs and lows in energy and hormones along with numerous problems like itching and allergies, eczema, dandruff, gas, bloating, belching, vaginal discharges, and sugar cravings.

Fortunately, the diet to eliminate yeast and fungus from your body is the same as the one needed for good hormonal functioning. Just getting rid of these chronic infections would improve your hormonal situation. But the diet laid out in this chapter does much more, directly promoting the production of beneficial hormones when you need them, and can prevent and address deficiencies.

ALCOHOL AND VINEGAR

These fermented products are also yeast-friendly and should be limited or avoided.

COFFEE AND TEA

Coffee and tea are diuretic. They create more urine, so we lose more water and become dehydrated. Dehydration causes many malfunctions in the body, one of which is the inability of the intestinal tract to secrete enough fluid in the digestive juices (hydrochloric acid from the stomach and pancreatic digestive enzymes from the pancreas) to sufficiently surround the food you take in and digest it efficiently. The caffeine in these substances makes the whole situation even worse. Most people can tolerate one cup of coffee or tea a day. Decaffeinated is always the better choice, especially if you are using thyroid hormones. No coffee whatsoever is even better. Herbal tea, provided it is not diuretic, is a good alternative.

THAT'S *WHAT* TO EAT . . . HERE'S *HOW*

*T*he Paleolithic diet our ancestors followed didn't mix too many kinds of food at one time. Here again, I think we should follow their example. Different foods require different acidity to digest properly. The more you mix different types of foods, the better your chances of having something in there in conditions not optimal for it. That means at least some of what you eat will sit there undigested, starting that whole yeast-infection cycle discussed above. Keep it simple.

Cook your meat at low temperatures. This kills any lurking microorganisms but prevents the fat from getting overheated. When fats get overheated, their structure changes, and they can become toxic and even carcinogenic. At the very least, substances are formed that can disturb digestion and cause fatigue.

Raw foods are good for you, but don't overburden your digestive tract with them late in the day when it is tired and slowing down. Raw foods are harder to digest than cooked ones, and if your gut can't handle them efficiently enough, they sit there undigested and that whole negative cycle begins. Give your body time to handle raw foods by not eating them in the late afternoon or evening.

That goes for fruit, too. It shouldn't be eaten raw after four or five o'clock. If you want it for dessert, it should be cooked, with no sugar added, like an apple baked with cinnamon, for example. And while we're on the subject of fruit—it should not be eaten in combination with other foods. In an empty stomach, fruit digests quickly. But when mixed with other foods, digestion slows down, and the high sugar content of fruit is especially bad for spurring on growth of yeast and bacteria. Eat fruit alone, half an hour before or three hours after other foods, especially grains (one to three hours in the stomach) and meat (three to nine hours in the stomach). It is fine to mix different types of fruit, with the exception of banana and melon, which should be eaten on their own. Fresh whole fruit is far better than juice, which is devoid of fiber and has concentrated sugar. If you find you have digestive trouble, you might need to avoid citrus fruits.

Finally, chew your food well and slowly. The first step of the digestive process takes place in your mouth . . . or it is *supposed* to. The way most of us eat nowadays, like you win some kind of medal for getting the most food in in the shortest amount of time, we severely shortchange the process. Great hunks of food arrive in our stomachs pretty much as they went into our mouths, with little of the digestive enzymes provided in saliva mixed in.

A WORD OF WARNING

If the diet described here is a radical change for you, your body will require a little while to adapt to it. For some people, this means a transition with some mild discomfort, like increased gas. For some people, it can be a rough first couple of weeks as the body detoxifies itself, and flulike symptoms can result. Stick with it, though, and by the third week you will feel fine and, in fact, much better than you did before eating in a way that supports your hormonal health.

EAT TO HEAL

Specific hormone deficiencies can call for specific dietary strategies. Most will be simple fine-tuning of the diet described above, although some, most notably thyroid hormones, sometimes require quite a different approach. We'll look at each hormone individually here, after a quick look at what the largest group of hormones—sex and adrenal hormones—have in common when it comes to diet.

SEX AND ADRENAL HORMONES

Animal proteins and fats are the key to countering a deficiency in any of the sex or adrenal hormones, which include estrogen, progesterone, testosterone, DHEA, aldosterone, pregnenolone, and cortisol. Numerous studies have shown the beneficial effect of these foods on the levels of sex hormones in the blood, and some show similar results on adrenal hormones. Those who eat meat, fish, and poultry have 30 to 40 percent more sex hormones than strict vegetarians. In India, in the purely vegetarian castes, women who have trouble getting pregnant are allowed to eat meat as long as necessary to increase their fertility (by increasing their levels of female sex hormones). A recent study showed that men aged forty to seventy whose diets were low in protein had less testosterone available in their bodies and lower muscle mass, small red blood cells, and lower bone density than men who got more protein.

You should, however, limit the amount of dairy products you consume. This is particularly important for women. The fungal infections described above often result from dairy-product consumption, and they disturb hormonal equilibrium, particularly that between estrogen and progesterone. Yeasts and fungi seem to especially love progesterone, but they do it irregularly, as I mentioned, so the estrogen-progesterone balance is continuously overthrown. The hormonal imbalance is very difficult to treat unless you first eliminate the fungal infection, which will require, at least, cleaning up the diet.

As for the specifics:

ACTH

To increase your ACTH levels naturally, eat more protein. Animal protein is especially helpful, particularly meat, poultry, fish, and eggs.

ALDOSTERONE

Eat more animal proteins (meat, poultry, fish, and eggs) and fats (meat, fatty fish, and eggs). Don't smoke, and keep caffeine and coffee (even decaf) to a minimum. Salt your food (with a light touch), as salt makes the aldosterone in your body work more efficiently.

CALCITONIN

Nondairy foods rich in calcium like shellfish, leafy greens, and beans will help boost the effects of calcitonin. You should also cut out caffeine and alcohol because they are linked to bone loss and low bone density. With calcitonin more so than other hormones, it is important to moderate the amount of protein you get; you don't want to be on a high-protein diet. Your bones need plenty of amino acids from protein, but metabolizing protein requires a lot of calcium, which can be leached from the bones when necessary. You want to hit the middle ground.

CORTISOL

Increase your intake of animal proteins, particularly meat, poultry, fish, and eggs, and healthful fats. People who are cortisol deficient often digest meat poorly; eating it might even make them nauseated, and they might avoid meat altogether as a result. If your cortisol level is low enough that you cannot tolerate meat, which you need to elevate your low cortisol levels, your deficiency is severe enough that you are going to need supplemental hormone. Barring that, cortisol levels that are only moderately low should improve with more meat, fish, eggs, and poultry in the diet.

Spicy and salty foods increase the effects of adrenal hormones, including cortisol. You should avoid sugar, especially when you are under stress, as sugar lowers the cortisol level. Unfortunately, low cortisol levels will make you crave sugar. If you do give in and have sugar, make sure it is only when you need momentary energy—to get you through a brief meeting, for instance—and not all day long.

DHEA

Avoid overcooked or superheated fats and increase animal proteins, especially meat, fish, poultry, and eggs. Avoid dairy products, however, as they can decrease DHEA levels and might cause digestive tract trouble besides.

Moderate fasting can help to increase DHEA levels.

Spicy and salty foods increase the effects of adrenal hormones, including DHEA.

BONUS FOODS
(excellent sources of the nutrients best for DHEA)

cod-liver oil	green, leafy vegetables	salmon
eggs	lobster	

EPO

Get plenty of fruits and vegetables. Every vegetable that contains a lot of water is good (that is, not the starchy vegetables). Make sure you eat enough in general. Don't overload the kidneys with too much meat. This is another exception to the general Hormone Solution rule and should look more like the diet that supports thyroid hormones, low in protein. Drink lots of water.

BONUS FOODS
(excellent sources of the nutrients best for EPO)

asparagus	kale	turnip greens
broccoli	oysters	watermelon
collard greens	salmon	white-meat chicken
eggs	spinach	
halibut	tuna	

ESTROGEN

For women who still have periods (and estrogen-producing ovaries), boost estrogen by making sure you get sufficient calories, particularly from proteins including meat, poultry, fish, and eggs, to produce hormones. Protein and healthful fats increase the amount and efficiency of sex hormones like estrogen. Limit whole grains to some extent, as large amounts of fiber can bind to estrogen and carry it out of the body. Use caffeine in moderation, if at all.

BONUS FOODS
(excellent sources of the nutrients best for estrogen)

beef	pork loin chop	tuna
eggs	salmon	white-meat chicken
halibut	spinach	

GROWTH HORMONE

Get lots of protein, especially from meat, poultry, fish, and eggs. A diet rich in protein also improves the effectiveness of growth hormone by providing lots of the amino acids the hormone needs to work in the skin, muscles, bones, and organs. Lose any excess weight. One in two people who reach a healthy body-mass index (BMI—see page 86)—a weight/height ratio—significantly increase their growth hormone secretion. Cut back on alcohol and coffee.

SCIENCE SAYS: PHYTOESTROGENS

Soy products have much the same effect on the body as does estrogen because they are rich in phytoestrogens (plant estrogens). New studies confirm estrogenic activity in the human body from these chemicals. But phytoestrogens also have anti-breast-cancer effects because they occupy estrogen receptors, thereby decreasing the breast-cancer-promoting effects of unopposed estrogen. However, relatively high doses of phytoestrogens, over 250 mg a day, are necessary to obtain clear beneficial effects, while the usual estrogen dose that most physicians prescribe for postmenopausal women is 100 mg daily.

INSULIN

Eat more fiber-rich vegetables.

BONUS FOODS
(excellent sources of the nutrients best for insulin)

apples	green, leafy vegetables	safflower oil
bananas	(especially spinach)	salmon
beef tenderloin	ground beef	shrimp
brown rice	halibut	soybean oil
cod-liver oil	liver	tuna
collard greens	lobster	watermelon
crab	oysters	white-meat chicken
eggs	pork loin chop	

MELATONIN

Melatonin is one of the exceptions to the protein rule; it works better with carbohydrates than proteins. If low melatonin is your only hormonal concern, you might want to follow a diet with more carbs and less protein. If, however, the more likely scenario occurs and melatonin is just one of the hormones that concern you, eat a balanced diet with carbs from fruits and vegetables and protein from meat and fish.

In any event, include a lot of melatonin-rich foods in your diet, including rice, small amounts of corn and oats, and fruits (especially bananas). Get generous amounts of cold-pressed vegetable oils rich in omega-6 fatty acids, but if your melatonin level is low, limited amounts of omega-3s (fish oils). Avoid caffeine and alcohol.

Melatonin levels improve with a hormone-friendly diet, but other lifestyle factors are even more important. Make sure you get lots of exposure to daylight, especially in the morning, and total darkness at night to increase the nocturnal secretion of melatonin. Avoid tranquilizers and alcohol, both of which can reduce the amount of melatonin released. So can stress, so learn to handle it constructively, since you can't avoid it altogether.

BONUS FOODS

(excellent sources of the nutrients best for melatonin)

bananas	corn	tomatoes
broccoli	corn tortillas	turnip greens
brown rice	oatmeal	
collard greens	spinach	

PREGNENOLONE

Increase your intake of animal proteins (meat, poultry, fish) and fats, including cholesterol (eggs, fish, and fatty meat), because they heighten the production of pregnenolone. Fish is a particularly good choice, as it provides both protein and healthful fats. Avoid overcooked or super-heated fats.

PROGESTERONE

Make sure you get sufficient calories, with plenty coming from protein, preferably animal protein (meat and poultry) and healthful fats.

TESTOSTERONE

Eat more protein from meat, fish, eggs, and poultry, and more healthful fats. Meat increases the levels and efficiency of sex hormones. Cut back on caffeine and avoid alcohol.

BONUS FOODS

(excellent sources of the nutrients best for testosterone)

beef	cod-liver oil	pork
chicken	eggs	salmon
	lobster	

THYROID

Thyroid hormones are another big exception to the rule. If your thyroid hormone level is low, eat more complex carbohydrates and limit meat and fats. Too much protein can decrease the conversion of T_4 into the active thyroid hormone T_3. What protein you get should come from small amounts of fish, eggs, and poultry; moderating meat; and avoiding dairy products. Milk contains a protein that can decrease thyroid hormone levels.

Begin with a focus on vegetables and fruits, which boost thyroid hormone levels, and perhaps work up to some grains. Fruit, in particular, increases thyroid hormones, and some studies show that grains and foods rich in iodine (ocean fish, shellfish) increase thyroid hormone levels. Because of the grain-yeast connection, however, it is best to limit grains.

You should also avoid caffeine.

All of that applies if thyroid hormones are your only concern. If other hormone levels are in question, too, you'll do better to follow the basic diet outlined above, although that will mean you won't be able to correct your thyroid hormone levels without supplements or that you might need more thyroid hormone supplements than you would on a thyroid-only diet.

BONUS FOODS
(excellent sources of the nutrients best for thyroid hormones)

apples	green, leafy vegetables	pineapple
bananas	kale	potatoes
brown rice	mangoes	spinach
collard greens	oranges	watermelon
grapefruits	peas	

VASOPRESSIN

Drink lots of water. Vasopressin keeps water in the body and works best with sufficient water intake.

The Hormone Solution Diet / 257

SO, NOW, WHAT DO I REALLY EAT?

On the Hormone Solution Diet, putting together a meal really shouldn't be difficult. It might be that you have to change your usual routine and steer clear of some foods you are in the habit of eating regularly, but you will be choosing from a bounty of delicious foods, and it is up to you whether you make them plain or fancy. Just to get you started, here are a week's worth of meals. You could follow them along as a program, if you so desired, but there is nothing magic about any one of these selections or the order they are in. If there's something that doesn't appeal to you, just skip it. And you might have to make adjustments for your particular hormonal situation or other health conditions or your family's tastes.

These are meant only to point you in the right direction anyway. If this diet doesn't mean big changes for you, you can just tinker with your current diet to get it right. Or if you are good with food, feel free to dream up your own combinations that fit into the guidelines in this chapter. Even if this is a more radical departure for you or you are hopeless in the kitchen, once you've done this for a little while, it will be easy to stretch your wings and take off on your own.

BREAKFAST IDEAS

1. Fruit salad or fresh melon
2. Scrambled eggs and bacon
3. Sliced turkey with rice cakes
4. Sprouted-bread toast with sugar-free jam or chocolate spread
5. Tuna sandwich on sprouted-grain bread or rice cakes
6. Soft-boiled egg with sprouted bread or rice cakes
7. Lightly dressed tossed salad or steamed vegetables

LUNCH IDEAS

1. Chopped salad with chicken
2. Fruits de mer (seafood soup) and a mixed-sprouts salad with lemon–olive oil dressing
3. Salad Niçoise
4. Grilled marinated tofu with mesclun greens
5. Red pepper frittata and guacamole

6. Chef's salad (no cheese)
7. Gazpacho and a turkey or roast beef wrap (in a sprouted-wheat tortilla)

DINNER IDEAS

1. Spice-rubbed salmon and vegetables with mashed potatoes (made with stock rather than milk)
2. Steamed vegetables (using cold-pressed oil) with shrimp, pork, chicken, beef, scallops, and/or tofu over rice, with avocado salad
3. Chateaubriand (or any steak) and dilled steamed new potatoes and asparagus with melted butter
4. Miso soup, sushi, or sashimi and steamed broccoli
5. Slow-roasted pork, roasted cauliflower, and tarragon carrots
6. Turkey breast, cinnamon-spiced acorn squash, and garlic green beans
7. Lamb chop, garlic green beans, and rice pilaf

CHAPTER EIGHTEEN

THE HORMONE SOLUTION
TREATMENT PLANS

By now you will have identified the hormones of most concern to you. This chapter reviews the treatment recommendations to discuss with your doctor as well as nutritional information you can use to balance your hormones on your own or improve the performance of the hormone supplements you use.

Because there will most likely be more than one hormone you'll be looking at, I suggest that you jot down the recommendations that are right for you. You'll then be able to fit all the pieces together into a cohesive plan for yourself and your doctor.

ACTH

TREATMENT

This treatment is rarely used. When it is, the usual course calls for ACTH injections of a slow-release form once or twice a week for several months, after which you switch to a combination of cortisol, DHEA, and aldosterone. Extremely serious cases may warrant as much as one injection a day of ACTH for a short time.

A word of warning: Excessive doses of ACTH can cause swollen face and shoulders, heartburn, weight gain, profuse sweating, nervousness, poor sleep, trembling, and palpitations.

NUTRITION PRESCRIPTION

Amino acids.

Supplement	Recommended Dosage Range	Instructions
ACTH	1–2 mg	injections once or twice a week
Amino Acids	increase protein intake (combats possible adverse effects of excessive cortisol production resulting from stimulation from the ACTH injections)	daily

ALDOSTERONE

TREATMENT

If you do have a deficiency, you'll most likely get a prescription for an aldosterone derivative, fludrocortisone. The usual dose is one 100 mcg pill taken in the morning.

A word of warning: Excessive doses can cause swelling due to water-retention in the hands, feet, and ankles, and, very rarely, high blood pressure. Aldosterone should be used only under medical supervision.

OTHER HORMONES TO WATCH OUT FOR

Deficiencies in cortisol and DHEA commonly accompany a lack of aldosterone.

NUTRITION PRESCRIPTION

Once you are following the Hormone Solution Diet and are eating healthful whole, natural, unprocessed foods, use salt at the table. Salt will increase aldosterone's effect (although too much might suppress aldosterone production).

Supplement	Recommended Dosage Range	Instructions
Aldosterone	50–100 mcg	take pills in the morning
Salt	2–3 g daily	salt your food lightly

DOCTOR, DOCTOR

I noticed a doctor in the audience at one of my seminars repeatedly opening and closing his eyes. I figured he either had some sort of tic, was irritated by something I was saying—or he had low blood pressure. He came up after I finished speaking, and I asked him if he felt his thinking was really focused only when he was lying down (a sign of insufficient blood pressure). When he said yes, I offered him a tablet of aldosterone. I am aldosterone-deficient myself and have used it to stay alert and energetic when I'm making presentations and am on my feet ten hours a day.

The next day, this doctor sought me out again just to report how, after all this time, his thought processes had cleared up with that single dose. He asked me for two more pills—just to hold him over through the end of the conference and until he could get home and get his own supply, he explained.

I was glad to have helped him and only felt bad that his simple and easily correctable problem had been overlooked for so long. One of the things I most enjoy about medicine is how such small things can have such a profound impact on people's lives.

CALCITONIN

TREATMENT

Calcitonin is usually given as a nasal spray and is taken every day. Before this spray was introduced, injections were the only option. They are still available and might be less expensive. Most are given three times a week.

A word of warning: Excessive doses of calcitonin can cause nausea, vomiting, lack of appetite, unwanted weight loss, nervousness, trembling, and palpitations. It is to be taken only under medical supervision.

OTHER HORMONES TO WATCH OUT FOR

Calcitonin is made and stored in the thyroid gland in specific calcitonin-producing cells, so having sufficient thyroid hormone levels is of particular importance. Although anyone can have a calcitonin deficiency, people who have undergone surgical removal of the thyroid gland, cutting off the supply of calcitonin, will need supplementation.

NUTRITION PRESCRIPTION

Amino acids. Calcium.

Supplement	Recommended Dosage Range	Instructions
Calcitonin	50–200 IU daily	nasal spray
Calcium	1,000–1,500 mg daily	
Amino Acids	150 g protein a day from meat, fish, poultry, and/or eggs	

CORTISOL

TREATMENT

If you are deficient, use prescription natural cortisol, typically 5 to 10 mg doses two or four times a day. Natural cortisol (or hydrocortisone) works better for mental complaints. Synthetic derivatives are much more powerful, especially against inflammation (though not as good as natural cortisol for small complaints). Prednisolone, methylprednisolone, and dexamethasone are usually prescribed in doses equivalent to 20 mg of natural cortisol. Too much cortisol is as harmful as too little, so doses and levels must be closely monitored.

If you get an infection or have a rheumatoid arthritis crisis, ask your doctor if you need to switch to a synthetic, at least for several days; their effects are longer-lasting. An infection or any other stress might mean you need a higher dose. (Don't treat yourself, however; follow your doctor's instructions.)

Unless you have androgenital or polycystic ovary syndromes, you should take dehydroepiandrosterone at the same time, as it prevents cortisol from "eating up" too much tissue.

A word of warning: As with all hormones, use only in case of recognized deficiency. Cortisol should be used under medical supervision. Signs of overdose (constant overexcitement, euphoria, a face swollen like a balloon—"moon face"—weight gain in the face and trunk, thinning skin, and/or a fatty "buffalo hump" on the back) should be addressed immediately.

OTHER HORMONES TO WATCH OUT FOR

Most people should take DHEA together with cortisol because it helps keep the activity of the cortisol in balance. So do androgens and growth hormone, so any deficiencies there should be corrected. These hormones control the amount of tissue cortisol burns to free energy.

The balance between melatonin and cortisol is crucial, so any deficiency in melatonin should also be corrected. Appropriate levels of thyroid hormone are also important here, as both can stimulate cortisol production. Finally, women should, if possible, avoid birth-control pills.

NUTRITION PRESCRIPTION

Vitamin E.

Supplement	Recommended Dosage Range	Instructions
Natural Cortisol	5–15 mg per dose two to four times a day	generally, a higher dose is used in the morning
DHEA	Women: 5–15 mg/day Men: 20–50 mg/day	
Vitamin E	100–400 IU daily	

DHEA

TREATMENT

In cases of deficiency, women will typically be prescribed between 5 and 30 mg of DHEA, and men 25 to 50 mg. DHEA is available over the counter, but you should talk to your doctor before starting oral DHEA.

Women are more likely to need and more likely to benefit from supplements than men.

If you take DHEA, keep a close watch for signs you are taking too much—greasy hair, oily skin, acne, and (in women) increased hair growth (which is rare).

OTHER HORMONES TO WATCH OUT FOR

Thyroid hormone and androgens (especially testosterone) stimulate DHEA production. Make sure to check for and remedy any deficiency.

NUTRITION PRESCRIPTION

Vitamin E.

Supplement	Recommended Dosage Range	Instructions
DHEA	Women: 5–25 mg Men: 25–50 mg	
Vitamin E	100–400 IU daily	

EPO

TREATMENT

If you have kidney disease with serious anemia, consider EPO injections. The normal course is 500 to 4,000 IU two or three times a week. The highest doses are used only in cases of severe anemia. Taking too much can make your blood too "thick" and cause it to coagulate too fast, a rare but very serious side effect that could lead to blood clots and stroke. If you use supplements, have your blood levels of EPO monitored.

OTHER HORMONES TO WATCH OUT FOR

Thyroid hormone, growth hormone, and the androgens support the kidneys (which make EPO).

NUTRITION PRESCRIPTION

Iron, folic acid, vitamin B_{12}.

Supplement	Recommended Dosage Range	Instructions
EPO	500–4,000 IU two to three times a week or 150 IU/day	
Iron	100–500 mg complexed iron or 10–80 mg elemental iron	
Folic Acid	5–10 mg daily	use for two to four months
Vitamin B_{12}	1,000–3,000 mcg over two weeks or 5,000 mcg via injection every two weeks	

HOW TO BUY HORMONES

Note: Natural forms of almost all these hormones are available, whether by prescription or over the counter. The hormones listed as available over the counter should be widely available. Any good health-food store will carry them. Choose only products from well-established, reputable firms.

Hormone	Prescription	Over the Counter
ACTH	✓	
Aldosterone	✓	
Calcitonin	✓	
Cortisol	✓	
DHEA		✓
EPO	✓	
Estrogen	✓	
Growth Hormone	✓	✓ (growth hormone secretagogues)
Insulin	✓	
Melatonin		✓
Pregnenolone		✓
Progesterone	✓	✓
Testosterone	✓	✓ (precursor: androstenedione)
Thyroid Hormones	✓	
Vasopressin	✓	

ESTROGEN

TREATMENT

For deficiency, use natural estrogen applied on the skin daily as a gel or from patches once or twice a week. (The gel is best before menopause; after menopause the patches are an acceptable option, although I still prefer the gel because it is more efficient and the doses can be more accurately personalized.) Taking any estrogen orally, even natural estrogen, puts you at risk of accumulating too much estrogen in the liver. That stimulates the production of too many binding proteins, which get not just the estrogen but also many other hormones, making them inactive, creating other deficiencies.

Anyone using estrogen should watch for signs of excess dosing, including tense and painful breasts, a swollen lower abdomen (or even the whole body), overly heavy or constantly painful periods, anxiety, jumpiness, irritability, and excessive emotionality.

OTHER HORMONES TO WATCH OUT FOR

Almost everyone taking estrogen should take progesterone as well, even women who have had their uteruses removed. Check for and correct any deficiencies in thyroid hormones, cortisol, growth hormone, progesterone, and androgens.

NUTRITION PRESCRIPTION

Vitamin B_6.

FURTHERMORE . . .

Avoid prolonged stress. Quit smoking.

Many women should avoid birth-control pills with low amounts of estrogen—20 mcg—as they can cause a deficiency. Unfortunately, the stronger pills present other problems, including risk of blood clots and the overproduction of binding proteins, as described earlier. The best idea is to limit the amount of time you use birth-control pills to two to five years—certainly not twenty years or more, as many women do.

Supplement	Recommended Dosage Range	Instructions
Estrogen	1–5 mg transdermal gel daily *or* 50–100 mcg patch twice a week	women who are not in menopause take estrogen for the first three weeks of a four-week cycle; after menopause, take it from the 1st to the 25th day of the month
Vitamin B_6	50–250 mg daily	
Progesterone	100–200 mg daily	women before menopause take it ten to fourteen days per menstrual cycle; after menopause, take it from the 13th to 25th day of the month for a period, or from the 1st to the 25th day of the month for no period

GROWTH HORMONE

TREATMENT

Once you establish that you do have a deficiency, the standard treatment is a small injection under the skin, which you give yourself every evening at bedtime. Adult doses vary from 0.02 to 0.4 mg per day. As a person who takes growth hormone, I am personally looking forward to the day, which should be in the near future, when growth hormone tablets that melt under the tongue are available.

Alternatively, or in addition, for those who still have the cells that secrete growth hormone (as most people under thirty-five do), you can take substances that stimulate the secretion of growth hormone. The amino acid arginine is one such substance, and taking seven grams a day divided into two to three doses should produce enough growth hormone. You can also use glutamine, which I like as well as arginine. Other options include leucine and lysine. GHB (gamma-hydroxybutyrate) is another powerful option, though what you take is actually its precursor furanone. Another choice that has found a lot of commercial success, at least, is pro-hGH, which contains a substance that inhibits somatostatin, a hormone that slows the secretion of growth hormone—a sort of "the enemy of my enemy is my friend" situation. All are available over the counter.

If you take growth hormone, watch out for signs you need to lower your dosage: swollen feet, pins and needles in the fingers, and carpal tunnel syndrome. These will appear after just two or three days of excess. Over the longer term, ten to thirty days, excessive muscle development, especially in the shoulders and thighs, and, rarely, pain in the joints should serve as serious warning signs.

Growth hormone is another one abused by some athletes. Doping usually involves 2 to 3 mg per day. You'll see that we're not talking anything like that when you compare that dosage level with the 0.25 to 0.5 mg the young adult body normally makes in a day, and that's the level we aim to maintain with supplements.

OTHER HORMONES TO WATCH OUT FOR

Growth hormone can stimulate the effects of thyroid hormones and androgens, notably testosterone, as well as slow down the adrenal glands, so you might require treatment in those areas or modification of the treatment you had been using.

Insulin, thyroid hormone, and the sex hormones also boost the effect of somatomedin C, making them important, too, for growth hormone production and effectiveness.

NUTRITION PRESCRIPTION

The amino acid arginine stimulates secretion of growth hormone (you need at least 7 g a day to get a meaningful result in terms of growth hormone). Glutamine, ornithine, and lysine are also helpful, as they stimulate the pituitary to free up its stored supply of growth hormone and make it available in the blood.

FURTHERMORE . . .

Get your exercise. Every time you exert yourself, growth hormone pours into the bloodstream. This is true, however, only for those still capable of making sufficient growth hormone—and for almost everyone over fifty or sixty years old, that becomes a real question mark.

Stop smoking, or at the very least cut back. Somatomedin C (which, remember, fulfills a great part of growth hormone action) decreases as the number of cigarettes increases. You know how so many heavy smokers have really wrinkled, parchment-like skin? That's in part an effect of insufficient growth hormone. Smoking already has more than enough recommending against it, but add to the list of things premature aging. You should also avoid marijuana; the "active ingredient" in it stops growth hormone secretion.

Supplement	Recommended Dosage Range	Instructions
Growth Hormone	0.02–0.4 mg daily	
Arginine	7–12 g daily	take at bedtime or one hour before exercise; arginine works best in young (20 to 35) and lean people
Glutamine	2 g at bedtime	works also in older adults (32 to 64)
Lysine	1–3 g at bedtime	works only in young adults (15 to 35), in combination with arginine

Supplement	Recommended Dosage Range	Instructions
Ornithine	2.5–5 g	works mainly in young (20 to 35) and lean people
Glycine	5–7 g	
Tryptophan	5–10 g	has a small growth hormone response; for best results, combine with vitamin B_6 (30 mg) and vitamin C (250 mg)
GHB (furanone)	0.5–1 g	
Niacin	0.2–1 g	with more than 0.8 g, you might experience "flush," especially in your face; works mainly in young (20 to 35) and lean adults; does not work in severely overweight people (more than 150 percent of their ideal weight)

INSULIN

TREATMENT

Talk to your doctor about whether you have insulin-resistant (type II) or insulin-deficient (type I or "juvenile") diabetes, and about specific dietary strategies and, in the latter case, insulin injections, along with the appropriate multiple hormone therapy (see below).

Anyone using insulin should be alert to signs of using too high a dose—excessive hunger, sudden drops in body temperature, sensitivity to cold, shivering, sleepiness, and hypoglycemia (low blood sugar). Over the long term, excess insulin will create too much fat on the stomach, hips, and thighs.

OTHER HORMONES TO WATCH OUT FOR

Transdermal estrogen and transdermal or injectable testosterone increase insulin production, so it is important to make sure you have sufficient levels in type I diabetes. For type II, growth hormone, androgens, and thyroid hormones are important, particularly in the way they reduce fat on the body and help optimize the action of insulin.

NUTRITION PRESCRIPTION

Chromium, vitamin E, magnesium, zinc, vitamin B_6, gamma-linoleic acid, and carnitine help move sugar from the blood into the cells, improving the action of insulin.

FURTHERMORE . . .

Exercise to lower blood sugar levels. Quit smoking, as tobacco use may increase both resistance to insulin (making it ineffective) and blood-sugar levels.

Supplement	Recommended Dosage Range	Additional Instructions (If any)
Insulin	5–50 U daily	follow your physician's instructions
Chromium	2–200 mg daily	take before meals
Vitamin E	400–800 mg daily	
Magnesium	350–450 mg daily	if the dose causes diarrhea, take after meals
Zinc	25 mg daily	take on an empty stomach or before bed
Vitamin B_6	50–100 mg daily	take with magnesium
Gamma-Linoleic Acid	500–2,000 mg daily	take with meals
Carnitine	100 mg daily	

MELATONIN

TREATMENT

Talk to your doctor about the supplemental dose that's right for you, usually between 0.05 and 5 mg. The lowest dose is about what your body would normally make. In extreme cases of poor sleep, the dose might go as high as 10 mg.

Whatever your usual dose of melatonin, you might want to double it for days when you are jet-lagged or after an especially stressful day.

Melatonin is so safe (no study has ever shown a serious side effect) that it is available over the counter in the United States. Still, if you use it, you should watch for signs of overdose and reduce your dose accordingly. Signs include a deep sleep that is too prolonged (until late in the morning, even after going to bed early); strong sleepiness in the morning; intense dreams and nightmares; difficulty in really waking up in the morning, no matter when you get up; and/or a short period (three to four hours) of very deep sleep followed by waking up in the middle of the night with inability to get back to sleep for many hours, and a "heavy" head in the morning.

OTHER HORMONES TO WATCH OUT FOR

Check for and correct any deficiencies in estrogen, growth hormone, and androgens.

NUTRITION PRESCRIPTION

Calcium and magnesium at bedtime; tryptophan at bedtime; niacin (vitamin B₃) and carnitine at bedtime.

FURTHERMORE . . .

Keep a moderate temperature (between 64 and 77 degrees) in the room where you sleep. Get a lot of light during the day, especially sunlight, but keep your room completely dark at night. (When you are traveling across time zones, get into the sun as soon as you arrive.)

Avoid (or use in moderation, following your doctor's advice) beta-blockers, benzodiazepines (especially at night), neuroleptics (especially during the day), clonidine (an antihypertensive), and lithium.

Supplement	Recommended Dosage Range	Instructions
Melatonin	0.05–5 mg daily	take at bedtime
Calcium	1,000–1,500 mg daily	take at bedtime
Magnesium	500 mg	take at bedtime
Tryptophan	1–4 g	take at bedtime
Niacin	100 mg	take at bedtime

PREGNENOLONE

TREATMENT

Pregnenolone dosages are usually in the range of 5 to 50 mg a day. If you have memory trouble, you'll probably need the full 50. For serious memory problems, the dose might go as high as 100 mg daily. Although this is available over the counter, do not take more than 25 mg a day unless you are under the supervision of a medical professional. Because all hormones are so interconnected—and this one in particular—I'd recommend working with your doctor in any event.

If you do use pregnenolone supplements, watch for signs you are getting too much, most of which are actually signs the pregnenolone is spurring too much production of the hormones derived from it. Beware of overexcited behavior and a swollen face (from too much cortisol), swollen hands and feet (too much aldosterone), and greasy hair (too much DHEA). These symptoms are especially likely in people under thirty-five whose bodies are still efficiently converting pregnenolone into other hormones, including cortisol, DHEA, progesterone, and aldosterone.

OTHER HORMONES TO WATCH OUT FOR

Check for and correct any deficiencies in somatomedin C and Aestosterone, which stimulate production of pregnenolone.

Supplement	Recommended Dosage Range	Instructions
Pregnenolone	5–100 mg daily	

PROGESTERONE

TREATMENT

Talk to your doctor about how to use natural progesterone. Before menopause, the typical plan is to take between 50 and 250 mg a day orally or vaginally (which spares the liver) from day fifteen to twenty-five of the cycle (taken with estrogen) or day eighteen to twenty-six (without estrogen), usually at night. (The first day of your period is the first day of the cycle.) After menopause, natural progesterone (with estrogen) from day thirteen to twenty-five of the month allows for a period (with estrogen taken from day one to twenty-five); take it from day one through twenty-five of the cycle for no period.

When using progesterone, look out for the signs of taking too much—sleepiness and dizziness when you get up in the morning, periodic depression, droopy breasts, low libido, sleeping too much or too long, or short menstrual cycles.

OTHER HORMONES TO WATCH OUT FOR

Check for and correct any deficiencies in cortisol, thyroid hormones, growth hormones, and somatomedin C, all of which contribute to ovulation and increase secretion of progesterone.

NUTRITION PRESCRIPTION

Take vitamin B_6 and magnesium.

FURTHERMORE . . .

Avoid situations stressful enough to disturb ovulation, thereby lowering progesterone secretion.

Supplement	Recommended Dosage Range	Instructions
Progesterone	50–250 mg daily	dose depends on what day of your menstrual cycle it is and whether you are menopausal
Vitamin B_6	50–250 mg daily	if you have bloating, use a dose from the high end of the range
Magnesium	150–500 mg daily (elemental)	

HORMONE DELIVERY METHODS

Note: Your local pharmacy will probably have at least one version of all the prescription hormones, with the possible exception of growth hormone. If they don't have the form that is best for you—natural versions are sometimes hard to find—try a compounding pharmacy (see Resources).

Hormone	Pill	Transdermal (patch, gel, or cream)	Injection	Other
ACTH			✓	
Aldosterone	✓			
Calcitonin			✓	✓ (nasal spray)
Cortisol	✓		✓	
DHEA	✓	✓		
EPO			✓	
Estrogen	✓	✓ (most desirable)	✓	
Growth Hormone			✓	

HORMONE DELIVERY METHODS (continued)

Hormone	Pill	Transdermal (patch, gel, or cream)	Injection	Other
Growth Hormone Secretagogues	✓	✓	✓	✓ (oral spray)
Insulin			✓	
Melatonin	✓			
Pregnenolone	✓			
Progesterone	✓ (more potent than transdermal)	✓	✓	✓ (vaginal suppository; more potent than oral form
Testosterone	✓	✓ (most desirable)	✓	
Thyroid Hormone	✓			
Vasopressin			✓	✓ (nasal)

TESTOSTERONE

TREATMENT

Young men are usually prescribed tablets (25 to 100 mg daily of mesterolon) or testosterone capsules (40 to 160 mg per day of decanoate)—which are used more in Europe—or gel to be smoothed on the skin—used more in the United States. Middle-aged men generally use a gel (50 to 400 mg/day transdermal) or injections (250 mg) of testos-

PRESCRIPTION SLIP: TESTOSTERONE

The newly FDA-approved AndroGel provides a dose only a fifth to a tenth of the strength of the forms most widely used before, so many men might need to use a lot of gel every day. But the convenience of the gel, which you use by simply rubbing it into the skin, and the ability to get a small dose if that is all you need, make this an important advance for hormone therapy. Compounding pharmacies can make gel of higher concentrations.

terone enanthate or testosterone cypionate (a shot every ten to twenty days). All except the first are natural forms of testosterone.

Women should use about a tenth to a fifth of the doses for men.

Men's bodies generally produce about 7 mg of testosterone daily. You can see why doping athletes can get into trouble taking 250 to 50,000 mg a day (by injection). Twenty to forty million American men are hypogonadal (low in testosterone)—and only 1 to 2 percent are treated.

Synthetic testosterone is available but does not completely mimic the effects of the natural substance.

You should be mindful of signs your dose is too high—overdeveloped muscles (à la Rambo), excess body odor, greasy hair, exaggerated aggression, or sexual desire that is disruptive or disturbing.

OTHER HORMONES TO WATCH OUT FOR

Check and correct any deficiencies in thyroid hormones, DHEA, and growth hormone.

NUTRITION PRESCRIPTION

Amino acids increase the effectiveness of testosterone in the body.

FURTHERMORE . . .

Men should have their prostate checked before taking testosterone.

Quit smoking.

Avoid (if possible) or use in moderation (following your doctor's instructions) beta-blockers, birth-control pills, and some anticholesterol medications.

Supplement	Recommended Dosage Range	Instructions
Testosterone	25–400 mg daily transdermal	proper dose depends on the form you take and your age (see above for details)
Amino Acids	10–20 g daily	eat a high-protein diet

THYROID HORMONES

TREATMENT

If you do need a thyroid supplement, your doctor will offer one of a few types of products. Most, as I've said, use only thyroxine, although better results are achieved by adding a little triiodothyronine to the mix. The natural conversion in the body of the nearly inactive precursor (thyroxine) into the active hormone (triiodothyronine) generally slows as we age. Most people with a deficiency need more help than the thyroxine alone can provide. Our bodies simply can't convert enough thyroxine, or can't do it fast enough. The combination, my first choice in therapies, is actually a more old-fashioned preparation, and it is available either in factory-made molecules or in a powder made from animal glands (with very tight quality control, necessarily).

Some doctors prescribe triiodothyronine alone, to be taken three or four times a day. If triiodothyronine is more powerful than thyroxine, you might think this is the best option of all. But determining the right dosage is very difficult. If you get a quick response, you also get a quick loss of effect. When you take mostly thyroxine and a little triiodothyronine, the body converts exactly what it needs, no more and no less.

Whatever you take, you should start with a small dose, increasing it every ten to fourteen days until you find the right level. You should avoid caffeine while you take thyroid hormones, as adequate levels of thyroid will make you very sensitive to the stimulant. You might find you need to decrease your dose in the summer, during stress, or when you are inactive and increase it in the winter and during periods of intense physical activity (which you should do only under the guidance of a health-care professional).

When taking thyroid hormones, as the more than nine million Americans who are hypothyroid should do, you need to be alert to signs you are taking too much and cut back accordingly. (Some estimates put the number higher still, at 30 to 40 percent of the population with low thyroid hormone levels.) Watch out for a heartbeat that is too hard and too fast, a feeling of suffocating, overheating, intense sweating, moist and humid skin, abnormal thirst, enormous appetite, unintentional weight loss, jumpiness, feverishness, poor sleep, and trembling fingers.

OTHER HORMONES TO WATCH OUT FOR

Check for and correct any deficiencies in melatonin, growth hormone, DHEA, androgens, and cortisol.

NUTRITION PRESCRIPTION

The amino acids tyrosine, cysteine, and methionine stimulate thyroid activity and change the weaker thyroxine to the more powerful tri-iodothyronine. Check for and correct any deficiencies in iron, selenium, and zinc.

FURTHERMORE . . .

Quit smoking.

Supplement	Recommended Dosage Range
Thyroid Hormones	45–300 mg daily desiccated thyroid *or* 50–350 mcg daily thyroxine
Tyrosine	0.5–1 g daily
Cysteine	200 mg three times daily
Methionine	1–5 g daily
Iron	10–80 mg (elemental)
Selenium	100–200 mcg
Zinc	10–50 mg daily
Copper	0.5–2 mg daily

PRESCRIPTION SLIP: DAILY DOSES FOR OVER-THE-COUNTER HORMONES

Supplement	Minimum	Maximum
Melatonin	0.05 mg	5 mg
Pregnenolone	5 mg	100 mg
DHEA (men)	20 mg	50 mg
DHEA (women)	5 mg	30 mg
Progesterone (oral/transdermal)	50 mg/100 mg	250 mg/500 mg

VASOPRESSIN

TREATMENT

You can take a synthetic derivative of vasopressin via nasal spray, 40 mcg three times a day (or via daily injection). Natural vasopressin can have even better benefits to memory than the synthetic version, but is available only to researchers at this time.

If you use the nasal spray, what you are actually getting is the vasopressin derivative desmopressin. The injection provides a different derivative, terlipressin. Both are synthetic and don't have as powerful an effect on the memory as natural forms, though they are the best currently available to the general public.

Whatever you take, watch for signs you are taking too much, primarily high blood pressure and bloating (swelling from fluid retention). Taking too much vasopressin can also cause signs of overdose of other hormones, because if you don't make enough urine, all hormones can accumulate in the blood when they would otherwise have been excreted.

NUTRITION PRESCRIPTION

Water.

Supplement	Recommended Dosage Range	Instructions
Vasopressin	10–30 mcg daily	three times a day, in 5 to 10 mcg doses, nasal spray
Water	2 liters daily	

RESOURCES

COMPOUNDING PHARMACIES

If you can't get the hormones you need at your local pharmacy, particularly natural preparations, compounding pharmacies are the solution. They work via mail order (unless you happen to be near one). You send in your doctor's prescription, they ship you the medicine (often overnight delivery)—very simple. Your insurance should cover anything bought this way that it would cover if you bought it at a local pharmacy. These are some of the best:

College Pharmacy
3505 Austin Bluffs Parkway,
    Suite 101
Colorado Springs, CO 80918
Phone: 800-888-9358
Fax: 800-556-5893

Kronos Pharmacy
Richard Fura
3675 S. Rainbow Boulevard, #103
Las Vegas, NV 89103
Phone: 800-723-7455
Fax: 702-873-6845

Lakeside Pharmacy
4632 Highway 58 N
Chattanooga, TN 37416
Phone: 800-523-1486
Fax: 877-890-8435
E-mail: don@lakesidepharmacy.com

University Compounding Pharmacy
Jerry Green
550 Washington Street
San Diego, CA 92103
Phone: 619-683-2005
Fax: 619-683-2008

Wellness Pharmacy
Gary R. Keel
4510 Hixson Pike
Hixson, TN 37343
Phone: 423-870-4241
Fax: 423-870-0553
E-mail: wellstar@cdc.net
Website: www.naturalwell.com

Women's International Pharmacy
5708 Mononda Drive
Madison, WI 53716
Phone: 800-279-5708
Fax: 800-279-8011

HORMONE TEST LABORATORY
(Including 24–hour urine)

AAL Reference Laboratories
1715 E. Wilshire Boulevard,
  Suite 715
Santa Anna, CA 92705
Phone: 800-522-2611
Fax: 714-972-9979
E-mail: inquire@aalrl.com
Website: www.aalrl.com

PHYSICIANS

EAQUALL can help you find a physician knowledgeable about natural hormones, multiple hormone therapy, and antiaging medicine. For example, the website lists doctors who have attended Dr. Hertoghe's hormone-therapy seminars.

95 Avenue Albert Giraud
B-1030 Brussels
Belgium
Fax: 32-2-732-57-43
E-mail: eaquall@busmail.net
Website: www.Eaquall.net

REFERENCES

CHAPTER 1. WHAT HORMONES MEAN TO YOU

Bermudez, F., et al. "High incidence of decreased serum triiodothyronine concentration in patients with nonthyroidal disease." *J Clin Endocrinol Metab.* 1975; 41: 28–40.

Hegstad, R., et al. "Aging and aldosterone." *Am J Med.* 1983; 74: 422–48.

Morer-Fargos, F., et al. "Die Testosteronansscheidung im harrn bei mannlichen individiren." *Acta Endocrinologica.* 1965; 491: 443–52.

Oventreich, N., et al. "Age changes and sex differences in serum DHEAs concentrations throughout adulthood." *J Clin Endocrinol Metab.* 1984; 59: 551–55.

Rudman, D., et al. "Impaired growth hormone secretion in the adult population." *J. Clin Invest.* 1981; 67: 1361–69.

Waldhauser, G., et al. "Alterations in nocturnal serum melatonin levels in humans with growth and aging." *J Clin Endocrinol Metab.* 1988; 66: 648–52.

Wiener, R., et al. "Age, sex and serum thyrotropin concentrations in primary hypothyroidism." *Acta Endocrinol Copenh.* 1991; 124 (4): 364–69.

CHAPTER 2. TEST YOURSELF

Abrahamssons, L., et al. "Catabolic effects and the influence on hormonal variables under treatment with gynodian-depot or DHEA oenanthate." *Maturitas.* 1981; 3: 225–34.

Angeli, A. "Effects of long-term, low-dose, time-specified melatonin administration on endocrine and cardiovascular variables in adult men." *J Pineal Res.* 1990; 9 (2): 113–24.

Berson, J. A., et al. "The effects of cortisone on the iodine accumulating function of the thyroid gland in euthyroid subjects." *J Clin Endocrinol Metab.* 1952; 12: 407.

Bian, X. P., et al. "Promotional role for glucocorticoids in the development of intracellular signaling: enhanced cardiac and renal adenylate cyclase reactivity to beta-adrenergic and non-adrenergic stimuli after low-dose fetal dexamethasone exposure." *J Dev Physiol.* 1992; 17 (6): 289–97.

Brixen, K., et al. "Effects of short-term growth hormone treatment on PTH, calcitriol, thyroid hormones, insulin and glucagon." *Acta Endocrinol.* 1992; 127: 331.

Cohen, A. M. "Interrelation of insulin activity and thyroid function." *Am J Physiol.* 1957; 188: 287.

Coleman, D. L., et al. "Therapeutic effects of DHEA metabolites in diabetes mutant mice." *Endocrinology.* 1984; 115 (1): 239–43.

Crespo, D., et al. "Interaction between melatonin and estradiol on morphological and morphometric features of MCF-7 human breast cancer cells." *J Pineal Res.* 1994; 16 (4): 215–22.

De Vroey, E., et al. "Het meervoudig deficiëntie syndrom." *Medical Trends,* March 1986.

Evans, W. S., et al. "Effects of in vivo gonadal hormone environment on in vitro hp GRF-40-stimulated GH release." *Am J Physiol.* 1985; 249: E276–80.

Gross, H. A., et al. "Effect of biologically active steroids on thyroid function in man." *J Clin Endocrinol Metab.* 1975; 33: 242.

Haffner, S. M., et al. "Decreased testosterone and dehydroepiandrosterone sulfate concentrations are associated with increased insulin and glucose concentrations in nondiabetic men." *Metabolism.* 1994; 43 (5): 599–603.

Hertoghe, Luc. "Over de inwendige sekretiën." *Exposition De Mensch.* 1936 (March 23): 31–37.

Hertoghe, T. "Growth hormone therapy in aging adults." In *Anti-Aging Medical Therapeutics,* R. M. Klatz, et al., eds. Marina Del Rey, California: Health Quest Publications, 1997; 10–28.

Hill, S. R., Jr., et al. "The effect of adrenocorticotropin and cortisone on thyroid function, thyroid-adrenocortical interrelationships." *J Clin Endocrinol Metab.* 1950; 10: 1375–400.

Janssen, J. O., et al. "Sexual dimorphism in the control of growth hormone secretion." *Endocr Rev.* 1985; 6: 128–50.

John, T. M., et al. "Influence of chronic melatonin implantation on circulating levels of catecholamines, growth hormone, thyroid hormone, glucose and free fatty acids in the pigeon." *Gen Comp Endocrinol.* 1990; 79 (2): 226–32.

Jolin, T., et al. "The different effects of thyroidectomy, KCIO4, and propylthiouracil on insulin secretion and glucose uptake in the rat." *Endocrinology.* 1974; 94: 1502.

Kalsbeek, A., et al. "Vasopressin and vasoactive intestinal peptide infused in the paraventricular nucleus of the hypothalamus elevate plasma melatonin levels." *J Pineal Res.* 1993; 15 (1): 46–52.

Miell, J. P., et al. "Effects of hypothyroidism and hyperthyroidism on insulin-like growth factors (IGFs) and growth hormone- and IGF-binding proteins." *J Clin Endocrinol Metab.* 1993; 76: 950–55.

Millard, W. J., et al. "Growth hormone secretion in the obese male rat:

modulation by the gonadal and thyroid axes." *Growth, Development & Ageing.* 1991; 55: 91–103.

Moller, J., et al. "Effects of growth hormone administration on fuel oxidation and thyroid function in normal man." *Metabolism.* 1992; 41: 728.

Murialdo, G., et al. "Circadian secretion of melatonin and thyrotropin in hospitalized aged patients." *Aging (Milano).* 1993; 5 (1): 39–46.

Peterson, R. E. "The miscible pool and turnover rate of adrenocortical steroids in men." *Recent Progr Horm Res.* 1959; 15: 231.

Regelson, W., et al. "DHEA the multifunctional steroid." *Annals NY Acad Sci.* 1994; 719: 564–75.

Romagnoli, E., et al. "Effect of estrogen deficiency on IGF-I plasma levels: relationship with bone mineral density in perimenopausal women." *Calcif Tissue. Int.* 1993; 53 (1): 1–6.

Schteingart, D. E. "Suppression of cortisol secretion by human growth hormone." *J Clin Endocrinol Metab.* 1980; 90: 721.

Terzolo, M., et al. "Effects of long-term, low-dose, time-specified melatonin administration on endocrine and cardiovascular variables in adult men." *J Pineal Res.* 1990; 9 (2): 113–24.

Thomas, R., et al. "Thyroid disease and reproductive function: a review." *Obstet Gynecol.* 1987; 70: 789.

Weaver, J. U., et al. "The effect of growth hormone replacement on cortisol metabolism and glucocorticoid sensitivity in hypopituitary adults." *Clin Endocrinol (Oxf).* 1994; 41 (5): 639–48.

Wortsmann, J., et al. "Abnormal testicular function in men with primary hypothyroidism." *Am J Med.* 1987; 82: 207.

CHAPTER 3. THE TOP FIFTEEN

Alba-Roth, J., et al. "Arginine stimulates growth hormone secretion by suppressing endogenous somatostatin secretion." *J Clin Endocrinol Metab.* 1988; 67: 1186–88.

Arthur, J. R., et al. "Selenium deficiency thyroid hormone metabolism and thyroid hormone deiodinases." *Am J Clin Nutr Suppl.* 1993; 57: 236S-9S.

Bringhurst, F. R., et al. "Hormones of the mineral metabolism. Calcitonin." In *Williams' Endocrinology,* 9th ed., vol 24. Philadelphia: W. B. Saunders Company, 1998; 1164–66.

Chan, V., et al. "Urinary triiodothyronine excretion as index of thyroid function." *Lancet.* 1972; 2 (7771): 253–56.

Chan, V., et al. "Urinary thyroxine excretion as an index of thyroid function." *Lancet.* 1972; 1 (7740): 4–6.

Chuang, J. I., et al. "Pharmacological effects of melatonin treatment on both locomotor activity and brain serotonin release in rats." *J Pineal Res.* 1994; 17 (1): 11–16.

De Lignières, B., et al. "Utilisation thérapeutique des estrogènes." In *Médecine de la Reproduction: gynécologie endocrinienne,* 3rd ed. Paris: Flammarion, 1997; 467–76.

Dillman, E., et al. "Hypothermia in iron deficiency due to altered tri-iodothyronine metabolism." *Am J Physiol.* 1980; 239: 377–81.

Dinu, M., et al. "The effects of vitamin D_2 on the lipid profile and on the platelet and cardiovascular activities in castrated or testosterone-treated male rats." *Rev Med Chir Soc Med Nat Iasi.* 1990; 94 (1): 123–27.

Dubbels, R., et al. "Melatonin in edible plants identified by radioim-munoassay and by high performance liquid chromatography-mass spectrometry." *J Pineal Res.* 1995; 18 (1): 28–31.

Falcon, J., et al. "Rhythmic secretion of melatonin by the superfused pike pineal organ: thermo- and photoperiod interaction." *Neuroendocrinology.* 1994; 60 (5): 535–43.

Gumbatov, N. B., et al. "State of the hypophyseal-gonadal system in patients with hypertension during long-term treatment with nadolol and anaprilin." *Kardiologia.* 1991; 31 (4): 15–18.

Hattori, A., et al. "Identification of melatonin in plants and its effects on plasma melatonin levels and binding to melatonin receptors in vertebrates." *Biochem Mol Biol Int.* 1995; 35 (3): 627–34.

Hertoghe, J. "Petits signes et dépistage de l'insuffisance thyroïdienne." *Merck Information* 1976; 2 (5): 3.

Hertoghe, T. *DHEA, l'hormone du mieux-vivre.* Paris: Presses du Châtelet, 2002.

Hertoghe, T. "DHEA: info ou intox?" *Le Monde Médical Hebdo.* 1995; 291: 12–15.

Hertoghe, T. "Growth hormone therapy in aging adults." In *Anti-Aging Medical Therapeutics,* ed. R. M. Klatz, et al. Marina Del Rey, California: Health Quest Publications, 1997; 10–28.

Hertoghe, T. "Thyroid Diagnosis and Treatment. Many conditions related to age reduce the conversion of thyroxine to triiodothyronine—a rationale for prescribing preferentially a combined T3 + T4 preparation in hypothyroid adults." *Anti-Aging Medical Therapeutics,* eds. R. M. Klatz and B. Goldman. Marina Del Rey, California: Health Quest Publications, 2000; 138–53.

Hertoghe, T. "Thyroid Diagnosis and Treatment. Poor reliability of the single plasma TSH-test for diagnosis of thyroid dysfunction and follow-up." *Anti-Aging Medical Therapeutics,* eds. R. M. Klatz and B. Goldman. Marina Del Rey, California: Health Quest Publications, 2000; 127–37.

Hertoghe, T., et al. "Considerable improvement of hypothyroid symptoms with two combined T_3–T_4 medication in patients still symptomatic with thyroxine treatment alone." In press.

Herxheimer, A. "Melatonin for preventing and treating jet lag." *Cochrane Database Syst Rev.* 2001; 1: CD001520.

Hill, S. R., Jr., et al. "The effect of adrenocorticotropin and cortisone on thyroid function: Thyroid-adrenocortical interrelationships." *J Clin Endocrinol.* 1950; 10: 1375–400.

Landin-Wilhelmsen, K., et al. "Serum insulin-like growth factor I in a random population sample of men and women: relation to age, sex, smoking habits, coffee consumption and physical activity, blood pressure and concentrations of plasma lipids, fibrinogen, parathyroid hormone and osteocalcin." *Clin Endocrinol (Oxf)*. 1994; 41 (3): 351–57.

Lecomte, P. "Insuffisances ovariennes primitives." In *Médecine de la Reproduction: gynécologie endocrinienne,* 3rd ed. Paris: Flammarion, 1997; 340–41, 346–51.

Orden, I., et al. "Thyroxine in unextracted urine." *Acta Endocrinol (Copenh).* 1987; 114: 503–8.

Orth, D. N., et al. "The adrenal cortex. Effects of glucocorticoids on diseases of the adrenal cortex. Hypofunction." In *Williams' Endocrinology,* 9th ed., vol 12. Philadelphia: W. B. Saunders Company, 1998; 544–63.

Orth, D. N., et al. "The adrenal cortex. Regulation of glucocorticoid secretion. Isolated ACTH deficiency." In *Williams' Endocrinology,* 9th ed., vol 12. Philadelphia: W. B. Saunders Company, 1998; 527–29.

Orth, D. N., et al. "The adrenal cortex. Treatment of adrenal insufficiency. Isolated mineral corticoid deficiency." In *Williams' Endocrinology,* 9th ed., vol 12. Philadelphia: W. B. Saunders Company, 1998; 560–65.

Pablos, M. I., et al. "Influence of lithium salts on chick pineal gland melatonin secretion." *Neurosci Lett.* 1994; 174 (1): 55–57.

Prettori, V., et al. "Hypothalamic action of delta-9-tetrahydrocannabinol to inhibit the release of prolactin and growth hormone in the rat." *Neuroendocrinology.* 1988; 47: 448–503.

Reiter, R., et al. "Mélatonine: faux miracle ou vraie révolution." 1st ed. Paris: First, 1995; 268–69.

Reiter, R. J., et al. *Melatonin: the discoveries that can help you.* New York: Bantam Books, 1995.

Roccak-Tebeka, B. *Progestatifs.* In *Médecine de la Reproduction: gynécologie endocrinienne.* 3rd ed. Paris: Flammarion, 1997; 481–507.

Rommel, T., et al. "Influence of chronic beta-adrenoreceptor blocker treatment on melatonin secretion and sleep quality in patients with essential hypertension." *J Neural Transm Gen Sect.* 1994; 95 (1): 39–48.

Sahelian, R. *Pregnenolone.* New York: Avery Publishing Group, 1997.

Thorner, M. O., et al. "The anterior pituitary. Corticotropin." In *Williams' Endocrinology,* 9th ed., vol. 16. Philadelphia: W. B. Saunders Company, 1998; 819–57.

Van Cauter, E., et al. "Demonstration of rapid light-induced advances and delays of the human circadian clock using hormonal phase markers." *Am J Physiol.* 1994; 266 (6, part 1): E953–63.

Watkins, P. J. "Clinical Presentation: why is diabetes so often missed?" In *ABC of Diabetes.* 4th ed. London: BMJ Publishing Group, 1998; 6–19.

Werner, S. C., et al. "Some effects of ACTH in chronic thyroiditis and myxedema." In *Proceedings of Second Clinical ACTH Conference,* ed. J. Mote. Vol. 2. Philadelphia: Blakiston, 1951; 521–28.

Youg, J. B., et al. "Catecholamines and the adrenal medulla. Erythropoietin." In *Williams' Endocrinology.* 9th ed., vol 13. Philadelphia: W. B. Saunders Company, 1998; 698.

Zanozdra, N. S., et al. "Effect of the treatment on hemodynamic indicators and plasma testosterone level in patients with juvenile hypertension." *Klin Med Mosk.* 1990; 68 (7): 89–92.

Zawilska, J. B. "Clonidine in vivo mimics the acute suppressive but not the phase-shifting effects of light on circadian rhythm of serotonin N-acetyltransferase activity in chick pineal gland." *J Pineal Res.* 1994; 17 (2): 63–68.

Zawilska, J. B., et al. "Clozapine and other neuroleptic drugs antagonize the light-evoked suppression of melatonin biosynthesis in chick retina: involvement of the D4-like dopamine receptor." *J Neural Transm Gen Sect.* 1994; 97 (2): 107–17.

Zimmermann, R. C., et al. "Urinary 6-hydroxymelatonin sulfate as a measure of melatonin secretion during acute tryptophan depletion." *Psychoneuroendocrinology.* 1993; 18 (8): 567–78.

CHAPTER 5. WEIGHT PROBLEMS
Overweight

Barrett-Connor, E., et al. "DHEA, DHEAs, obesity, waist-hip ratio, and non-insulin-dependent diabetes in postmenopausal women: the Rancho Bernardo Study." *J Clin Endocrinol Metab.* 1996; 81 (1): 59–64.

Barrett-Connor, E., et al. "Endogenous sex hormones and cardiovascular disease in men. A prospective population-based study." *Circulation.* 1988; 78: 539–45.

Blaicher, W., et al. "Melatonin in postmenopausal females." *Arch Gynecol Obstet.* 2000; 263 (3): 116–18.

Chopra, I. J., et al. "Circulating thyroid hormones in thyrotropin in adult patients with protein-calorie malnutrition." *J Clin Endocrinol Metab.* 1975; 40: 221–27.

Chmouliovsky, L., et al. "Beneficial effect of hormone replacement therapy on weight loss in obese menopausal women." *Maturitas.* 1999; 32 (3): 147–53.

Cruz, M. L., et al. "Effects of triiodothyronine administration on dietary (14C)triolein partitioning between deposition in adipose tissue and oxidation to (14C)CO2 in ad libitum-fed or food-restricted rats." *Biochim Biophys Acta.* 1993; 1168 (2): 205–12.

Davis, S. R., et al. "Effects of estradiol with and without testosterone on body composition and relationships with lipids in postmenopausal women." *Menopause.* 2000; 7 (6): 395–401.

De Pergola, G. "The adipose tissue metabolism: role of testosterone and dehydroepiandrosterone." *Int J Obes Relat Metab Disord.* 2000; 24 (Suppl 2): S59–63.

De Pergola, G., et al. "Body fat accumulation is possibly responsible for lower dehydroepiandrosterone circulating levels in premenopausal obese women." *Int J Obes Relat Metab Disord.* 1996; 20 (12): 1105–10.

De Pergola, G., et al. "Low dehydroepiandrosterone circulating levels in premenopausal obese women with very high body mass index." *Metabolism.* 1991; 40 (2): 187–90.

Diamond, P., et al. "Metabolic effects of 12-month percutaneous dehydroepiandrosterone replacement therapy in postmenopausal women." *J Endocrinol.* 1996; 150 (Suppl): S43–50.

Exton, J. H. *Regulation of glucocorticoid hormone action.* New York: Springer-Verlag, 1979; 535–46.

Flegal, K. M., et al. "Overweight and obesity in the United States: prevalence and trends, 1960–1994." *Int J. Obes Relat Metab Disord.* 1998; 22 (1): 39–47.

Garvey, W. T., et al. "Expression of a glucose transporter gene cloned from brain in cellular models of insulin resistance: dexamethasone decreases transporter mRNA in primary cultured adipocytes." *Mol Endocrinol.* 1989; 3: 1132–41.

Giagulli, V. A., et al. "Pathogenesis of the decreased androgen levels in obese men." *J Clin Endocrinol Metab.* 1994; 79 (4): 997–1000.

Hassager, C., et al. "Estrogen/proestagen therapy changes soft tissue body composition in postmenopausal women." *Metabolism.* 1989; 38 (7): 662–65.

Hausberger, F. X., et al. "Castration-induced obesity in mice." *Acta Endocrinol.* 1966; 53: 571–83.

Hautanen, A., et al. "Altered adrenocorticotropin and cortisol secretion in abdominal obesity: implications for the insulin resistance syndrome." *J Intern Med.* 1993; 234 (5): 461–69.

Hertoghe, T. "The beneficial effects of hormone replacement therapies on obesity." *Anti-Aging Medical Therapeutics,* eds. R. M. Klatz and B. Goldman. Marina Del Rey, California: Health Quest Publications, 2001.

Iranmanesh, A., et al. "Age and relative adiposity are specific negative determinants of the frequency and amplitude of growth hormone (GH) secretory bursts and the half-life of endogenous GH in healthy men." *J Clin Endocrinol Metab.* 1991; 73 (5): 1081–88.

Jacubinovicz, D., et al. "Disparate effects of weight reduction by diet on serum DHEA in obese men and women." *J Clin Endocrinol Metab.* 1993; 80 (11): 3373–76.

Jungmann, E., et al. "Somatomedin C level and stimulation of growth hormone and adrenal cortex function by administration of releasing hormones and physical exertion in patients with obesity." *Med Klin.* 1991; 86 (5): 237–40.

Khaw, K. T., et al. "Lower endogenous androgens predict central adiposity in men." *Ann Epidemiol.* 1992; 2 (5): 675–82.

Kritz-Silverstein, D., et al. "Long-term postmenopausal hormone use, obesity and fat distribution in older women." *JAMA.* 1996; 276 (1).

Leenen, R., et al. "Visceral fat accumulation in relation to sex hormones in obese men and women undergoing weight loss therapy." *J Clin Endocrinol Metab.* 1994; 78 (6): 1515–20.

Lew, E. A., et al. "Variations in mortality by weight among 750,000 men and women." *J Chron Dis.* 1979; 32: 563–76.

Marcus, M. A., et al. "Insulin sensitivity and serum triglyceride level in obese white and black women: relationship to visceral and truncal subcutaneous fat." *Metabolism.* 1999; 48 (2): 194–99.

Marin, P. "Metabolic and gastrointestinal drugs: testosterone and regional fat distribution." *Obesity Res* 1995; 3 (suppl. 4): 6095–125.

Marin, P., et al. "Assimilation and mobilization of triglycerides in subcutaneous abdominal and femoral adipose tissue in vivo in men: effects of androgens." *J Clin Endocrinol Metab.* 1995; 80 (1): 239–43.

Marin, P., et al. "Cortisol secretion in relation to body fat distribution in obese premenopausal women." *Metabolism.* 1992; 41 (8): 882–86.

Marin, P., et al. "Low concentrations of insulin-like growth factor-I in abdominal obesity." *Int J Obes Relat Metab Disord.* 1993; 17 (2): 83–89.

Mohan, P. F., et al. "Effects of DHEA treatment in rats with diet-induced obesity." *Nutrition Pharmacology & Toxicology.* 1990: 1103–14.

Munzer, T., et al. "Effects of GH and/or sex steroid administration on abdominal subcutaneous and visceral fat in healthy aged women and men." *J Clin Endocrinol Metab.* 2001; 86 (8): 3604–10.

Nestler, J. E., et al. "DHEA reduces serum low density lipoprotein levels and body fat but does not alter insulin sensitivity in normal men." *J Clin Endocrinol Metab.* 1988; 66 (1): 57–61.

Nicoloff, J. T., et al. "Altered peripheral thyroxine metabolism in severe obesity." *Clin Res.* 1966; 14: 148.

Niskonen, L., et al. "The effects of weight loss on insulin sensitivity, skeletal muscle composition and capillary density in obese non-diabetic subjects." *Int J Obes Relat Metab Disord.* 1996; 20 (2): 154–60.

Porter, J., et al. "The effect of discontinuing DHEA supplementation on Zucher rat food disord." *Int J Obes Relat Metab.* 1995; 19 (7): 480–88.

Rebuffe-Scrive, M., et al. "Effect of testosterone on abdominal adipose tissue in men." *Int J Obes.* 1991; 15 (11): 791–95.

Rosenbaum, M., et al. "Effects of systemic growth hormone (GH) administration on regional adipose tissue in children with non-GH-deficient short stature." *J Clin Endocrinol Metab.* 1992; 75 (1): 151–56.

Salomen, F., et al. "Physiological role of growth hormone in adult life." In *Diagnosis and treatment of impaired growth hormone secretion,* ed. H. Flodh. Dorchester: Henry Ling Ltd., 1987; 158–62.

Sandhu, G. S., et al. "Effect of L-thyroxine (LT4) and D-thyroxine (DT4) on cardiac function and high-energy phosphate metabolism: a 31P NMR study." *Magn Reson Med.* 1991; 18 (1): 237–43.

Schmitt, T., et al. "Unresponsiveness to exogenesis TSH in obesity." *Int J. Obesity.* 1977; 1: 185–90.·

Seidell, J. C., et al. "Visceral fat accumulation in men is positively associated with insulin, glucose, and C-peptide levels, but negatively with testosterone levels." *Metabolism.* 1990; 39 (9): 897–901.

Sorensen, M. B., et al. "Obesity and sarcopenia after menopause are reversed by sex hormone replacement therapy." *Obes Res.* 2001; 9 (10): 622–26.

Svec, F., et al. "Synergestic effect of DHEA and fenfluramine on Zucher rat food intake and selection: the obesity research program." *Ann NY Acad Sci.* 1995; 774: 332–34.

Tofovic, S. P., et al. "2-Hydroxyestradiol attenuates the development of obesity, the metabolic syndrome, and vascular and renal dysfunction in obese ZSF1 rats." *J Pharmacol Exp Ther.* 2001; 299 (3): 973–77.

Veldhuis, J. D., et al. "Dual effects in pulsatile growth hormone secretion and clearance subserve the hyposomatotropism of obesity in man." *J Clin Endocrinol Metab.* 1991; 72: 51–59.

Villareal, D. T., et al. "Effects of DHEA replacement on bone mineral density and body composition in elderly women and men." *Clin Endocrinol (Oxf).* 2000; 53 (5): 561–68.

Wolden-Hanson, T., et al. "Daily melatonin administration to middle-aged male rats suppresses body weight, intraabdominal adiposity, and plasma leptin and insulin independent of food intake and total body fat." *Endocrinology.* 2000; 141 (2): 487–97.

Zumoff, B., et al. "Plasma free and non-sex-hormone-binding-globulin-bound testosterone are decreased in obese men in proportion to their degree of obesity." *J Clin Endocrinol Metab.* 1990; 71 (4): 929–31.

Underweight

Argente, J., et al. "Multiple endocrine abnormalities of the growth hormone and insulin-like growth factor axis in patients with anorexia nervosa: effect of short- and long-term weight recuperation." *J Clin Endocrinol Metab.* 1997; 82 (7): 2084–92.

Bhasin, S., et al. "Testosterone dose-response relationships in healthy young men." *Am J Physiol Endocrinol Metab.* 2001; 281 (6): E1172–81.

Fairfield, W. P., et al. "Effects of testosterone and exercise on muscle leanness in eugonadal men with AIDS wasting." *J Appl Physiol.* 2001; 90 (6): 2166–71.

Geyelin, H. R., et al. *J Metab Res.* 1922; 767–91.

Grinspoon, S., et al. "Effect of androgen administration in men with the AIDS wasting syndrome. A randomized, double-blind, placebo-controlled trial." *Ann Intern Med.* 1998; 129 (1): 18–26.

Grinspoon, S., et al. "Loss of lean body and muscle mass correlates with androgen levels in hypogonadal men with acquired immunodeficiency syndrome and wasting." *J Clin Endocrinol Metab.* 1996; 8 (11): 4051–58.

Hassager, C., et al. "Collagen synthesis in postmenopausal women during therapy with anabolic steroid or female sex hormones." *Metabolism.* 1990; 39 (11): 1167–69.

"Hormonal regulation of the differentiation of rat preadipocytes." *Nutr Rev.* 1988; 46: 235–36.

Jacobson, L. "Glucocorticoid replacement but not corticotropin-releasing hormone deficiency, prevents adrenalectomy-induced anorexia in mice." *Endocrinology.* 1999; 140 (1): 310–17.

Krentz, A. J., et al. "Anthropometric, metabolic, and immunological effects of recombinant human growth hormone in AIDS and AIDS-related complex." *J Acquir Immune Defic Syndr.* 1993; 6 (3): 245–51.

Lieberman, S. A., et al. "Anabolic effects of recombinant insulin-like growth factor-1 in cachectic patients with the acquired immunodeficiency syndrome." *J Clin Endocrinol Metab.* 1994; 78 (2): 404–10.

Meyer, N. A., et al. "Combined IGF-1 and growth hormone improves weight loss and wound healing in burned rats." *J Trauma.* 1996; 1 (6): 1008–12.

Miller, K., et al. "Transdermal testosterone administration in women with acquired immuno deficiency wasting syndrome: a pilot study." *J Clin Endocrinol Metab.* 1998; 83 (8): 717–25.

Mulligan, K., et al. "Anabolic effects of recombinant human growth hormone in patients with wasting associated with human immunodeficiency virus infection." *J Clin Endocrinol Metab.* 1993; 77 (4): 956–62.

Rizza, R. A., et al. "Dose-response characteristics for the effects of insulin on production and utilization of glucose in man." *Am J Physiol.* 1981; 240 (6): E630–39.

Sipila, S., et al. "Effects of hormone replacement therapy and high-impact physical exercise on skeletal muscle in post-menopausal women: a randomized placebo-controlled study." *Clin Sci (Lond).* 2001; 101 (2): 147–57.

Twycross, R. "The risks and benefits of corticosteroids in advanced cancer." *Drug Saf.* 1994; 11 (3): 163–78.

CHAPTER 6. THE BEAUTY PRESCRIPTION: CARING FOR YOUR SKIN AND HAIR
Skin

Andersson, S. "Steroidogenic enzymes in skin." *Eur J Dermatol.* 2001; 11 (4): 293–95.

Araneo, B. A., et al. "Dehydroepiandrosterone reduces progressive dermal ischemia caused by thermal injury." *J Surg Res.* 1995; 59 (2): 250–62.

Baulieu, E. E., et al. "Dehydroepiandrosterone (DHEA), DHEA sulfate, and aging: contribution of the DHEAge Study to a sociobiomedical issue." *Proc Natl Acad Sci USA.* 2000; 97 (8): 4279–84.

Black, M. M., et al. "Skin collagen and thickness in Cushing's syndrome." *Arch Dermatol Forsch.* 1973; 246 (4): 365–68.

Bolognia, J. L. "Aging skin." *Am J Med.* 1995; 98 (1A): 995–1035.

Brincat, M., et al. "Long-term effects of the menopause and sex hormones on skin thickness." *Br J Obstet Gynaecol.* 1985; 92: 256–59.

Deplewski, D., et al. "Growth hormone and insulin-like growth factors have different effects on sebaceous cell growth and differentiation." *Endrocrinology.* 1999; 140 (9): 4089–94.

Feinhold, K. R., et al. "Endocrine-skin interactions. Cutaneous manifestations of pituitary disease, thyroid disease, calcium disorders and diabetes." *J Am Acad Dermatol.* 1987; 17 (6): 921–40.

Gaher, A., et al. "Effect of anti-IGF-1 on epidermal proliferation of human skin transplanted into nude mice treated with growth hormone." *Endocrinology.* 1994; 134 (1): 229–32.

Gilpin, D. A., et al. "Recombinant human growth hormone accelerates wound healing in children with large cutaneous burns." *Ann Surg.* 1994; 220 (1): 19–24.

Giltay, E. J., et al. "Effects of sex steroid deprivation/administration on hair growth and skin sebum production in transsexual males and females." *J Clin Endocrinol Metab.* 2000; 85 (8): 2913–21.

Gower, D. B., et al. "Comparison of 16-androstene steroid concentrations in sterile apocrine sweat and axillary secretions: interconversions of 16-androstenes by the axillary microflora—a mechanism for axillary odour production in man?" *J Steroid Biochem Mol Biol* 1994; 48 (4): 409–18.

Hassager, C., et al. "Collagen synthesis in postmenopausal women during therapy with anabolic steroid or female sex hormones." *Endocrinology.* 1990; 1167–69.

Hertoghe, E. "Le myxoedème fruste." *Bulletin de l'Académie Royale de Médecine.* Brussels: Ed Hayez, 1899; 24–25.

Heymann, W. "Cutaneous manifestations of thyroid disease." *J Am Acad Dermatol.* 1992; 26: 885–902.

Imperato-McGinley, J. J., et al. "The androgen control of sebum production. Studies of subjects with dihydrotestosterone deficiency and complete androgen insensitivity." *J Clin Endocrinol Metab.* 1993; 76: 524–28.

Jacobson, E., et al. "Age-related changes in sebaceous wax external secretion rates in men and women." *J Invest Dermatol* 1985; 85: 473–85.

Jorgensen, O., et al. "Influence of sex hormones on granulation tissue formation and on healing of linear wounds." *Arch Chirurg Scandinav.* 1962; 124: 1–10.

Kolbe, L., et al. "Corticosteroid-induced atrophy and barrier impairment measured by non-invasive methods in human skin." *Skin Res Technol.* 2001; 7 (2): 73–77.

Lund, P., et al. "The effect of L-Thyroxine treatment on skin accumulation of acid glycosaminoglycans in primary myxoedema." *Acta Endocrinol (Copenh).* 1986; 113 (1): 56–58.

Mullin, G. E., et al. "Cutaneous signs of thyroid disease." *Am Fam Physician.* 1989; 34 (4): 93–98.

Niepomniszcze, H., et al. "Skin disorders and thyroid diseases." *J Endocrinol Invest.* 2001; 24 (8): 628–38.

Noble, D. E., et al. "Localization of the growth hormone receptor/binding protein in skin." *Endocrinol.* 1990; 126 (3): 467–71.

Nuutinen, P., et al. "Glucocorticoid action on skin collagen: overview on clinical significance and consequences." *J Eur Acad Dermatol Venereol.* 2001; 15 (4): 361–62.

Osclund, H., et al. "Alterations in the cross-links of skin collagen of rats treated with synthetic growth hormone." *Connect Tissue Res.* 1991; 26 (1–2): 65–75.

Phillips, T. J., et al. "Hormonal effects on skin aging." *Clin Geriatr Med.* 2001; 17 (4): 661–72.

Pichi, Pe., et al. "Sebaceous gland suppression with ethinyl estradiol and diethylstilbestrol." *Arch Derm.* 1973; 108 (2): 210–14.

Rabbidsi, G., et al. "Relationship between ground substance and hormones in skin aging." *G ltal Derm Minerva Derm.* 1973; F108 (1): 59–64.

Savuas, M., et al. "Type III collagen content in the skin of postmenopausal women receiving oestradiol and testosterone implants." *Br J Obstet Gynaecol.* 1993; 100 (2): 154–56.

Seyer-Hansen, M., et al. "Influence of bio-synthetic human growth hormone on the biomechanical strength development in skin incisional wounds of diabetic rats." *Eur Surg Res.* 1993; 25 (3): 162–68.

Shuster, J., et al. "The influence of age and sex on skin thickness, skin collagen and density." *Br J Dermatol.* 1975; 93: 639–43.

Tayama, K., et al. "Development of pigmented scales on rat skin: relation to age, sex, strain and hormonal effect." *Lab Anim Sci.* 1994; 44 (3): 240–44.

Therndon, D. N., et al. "Characterization of growth hormone enhanced donor site healing in patients with large cutaneous burns." *Ann Surg.* 1995; 221 (6): 649–56.

Thiboutot, D. M. "Dermatological manifestations of endocrine disorders." *J Clin Endoc Metab.* 1995; 80: 3082–87.

Yamamoto, A., et al. "Sebaceous gland activity and urinary androgen levels in children." *J Dermatol Sci.* 1992; 4 (2): 98–104.

Hair

Bruno, O. D., et al. "Thyroid gland function and autoimmunity in children with alopecia universalis." *Medicine B Aires.* 1985; 45 (1): 25–28.

Choudhry, R., et al. "Localization of androgen receptors in human skin by immunohistochemistry: implications for the hormonal regulation of hair growth, sebaceous glands and sweat glands." *J Endocrinol.* 1992; 133 (3): 467–75.

Fazekas, A. G., et al. "The metabolism of DHEA by human scalp hair follicles." *J Clin Endocrinol Metab.* 1973; 36: 582.

Hamilton, J. B. "Increased levels of circulating testosterone can cause scalp hair loss in susceptible individuals." *Amer J Anat.* 1992; 71: 451.

Hertoghe, E. "Le myxoedème fruste." *Bulletin de l'Académie Royale de Médecine de Belgique.* Brussels: Ed Hayez, 1899; 21–25.

Knussmann, R., et al. "Relationship between sex hormones level and characters of hair and skin in healthy young men." *Am J Phys Anthropol.* 1992; 88 (1): 59–67.

Lutz, G., et al. "Value of pathologic thyroid glands finding in alopecia areata." *Z Hautkr.* 1987; 62 (17): 1253–61.

Mohn, M. P. "The effects of different hormonal states on the growth of hair in rats." In Montagna W., et al., eds. *The biology of hair growth.* New York: Academic Press, 1958; 355.

Oh, H. S., et al. "An estrogen receptor pathway regulates the telogen anagen hair follicles transition and influences epidermal cell proliferation." *Proc Natl Acad Sci USA.* 1996; 93 (22): 125–30.

Perloff, W. H. "Hirsutism: a manifestation of juvenile hypothyroidism." *JAMA.* 1955; 157: 161.

Relli, E. P., et al. "Stimulating effect of adrenalectomy on hair growth and melanin deposition in rats fed diets adequate and deficient in the filtrate factors of vitamin B." *Endocrinology.* 1993; 32 (1): 1–12.

Rook, A. "Endocrine influences on hair growth." *Br Med J.* 1965; 1: 609.

Rose, J. "ACTH but not alpha-MSH as a mediator of adrenalectomy induced hair growth in mink." *J Invest Dermatol.* 1998; 110 (4): 456–57.

Sawaya, M. E., et al. "Glucocorticoid regulation of hair growth in alopecia areata." *J Invest Dermatol.* 1995; 104 (5 suppl): 305.

Schweikert, H. V., et al. "Regulation of human hair growth by steroid hormones II Androstenedione metabolism in isolated hairs." *J Clin Endocrinol Metab.* 1974; 39: 1012.

Smith, J. G., et al. "Hair rats of the human scalp in thyroid disease." *J Invest Dermatol.* 1959; 32: 35.

Van Schoor, J. "Een vrouw met alopecia totalis en multipele endocrine uitval." *Ned Tijdsch Gen.* 1989; 133 (25): 946–49.

CHAPTER 7. SMOOTH JOINTS

Allebeck, P., et al. "Do oral contraceptives reduce the incidence of rheumatoid arthritis?" *Scand J Rheumatol.* 1984; 13: 140–46.

Allen, R. C., et al. "Insulin-like growth factor and growth hormone secretion in juvenile chronic arthritis." *Ann Rheum Dis.* 1991; 50 (9): 602–6.

Aschoff, L. *Lectures on Pathology.* New York: Ed Hoeber, 1924; 5: 101.

Bennett, R. M., et al. "Low levels of somatomedin C in patients with the fibromyalgia syndrome. A possible link between sleep and muscle pain." *Arthritis Rheum.* 1992; 35 (10): 1113–16.

Bland, J. H., et al. "Rheumatic syndromes of myxedema." *N Engl J Med.* 1970; 282 (21): 1171–74.

Carette, S., et al. "Fibromyalgia and sex hormones." *J Rheumatol.* 1992; 9 (5): 831.

Carette, S., et al. "Fibrosis and primary hypothyroidism." *J Rheumatol.* 1988; 15: 1418–21.

Citera, G., et al. "The effect of melatonin in patients with fibromyalgia: a pilot study." *Clin Rheumatol.* 2000; 19 (1): 9–13.

Cutolo, M., et al. "The hypothalamic-pituitary-adrenocortical and gonadal axis function in rheumatoid arthritis." *Z Rheumatol.* 2000; 59 (Suppl 2): II/65–69.

Dailey, M. P., et al. "Polymyalgia rheumatic begins at 40." *Arch Int Med.* 1979; 139: 743–74.

Dessein, P. H., et al. "Hyposecretion of the adrenal androgen dehydroepiandrosterone sulfate and its relation to clinical variables in inflammatory arthrosis." *Arthrosis Res.* 2001; 3 (3): 183–88.

Dessein, P. H., et al. "Hyposecretion of adrenal androgens and the relation of serum adrenal steroids, serotonin and insulin-like growth factor-1 to clinical features in women with fibromyalgia." *Pain.* 1999; 83 (2): 313–19.

Dorwart, B. B., et al. "Joint effusions, chondrocalcinosis and other traumatic manifestations in hypothyroidism." *Am J Med.* 1975; 59: 780.

Ehrlich, H. P., et al. "Effects of vitamin A and glucocorticoids upon inflammation and collagen synthesis." *Ann Surg.* 1973; 177: 222–27.

Everitt, A. V. In *Hypothalamus, pituitary and ageing.* Springfield, Illinois: Thomas; 68.

Fauci, A. S. "Immunosuppressive and anti-inflammatory effects of glucocorticoids." In Baxter, J. D., et al., eds. *Glucocorticoid Hormone Action.* New York: Springer-Verlag, 1979; 449–65.

Frymoyer, J. W., et al. "Carpal-tunnel syndrome in patients with myxedematous arthropathy." *J Bone Joint Surg* (Am). 1973; 55: 78–82.

Golding, D. N. "Hypothyroidism presenting with musculo-skeletal symptoms." *Ann Rheum Dis.* 1970; 29: 10–14.

Healey, L. A. "Polymyalgia rheumatica." In Hollander, J. L., et al., eds. *Arthritis and Allied Conditions,* 8th ed., Philadelphia: Lea and Febiger, 1972; 885–89.

Heikkila, R., et al. "Serum androgen-anabolic hormones and the risk of rheumatoid arthritis." *Ann Rheum Dis.* 1998; 57 (5): 281–85.

Henderson, E., et al. "Pregnenolone." *J Clin Endocrinol.* 1950; 10: 455–74.

Hill, S. R., Jr., et al. "The role of the endocrine glands in the rheumatic diseases." In Hollander, J. L. ed. *Arthritis and Allied Conditions,* 7th ed., Philadelphia: Lea & Febiger, 1966; 597–605.

Holmdahl, R., et al. "Female sex hormones suppress development of collagen-induced arthritis in mice." *Arthritis Rheum.* 1986; 29: 1501–9.

Holmdahl, R., et al. "Oestrogen is a potent immunomodulator of murine experimental rheumatoid arthritis." *Br J Rheum.* 1989; 28 (suppl 1): 54.

Jefferies, W. M. "Hypothyroidism with high circulating T_3." *Safe Use of Cortisone.* Springfield, Illinois: Thomas, 1981; 154–56.

John, T. M., et al. "Melatonin replacement nullifies the effect of light-induced functional pinealectomy on nociceptive rhythm in the rat." *Physiol Behav.* 1994; 55 (4): 735–39.

Kantrowitz, F., et al. "Corticosteroids inhibit prostaglandin production by rheumatoid synovia." *Nature.* 1975; 258: 737–39.

Kelly, W. K., et al. "Prospective evaluation of hydrocortisone and suramin in patients with androgen-independent prostate cancer." *J Clin Oncol.* 1995; 13 (9): 2208–13.

Khalkhali-Ellis, Z., et al. "Reduced levels of testosterone and dehydroepiandrosterone sulphate in the serum and synovial fluid of juvenile rheumatoid arthritis patients correlates with disease severity." *Clin Exp Rheumatol.* 1998; 16 (6): 753–56.

Klappenberg, M., et al. "Slechts beperkt effect van behandeling van schilklierstoonissen op klachten van het bewegingsapparaat." *Ned Tijschr Geneesk.* 1992; 136 (1): 21–25.

Krane, S. M., et al. "The skeletal system." Ingbar, S., et al., eds. In *Werner's the Thyroid.* Philadelphia: Lippincott Company, 1986; 1205.

Martens, H. F., et al. "Decreased testosterone levels in men with rheumatoid arthritis: effect of low dose prednisone therapy." *J Rheumatol.* 1994; 21 (8): 1427–31.

Masi, A. T. "Sex hormones and rheumatoid arthritis: cause or effect relationships in a complex pathophysiology?" *Clin Exp Rheumatol.* 1995; 13 (2): 227–40.

Matteo, L., et al. "Sex hormones status and bone mineral density in men with rheumatoid arthritis." *J Rheumatol.* 1995; 22 (8): 1455–60.

McGavack, T., et al. "The use of pregnenolone in various clinical disorders." *J Clin Endocrinol.* 1951; 11: 559–77.

Mielants, H., et al. "Invloed van de sekssteroiden op reumatische auto-immuunziekten." *TijdschrGeneesk.* 1991; 47 (18): 1203–10.

Monroe, R. T. "Chronic arthritis in hyperthyroidism and myxedema." *N Engl J Med* 1935; 121: 1074.

Neidel, J. "Changes in systemic levels of insulin-like growth factors and their binding proteins in patients with rheumatoid arthritis." *Clin Exp Rheumatol.* 2001; 19 (1): 81–84.

Ornat, SIa. "The effect of aurotherapy on the content of corticotropin, cortisol, aldosterone and insulin in the blood serum of rheumatoid arthritis patients." *Vrach Delo.* 1991; (1): 61–65.

Roberts, E., et al. "Oral DHEA in multiple sclerosis: Results of a phase one, open study." *Dans: The Biological Role of DHEA.* Berlin: Walter de Gruyter, 1990; 81–93.

Robinzon, B., et al. "Should dehydroepiandrosterone replacement therapy be provided with glucocorticoids?" *Rheumatology (Oxf).* 1999; 38 (6): 488–95.

Ross, D. S. "Hyperthyroidism, thyroid hormone therapy, and bone." *Thyroid.* 1994; 4 (3): 319–26.

Royal College of General Practitioners: *Oral contraceptives and health, interim report.* London: Pitman Medical, 1974.

Sambrook, P., et al. "Postmenopausal bone loss in rheumatoid arthritis: effect of estrogens and androgens." *J Rheumatol.* 1992; 19 (3): 357–61.

Sambrook, P. N., et al. "Sex hormone status and osteoporosis in postmenopausal women with rheumatoid arthritis." *Arthritis Rheum.* 1988; 31: 973–78.

Schlaghecke, R., et al. "Effects of glucocorticoids in rheumatoid arthritis. Diminished glucocorticoid receptors do not result in glucocorticoid resistance." *Arthritis Rheum.* 1994; 37 (8): 1127–31.

Slocumb, C. H. "Cortisone and related steroids in the treatment of rheumatoid arthritis." *Med Clin North Am.* 1961; 45: 1209–18.

Smith, T. J. "Dexamethasone regulation of glycosaminoglycan synthesis in cultured human skin fibroblasts. Similar effects of glucocorticoid and thyroid hormones." *J Clin Invest.* 1984; 74: 2157–63.

Sterling, K. M., et al. "Dexamethasone decreases the amounts of type 1 procollagen mRNAs in vivo and in fibroblast cell cultures." *J Biol Chem.* 1983; 258: 7644–47.

Straub, R. H., et al. "High prolactin and low dehydroepiandrosterone sulphate serum levels in patients with severe systemic sclerosis." *Br J Rheumatol.* 1997; 36 (4): 426–32.

Straub, R. H., et al. "Replacement therapy with DHEA plus corticosteroids in patients with chronic inflammatory diseases—substitutes of adrenal and sex hormones." *Z Rheumatol.* 2000; 59 (Suppl 2): II/108–18.

Suzuki, T., et al. "Low serum levels of DHEA may cause deficient IL-2 production by lymphocytes in patients with SLE." *Clin Exp Immunol.* 1995; 99 (2): 251–55.

Twycross, R. "The risks and benefits of corticosteroids in advanced cancer." *Drug Saf.* 1994; 11 (3): 163–78.

Van Vollenhoven, R. F., et al. "An open study of DHEA in SLE." *Arthritis Rheum.* 1994; 37 (9): 1305–12.

Vandenbroucke, J. P., et al. "Noncontraceptive hormones and rheumatoid arthritis in perimenopausal and postmenopausal women." *JAMA.* 1986; 255 (10): 1299–1303.

Vassali, J. D., et al. "Macrophage plasminogen activator: modulation of enzyme production by anti-inflammatory steroids, mitotic inhibitors, and cyclic nucleotides." *Cell.* 1976; 8: 271–81.

von Knorring, L., et al. "Idiopathic pain and depression." *Qual Life Res.* 1994; 3 (Suppl 1): 557–68.

Werb, Z. "Biochemical actions of glucocorticoids on macrophages in culture. Specific inhibition of elastase, collagenase and plasminogen activator secretion and effects on other metabolic functions." *J Exp Med.* 1978; 147: 1695–1712.

West, S. K., et al. "Melatonin levels are decreased in rheumatoid arthritis." *J Basic Clin Physiol Pharmacol.* 1992; 3 (1): 33–40.

Zweifach, B. W., et al. "The influence of the adrenal cortex on the terminal vascular bed." *Ann NY Acad Sci.* 1953; 56: 626–33.

CHAPTER 8. RIGHT DOWN TO THE BONE

Adlin, E. V., et al. "Bone mineral density in postmenopausal women treated with L-thyroxine." *Am J Med.* 1991; 90 (3): 360–66.

Baulieu, E. E., et al. "Dehydroepiandrosterone (DHEA), DHEA sulfate, and aging: contribution of the DHEAge Study to a sociobiomedical issue." *Proc Natl Acad Sci USA.* 2000; 97 (8): 4279–84.

Brixen, K., et al. "A short course of recombinant human growth hormone treatment stimulates osteoblasts and activates bone remodeling in normal human volunteers." *J Bone Miner Res.* 1990; 5 (6): 609–18.

Buchanan, J. R., et al. "Effect of excess endogenous androgens on bone density in young women." *J Clin Endocrinol Metab.* 1988; 67 (5): 937.

Buckley, L. M., et al. "Effects of low dose corticosteroids on the bone mineral density of patients with rheumatoid arthritis." *J Rheumatol.* 1995; 22 (6): 1055–59.

Clemmesen, B., et al. "Human growth hormone and growth hormone releasing hormone: a double-masked, placebo-controlled study of their effects on bone metabolism in elderly women." *Osteoporos Int.* 1993; 6: 330–36.

Degerbland, M., et al. "Potent effect of recombinant growth hormone on bone mineral density and body composition in adults with panhypopituitarism." *Acta Endocrinol (Copenh).* 1992; 126 (5): 387–93.

Deutsch, S., et al. "The correlation of serum estrogens and androgens with bone density in the late postmenopause." *Int J Gynaecol Obstet.* 1987; 25 (3): 217–22.

Dhillon, V. B., et al. "Assessment of the effect of oral corticosteroids on bone mineral density in systemic lupus erythematosus: a preliminary study with dual energy x ray absorptiometry." *Ann Rheum Dis.* 1990; 49 (8): 624–26.

Diamond, T., et al. "Effects of testosterone and venesection on spinal and peripheral bone mineral in six hypogonadal men with hemochromatosis." *J Bone Miner Res.* 1991; 6 (1): 39–43.

Eriksen, E. F., et al. "Growth hormone and insulin-like growth factors as anabolic therapies for osteoporosis." *Horm Res.* 1993; 40 (1–3): 95–98.

Eulry, F., et al. "Bone density in differentiated cancer of the thyroid gland treated by hormone-suppressive therapy." Study based on fifty-one cases. *Rev Rhum Mal Osteoartic.* 1992; 59 (4): 247–52.

Fingerova, H., et al. "Reduced serum dehydroepiandrosterone levels in postmenopausal osteoporosis." *Ceska Gynekol.* 1998; 63 (2): 110–13.

Firestein, G. S., et al. "Gene expression (collagenase, tissue inhibitor of metalloproteinases, complement, and HLA-DR) in rheumatoid arthritis and osteoarthritis synovium. Quantitative analysis and effect of intraarticular corticosteroids." *Arthritis Rheum.* 1991; 34 (9): 1094–105.

Foldes, J., et al. "Decreased serum IGF-I and dehydroepiandrosterone sulphate may be risk factors for the development of reduced bone mass in postmenopausal women with endogenous subclinical hyperthyroidism." *Eur J Endocrinol.* 1997; 136 (3): 277–81.

Garnero, P., et al. "Biochemical markers of bone turnover, endogenous hormones and the risk of fractures in postmenopausal women: the OFELY study." *J Bone Miner Res.* 2000; 15 (8): 1526–36.

Grant, D. J., et al. "Suppressed TSH levels secondary to thyroxine replacement therapy are not associated with osteoporosis." *Clin Endocrinol (Oxf).* 1993; 39 (5): 529–33.

Holmes, S. J., et al. "Reduced bone mineral density in patients with adult onset growth hormone deficiency." *J Clin Endocrinol Metab.* 1994; 78 (3): 669–74.

Hyer, S. L., et al. "Growth hormone deficiency during puberty reduces adult bone mineral density." *Arch Dis Child.* 1992; 67 (12): 1472–74.

Inoh, H., et al. "Correlation between the age of pinealectomy and the development of scoliosis in chickens." *Spine.* 2001; 26 (9): 1014–21.

Kenny, A. M., et al. "Effects of transdermal testosterone on bone and muscle in older men with low bioavailable testosterone levels." *J Gerontol A Biol Sci Med Sci.* 2001; 56 (5): M266–72.

Laan, R. F., et al. "Differential effects of glucocorticoids on cortical appendicular and cortical vertebral bone mineral content." *Calcif Tissue Int.* 1993; 52 (1): 5–9.

Labrie, F., et al. "Effect of 12-month dehydroepiandrosterone replacement therapy on bone, vagina, and endometrium in postmenopausal women." *J Clin Endocrinol Metab.* 1997; 82 (10): 3498–505.

Lau, E. M., et al. "Risk factors for hip fracture in Asian men and women: the Asian osteoporosis study." *J Bone Miner Res.* 2001; 16 (3): 572–80.

Maestroni, G. J. "Neurohormones and catecholamines as functional components of the bone marrow microenvironment." *Ann NY Acad Sci.* 2000; 917: 29–37. Review.

Mann, D. R., et al. "Preservation of bone mass in hypogonadal female monkeys with recombinant human growth hormone administration." *J Clin Endocrinol Metab.* 1992; 74 (6): 1263–69.

Melton, L. J., 3d., et al. "Fractures following thyroidectomy in women: a population-based cohort study." *Bone.* 2000; 27 (5): 695–700.

Minaire, P., et al. "Acute osteoporosis in paraplegic patients: pathophysiology and effects of treatment with calcitonin or dichlorodimethylene diphosponate." In Menczel, J., et al., eds. *Osteoporosis.* New York: Wiley, 1982; 421–28.

Mishra, K. K., et al. "A study on physiological changes in essential hypertension and rheumatoid arthritis with reference to the levels of cortisol, blood glucose, triglycerides and cholesterol." *Indian J Physiol Pharmacol.* 1995; 39 (1): 68–70.

Mortola, J. F., et al. "The effect of oral DHEA on endocrine-metabolic parameters in postmenopausal women." *J Clin Endocrinol Metab.* 1990; 71 (3): 696–704.

Nagant de Deuxchaisnes, C., et al. "New modes of administration of salmon calcitonin in Paget's disease." *Clin Orthop Rel Res.* 1987; 217: 56–71.

Nowata, H., et al. "Aromatase in bone cell: association with osteoporosis in postmenopausal women." *J Steroid Biochem Mol Biol.* 1995; 53 (1–6): 165–74.

"Osteoporosis contribution to modern management." The proceedings of a Symposium held at the XVIIth Congress of Rheumatology, Rio de Janeiro, September 1989. Ed. B.E.C. Nordin. Novartis, New Jersey: The Parthenon Publishing Group, 1990.

Ostrowska, Z., et al. "Assessment of the relationship between dynamic pattern of nighttime levels of melatonin and chosen biochemical markers of bone metabolism in a rat model of postmenopausal osteoporosis." *Neuroendocrinol Lett.* 2001; 22 (2): 129–36.

Overgaard, K., et al. "Effect of salcatonin given intranasally on early postmenopausal bone loss." *Br Med J.* 1989; 299: 477–79.

Overgaard, O., et al. "Effect of salcatonin given intranasally on bone mass and fracture rates in established osteoporosis: a dose-response study." *Br Med J.* 1992; 305: 556–61.

Pun, K. K., et al. "Analgesic effect of intranasal salmon calcitonin in the treatment of osteoporotic vertebral fractures." *Clin Therapeutics.* 1989; 11 (2): 205–9.

Ribot, C., et al. "Bone mineral density and thyroid hormone therapy." *Clin Endocrinol (Oxf).* 1990; 33 (2): 143–53.

Rozenberg, S., et al. "Age, steroids and bone mineral content." *Maturitas.* 1990; 12: 137–43.

Sadat-Ali, M., et al. "Adolescent idiopathic scoliosis. Is low melatonin a cause?" *Joint Bone Spine.* 2000; 67 (1): 62–64.

Sambrook, P., et al. "Postmenopausal bone loss in rheumatoid arthritis: effect of estrogen and androgens." *J. Rheumatol.* 1992; 19 (3): 357–61.

Sambrook, P. N., et al. "Sex hormone status and osteoporosis in postmenopausal women with rheumatoid arthritis." *Arthritis Rheum.* 1988; 31 (8): 973–78.

Sandyk, R., et al. "Is postmenopausal osteoporosis related to pineal gland functions?" *Int J Neurosci.* 1992; 62 (3–4): 215–25.

Snyder, P. J., et al. "Effects of testosterone replacement in hypogonadal men." *J Clin Endocrinol Metab.* 2000; 85 (8): 2670–77.

Soskolne, W. A., et al. "The biphasic effect of triiodothyronine compared to bone resorbing effect of PTH on bone modelling of mouse long bone in vitro." *Bone.* 1990; 11 (5): 301–7.

Stall, G. M., et al. "Accelerated bone loss in hypothyroid patients overtreated with L-thyroxine." *Ann Intern Med.* 1990; 113 (4): 265–69.

Svanberg, E., et al. "Anabolic effects of rhIGF-I/IGFBP-3 in vivo are influenced by thyroid status." *Eur J Clin Invest.* 2001; 31 (4): 329–36.

Taelman, P., et al. "Reduced forearm bone mineral content and biochemical evidence of increased bone turnover in women with euthyroid goitre treated with thyroid hormone." *Clin Endocrinol (Oxf).* 1990; 33 (1): 107–17.

Taggart, H. M., et al. "Deficient calcitonin response to calcium stimulation in postmenopausal osteoporosis." *Lancet.* 1982; 1: 475–78.

Tannirandorn, P., et al. "Drug-induced bone loss." *Osteoporos Int.* 2000; 11 (8): 637–59. Review.

van den Beld, A. W., et al. "Measures of bioavailable serum testosterone and estradiol and their relationships with muscle strength, bone density, and body composition in elderly men." *J Clin Endocrinol Metab.* 2000; 85 (9): 3276–82.

Vander Veen, E. A., et al. "Growth hormone (replacement) therapy in adults: bone and calcium metabolism." *Horm Res.* 1990; 33 (Suppl 4): 65–68.

Vandewighe, M., et al. "Short- and long-term effects of growth hormone treatment on bone turnover and bone mineral content in adult growth hormone-deficient males." *Clin Endocrinol (Oxf).* 1993; 39 (4): 409–15.

Villareal, D. T., et al. "Effects of DHEA replacement on bone mineral density and body composition in elderly women and men." *Clin Endocrinol (Oxf)*. 2000; 53 (5): 561–68.

Watts, N. B., et al. "Comparison of oral estrogens and estrogens plus androgen on bone mineral density, menopausal symptoms, and lipid-lipoprotein profiles in surgical menopause." *Obstet Gynecol*. 1995; 85 (4): 529–37.

Wimalawansa, S. J., et al. "The effect of percutaneous oestradiol and low dose human calcitonin on postmenopausal vertebral bone loss." *Osteoporosis*. 1987; 528–32.

Wuster, C., et al. "Decreased serum levels on insulin-like growth factors and IGF binding protein 3 in osteoporosis." *J Intern Med*. 1993; 234 (3): 249–55.

CHAPTER 9. MATTERS OF THE HEART
Atherosclerosis

Bernini, G. P., et al. "Influence of endogenous androgens on carotid wall in postmenopausal women." *Menopause*. 2001; 8 (1): 43–50.

de Kleijn, M. J., et al. "Hormone replacement therapy in perimenopausal women and 2-year change of carotid intima-media thickness." *Maturitas*. 1999; 32 (3): 195–204.

Hayashi, T., et al. "Dehydroepiandrosterone retards atherosclerosis formation through its conversion to estrogen: the possible role of nitric oxide." *Arterioscler Thromb Vasc Biol*. 2000; 20 (3): 782–92.

Mullick, A. E., et al. "Chronic estradiol treatment attenuates stiffening, glycoxidation, and permeability in rat carotid arteries." *Am J Physiol Heart Circ Physiol*. 2001; 281 (5): H2204–10.

Smith, J. C., et al. "The effects of induced hypogonadism on arterial stiffness, body composition, and metabolic parameters in males with prostate cancer." *J Clin Endocrinol Metab*. 2001; 86 (9): 4261–67.

Tremollieres, F. A., et al. "Effect of hormone replacement therapy on age-related increase in carotid artery intima-media thickness in postmenopausal women." *Atherosclerosis*. 2000; 153 (1): 81–88.

Walsh, B. A., et al. "17beta-estradiol acts separately on the LDL particle and artery wall to reduce LDL accumulation." *J Lipid Res*. 2000; 41 (1): 134–41.

Walsh, B. A., et al. "17beta-estradiol reduces tumor necrosis factor-alpha-mediated LDL accumulation in the artery wall." *J Lipid Res*. 1999; 40 (3): 387–96.

Cholesterol

Abdu, T. A., et al. "Coronary risk in growth hormone deficient hypopituitary adults: increased predicted risk is due largely to lipid profile abnormalities." *Clin Endocrinol (Oxf)*. 2001; 55 (2): 209–16.

Aoyama, H., et al. "Effects of melatonin on genetic hypercholesterolemia in rats." *Atherosclerosis*. 1988; 69: 269–72.

Bengtsson, B. A., et al. "Treatment of adults with growth hormone deficiency with recombinant human GH." *J Clin Endocrinol Metab*. 1993; 76: 309–17.

Elder, J., et al. "The relationship between serum cholesterol and serum thyrotropin, thyroxine and triiodothyronine concentrations in suspected hypothyroidism." *Ann Clin Biochem.* 1990; 27 (Pt 2): 110–13.

Franklyn, J. A., et al. "Thyroxine replacement therapy and circulations rapid concentrations." *Clin Endocrinol (Oxf).* 1993; 38 (5): 453–59.

Freedman, D. S., et al. "Relation of serum testosterone levels to high density lipoprotein cholesterol and other characteristics in men." *Arterioscler Thromb.* 1991; 11 (2): 307–15.

Friedl, K. E., et al. "High-density lipoprotein cholesterol is not decreased if an aromatizable androgen is administered." *Metabolism.* 1990; 39 (1): 69–74.

Furman, R. H., et al. "Effect of androgens and estrogens on serum lipids and the composition and concentration of serum lipoproteins in normolipemic and hyperlipidemic states." *Proc Biochem Pharmacol.* 1967; 12: 215–49.

Houser, S. L., et al. "Serum lipids and arterial plaque load are altered independently with high-dose progesterone in hypercholesterolemic male rabbits." *Cardiovasc Pathol.* 2000; 9 (6): 317–22.

Hromadova, M., et al. "Alterations of lipid metabolism in men with hypotestosteronemia." *Horm Metab Res.* 1991; 23 (8): 392–94.

Khaw, K. T., et al. "Endogenous sex hormones, high density lipoprotein cholesterol, and other lipoprotein fractions in men." *Arterioscler Thromb.* 1991; 11 (3): 489–94.

Marek, J. "The significance of ovarian and testicular steroids in lipid metabolism and atherogenesis." *Vnitr Lek.* 1992; 38 (9): 913–20.

Mori, N., et al. "Anti-hypercholesterolemic effect of melatonin in rats." *Japanese Society of Pathology.* 1989; 39: 613–18.

Mori, W., et al. "Melatonin protects rats from injurious effects of glucocorticoid, dexamethasone." *Jap Exp Med.* 1984; 54 (6): 255–61.

Mortola, J. F., et al. "The effects of oral dehydroepiandrosterone on endocrine-metabolic parameters in postmenopausal women." *J Clin Endocrinol Metab.* 1990; 71 (3): 696–704.

Nagata, C., et al. "Association of dehydroepiandrosterone sulfate with serum HDL-cholesterol concentrations in post-menopausal Japanese women." *Maturitas.* 1998; 31 (1): 21–27.

Nestler, J. E., et al. "Dehydroepiandrosterone reduces serum low density lipoprotein levels and body fat but does not alter insulin sensitivity in normal men." *J Clin Endocrinol Metab.* 1988; 66 (1): 57–61.

Okamoto, K. "Distribution of dehydroepiandrosterone sulfate and relationships between its level and serum lipid levels in a rural Japanese population." *J Epidemiol.* 1998; 8 (5): 285–91.

Okamoto, K. "Relationship between dehydroepiandrosterone sulfate and serum lipid levels in Japanese men." *J Epidemiol.* 1996; 6 (2): 63–67.

Pierpaoli, W., et al. "The pineal control of aging: the effects of melatonin and pineal grafting on the survival of older mice." *Ann NY Acad Sci.* 1991; 621: 291–313.

Reiter, R. "Protecting your heart." In *Melatonin: Breakthrough discoveries that can help you.* New York: Bantam Books, 1995; 106–22.

Russel-Jones, D. L., et al. "The effect of growth hormone replacement on serum lipids, lipoproteins, apolipoproteins and cholesterol precursors in adult growth hormone deficient patients." *Clin Endocrinol (Oxf).* 1994; 41 (3): 345–50.

Shapiro, J., et al. "Testosterone and other anabolic steroids as cardiovascular drugs." *Am J Ther.* 1999; 6 (3): 167–74.

Whitsel, E. A., et al. "Intramuscular testosterone esters and plasma lipids in hypogonadal men: a meta-analysis." *Am J Med.* 2001; 111 (4): 261–69.

High Blood Pressure

Christiaansen, J. S., et al. "Kidney function and size in normal subjects before and during growth hormone administration for one week." *Eur J Clin Invest.* 1981; 11: 487–90.

Chuang, J. I., et al. "Melatonin decreases brain serotonin release, arterial pressure and heart rate in rats." *Pharmacology.* 1993;.47 (2): 91–97.

Crane, M. G., et al. "Hypertension, oral contraceptive agents and conjugated estrogens." *Ann Intern Med.* 1971; 74: 13–21.

Dulchavsky, S. A., et al. "Triiodothyronine (T_3) improves cardio-vascular function during hemorrhagic shock." *Circ Shock.* 1993; 39 (1): 68–73.

Fagard, R. "The role of exercise in blood pressure control: supportive evidence." *J Hypertension.* 1995; 13: 1223–27.

Falkheden, T., et al. "Renal function and kidney size following hypophysectomy in man." *Acta Endocrinol (Copenh).* 1965; 48: 348.

Fish, I. R., et al. "Oral contraceptives and blood pressure." *J Am Med Assoc.* 1977; 237: 2499–503.

Fuller, H. Jr., et al. "Myxedema and hypertension." *Postgrad. Med.* 1966; 40: 425–28.

Gerhard, M., et al. "Estradiol therapy combined with progesterone and endothelium-dependent vasodilation in postmenopausal women." *Circulation.* 1998; 98 (12): 1158–63.

Holmes, S. W., et al. "The effect of melatonin on pinealectomy-induced hypertension in a rat." Proceedings of the B. P. S. 1975; 306.

Hughes, G. S., et al. "Fish oil produces an atherogenic lipid profile in hypertensive men." *Atherosclerosis.* 1990; 84 (2–3): 229–37.

Johannes, C. B., et al. "Relation of dehydroepiandrosterone and dehydroepiandrosterone sulfate with cardiovascular disease risk factors in women: longitudinal results from the Massachusetts Women's Health Study." *J Clin Epidemiol.* 1999; 52 (2): 95–103.

Kapitola, J. "Hemodynamic effects of dehydroepiandrosterone in rats." *Agressologie.* 1972; 13 (4): 247–51.

Kornhauser, C., et al. "The effect of hormone replacement therapy on blood pressure and cardiovascular risk factors in menopausal women with moderate hypertension." *J Hum Hypertens.* 1997; 11 (7): 405–11.

Landin-Wilhelmsen, K., et al. "Serum insulin-like growth factor I in a random population sample of men and women: relation to age, sex, smoking habits, coffee consumption and physical activity, blood pressure and concentrations of plasma lipids, fibrinogen, parathyroid hormone and osteocalcin." *Clin Endocrinol (Oxf).* 1994; 41 (3): 351–57.

Laragh, J. H. "Oral contraceptive-induced hypertension. Nine years later." *Am J Obstet Gynecol.* 1976; 126: 141–47.

Lusardi, P., et al. "Effect of bedtime melatonin ingestion on blood pressure of normotensive subjects." *Blood Press Monit.* 1997; 2 (2): 99–103.

Menof, P. "New method for control of hypertension." *S Afr Med J.* 1950; 24: 172.

Nowaczynski, W., et al. "Further evidence of altered adrenocortical function in hypertension. Dehydroepiandrosterone excretion rate." *Can J Biochem.* 1968; 46: 1031–38.

Reiter, R. "Protecting your heart." In *Melatonin: Breakthrough discoveries that can help you.* New York: Bantam Books, 1995; 106–22.

Satake, N., et al. "Vasorelaxing action of melatonin in rat isolated aorta; possible endothelium dependent relaxation." *Gen Pharmacol.* 1991; 22 (6): 1127–33.

Tseng, K. H., et al. "Concurrent aortic and mitral valve echocardiography permits measurement of systolic time intervals as an index of peripheral tissue thyroid functional status." *J Clin Endocrinol Metab.* 1989; 69 (3): 633–38.

Tuev, A. V., et al. "Several indicators of hormonal homeostasis (hypophysis-gonads) in patients with hypertension." *Ross Med Zh.* 1992; 3: 10–13.

Worboys, S., et al. "Evidence that parenteral testosterone therapy may improve endothelium-dependent and -independent vasodilation in post-menopausal women already receiving estrogen." *J Clin Endocrinol Metab.* 2001; 86 (1): 158–61.

Yanal Shafagoj, et al. "DHEA prevents dexamethasone-induced hypertension in rats." *Am Physiol.* 1992; 263 (2 pt): E201–3.

Yue, P., et al. "Testosterone relaxes rabbit coronary arteries and aorta." *Circulation.* 1995; 91 (4): 1154–60.

Low Blood Pressure

Bou-Holaigah, I., et al. "The relationship between neurally mediated hypotension and the chronic fatigue syndrome." *JAMA.* 1995; 274 (12): 961–67.

Sudsuang, R., et al. "Effect of Buddhist meditation on serum cortisol and total protein levels, blood pressure, pulse rate, lung volume and reaction time." *Physiol Behav.* 1991; 50 (3): 543–58.

Sutherland, D. H. A., et al. "Hypertension, increased aldosterone secretion and low plasma renin activity relieved by dexamethazone." *Can Med Assoc J.* 1966; 95: 1109–19.

Walker, B. R., et al. "Glucocorticoids and blood pressure: a role for the cortisol/cortisone shuttle in the control of vascular tone in man." *Clin Sci Colch.* 1992; 83 (2): 171–78.

Wong, K. S., et al. "Effects of blood pressure and salt preference in normal humans." *JA Clin Exp Pharmacol Physiol.* 1993; 20 (2): 121–26.

Yamakado, M., et al. "Extrarenal role of aldosterone in the regulation of blood pressure." *Am J Hypertens.* 1988; 1: 276–79.

The Heart

Alexandersen, P., et al. "The relationship of natural androgens to coronary heart disease in males: a review." *Atherosclerosis.* 1996; 125 (1): 1–13.

Barnes, B. O., et al. *Hypothyroidism.* New York: Harper & Row Publishers, 1976; 155–96.

Barrett-Connor, E. "A prospective study of DHEAs, mortality and cardiovascular disease." *N Engl J Med.* 1986; 315 (24): 1519–24.

Barrett-Connor, E., et al. "The epidemiology of DHEAs and cardiovascular disease." *Ann NY Acad Sci.* 1995; 774: 259–70.

Beekman, R. E., et al. "Thyroid status and beta-agonistic effects on cytosolic calcium concentrations in single rat cardiac myocytes activated by electrical stimulation on high-K+ depolarization." *Biochem J.* 1990; 268 (3): 563–69.

Berk, B. C., et al. "Pharmacologic roles of heparin and glucocorticoids to prevent restenosis after coronary angioplasty." *J Am Coll Cardiol.* 1991; 17 (6 suppl B): 111B–117B.

Bian, X. P., et al. "Promotional role for glucocorticoids in the development of intracellular signalling: enhanced cardiac and renal adenylate cyclase reactivity to beta-adrenergic and non-adrenergic stimuli after low-dose fetal dexamethasone exposure." *J Dev Physiol.* 1992; 17 (6): 289–97.

Brugger, P., et al. "Impaired nocturnal secretion of melatonin in coronary heart disease." *Lancet.* 1995; 345 (8962): 1408.

Bush, T. L., et al. "Cardiovascular mortality and noncontraceptive use of estrogen in women: Results from the lipid Research Clinics Program Follow-up Study." *Circulation.* 1987; 75: 1102–9.

Chen, F. P., et al. "Effects of hormone replacement therapy on cardiovascular risk factors in postmenopausal women." *Fertil Steril.* 1998; 69 (2): 267–73.

Cittadini, A., et al. "Impaired cardiac performance in GH deficient adults and its improvement after GH replacement." *Am J Physiol.* 1994; 267 (2 Pt 1): E219–25.

Conti, E., et al. "Markedly reduced insulin-like growth factor-1 in the acute phase of myocardial infarction." *J Am Coll Cardiol.* 2001; 38 (1): 26–32.

Criqui, M. H., et al. "Postmenopausal estrogen use and mortality: Results from a prospective study in a defined, homogeneous community." *Am J Epidemiol.* 1988; 128: 606–14.

Czarnecki, C. M. "Influence of exogenous T_4 on bodyweight, feed consumption, T_4 levels, and myocardial glycogen in furazolidonefed turkey poults." *Avian Dis.* 1991; 35 (4): 930–36.

Dazai, Y., et al. "Direct effect of thyroid hormone on left ventricular myocardial relaxation." *Jpn Circ J.* 1992; 56 (4): 334–42.

Del Rio, G., et al. "Effect of estradiol on the sympathoadrenal response to mental stress in normal men." *J Clin Endocrinol Metab.* 1994; 79 (3): 836–40.

Ducceschi, V., et al. "Estrogens, left ventricular function and coronary circulation: what are the possibilities of therapeutic use?" *Minerva Cardioangiol.* 1995; 43 (4): 135–43.

Edwards, E. A., et al. "Testosterone propionate as a therapeutic agent in patients with organic disease of the peripheral vessels." *N Engl J Med.* 1939; 220: 865.

Ersley, A. J. "Erythropoietin." *N Engl J Med.* 1991; 324 (19): 1339–43.

Eschbach, J. W., et al. "Correction of the anemia of end-stage renal disease with recombinant human erythropoietin: results of a combined Phase I and II clinical trial." *N Engl J Med.* 1987; 316: 73–78.

Fazio, S., et al. "A preliminary study of growth hormone in the treatment of dilated cardiomyopathy." *N Eng J Med.* 1996; 334 (13): 809–14.

Feldman, H. A., et al. "Low dehydroepiandrosterone and ischemic heart disease in middle-aged men: prospective results from the Masschusetts Male Aging Study." *Am J Epidemiol.* 2001; 153 (1): 79–89.

Feldman, H. A., et al. "Low dehydroepiandrosterone sulfate and heart disease in middle-aged men: cross-sectional results from the Massachusetts Male Aging Study." *Ann Epidemiol.* 1998; 8 (4): 217–28.

Frey, F. J., et al. "Glucocorticoids and infection." *Schweiz Med Wochenschr.* 1992; 122 (5): 137–46.

Gotthardt, U., et al. "Cortisol, ACTH, and cardiovascular response to a cognitive challenge paradigm in aging and depression." *Am J Physiol.* 1995; 268 (4 Pt 2): R865–73.

Grad, B. R., et al. "The role of melatonin and serotonin in aging: update." Published erratum appears in *Psychoneuroendocrinology.* 1993; 18 (7): 541.

Grodstein, F., et al. "A prospective, observational study of postmenopausal hormone therapy and primary prevention of cardiovascular disease." *Ann Intern Med.* 2000; 133 (12): 933–41.

Hanke, H., et al. "Estradiol concentrations in premenopausal women with coronary heart disease." *Coron Artery Dis.* 1997; 8 (8–9): 511–15.

Herrington D. "DHEA and atherosclerosis." *Ann NY Acad Sci.* 1999; 774: 271–80.

Herrington, O., et al. "Plasma DHEA and DHEAs in patients undergoing diagnostic coronary angiography." *J Am Coll Cardiol.* 1990; 16: 862–70.

Hulley, S., et al. "Randomized trial of estrogen plus progestin for secondary prevention of coronary heart disease in postmenopausal women. Heart and Estrogen/progestin Replacement Study (HERS) Research Group." *JAMA.* 1998; 280 (7): 605–13.

Israel, N. "An effective therapeutic approach to atherosclerosis illustrating harmlessness of prolonged use of thyroid hormone in coronary disease." *Am J Dig Dis.* 1955; 22: 161–68.

Jansson, J. H., et al. "Von Willebrand factor, tissue plasminogen activator, and dehydroepiandrosterone sulphate predict cardiovascular death in a 10-year follow-up of survivors of acute myocardial infarction." *Heart.* 1998; 80 (4): 334–37.

Johannes, C. B., et al. "Relation of dehydroepiandrosterone and dehydroepiandrosterone sulfate with cardiovascular disease risk factors in women: longitudinal results from the Massachusetts Women's Health Study." *J Clin Epidemiol.* 1999; 52 (2): 95–103.

Kinson, G. A., et al. "Influences of anabolic androgens on cardiac growth and metabolism in the rat." *Can J Physiol Pharmacol.* 1991; 69 (11): 1698–704.

Kreze, A., Jr., et al. "Dehydroepiandrosterone, dehydroepiandrosterone-sulfate and insulin in acute myocardial infarct." *Vnitr Lek.* 2000; 46 (12): 835–38.

Krieg, M., et al. "Demonstration of a specific androgen receptor in rat heart muscle: relationship between binding, metabolism, and tissue levels of androgens." *Endocrinology.* 1978; 1686–94.

Lesser, M. A. "Testosterone propionate therapy in one hundred cases of angina pectoris." *J Clin Endocrinol Metab.* 1946; 549–57.

Minshall, R. D., et al. "Ovarian steroid protection against coronary artery hyperactivity in Rhesus Monkey." *J Clin Endocrinol Metab.* 1988; 83: 649–59.

Mitchell, L. E., et al. "Evidence for an association between dehydroepiandrosterone sulfate and nonfatal, premature myocardial infarction in males." *Circulation.* 1994; 89 (1): 89–93.

Möller, J. *Cholesterol: interactions with testosterone and cortisol in cardiovascular diseases.* Berlin Heidelberg: Springer-Verlag, 1987.

Palmen, M., et al. "Cardiac remodeling after myocardial infarction is impaired in IGF-1 deficient mice." *Cardiovasc Res.* 2001; 50 (3): 516–24.

Pepine, C. J., et al. "A controlled trial of corticosteroids to prevent restenosis after coronary angioplasty. M-HEART Group." *Circulation.* 1990; 81 (6): 1753–61.

Petiti, D. B., et al. "Noncontraceptive estrogens and mortality: Long-term follow-up of women in the Walnut Creek study." *Obstet Gynecol.* 1987; 70 (3 Pt 1): 289–93.

Pirpiris, M., et al. "Hydrocortisone-induced hypertension in men. The role of cardiac output." *Am J Hypertens.* 1993; 6 (4): 287–94.

Rosano, G. M., et al. "Acute anti-ischemic effect of testosterone in men with coronary artery disease." *Circulation.* 1999; 99 (13): 1666–70.

Rosano, G. M., et al. "Natural progesterone, but not medroxyprogesterone acetate, enhances the beneficial effect of estrogen on exercise-induced myocardial ischemia in postmenopausal women." *J Am Coll Cardiol.* 2000; 36 (7): 2154–59.

Rosen, T., et al. "Premature mortality due to cardiovascular disease in hypopituitarism." *Lancet.* 1990; 336: 285–88.

Rouleau, J. R., et al. "Effect of estrogen replacement therapy on distribution of myocardial blood flow in female anesthetized rabbits." *Jr Am J Physiol Heart Circ Physiol.* 2001; 281 (3): H1407–12.

Seeger, H., et al. "Effect of medroxyprogesterone acetate and norethisterone on serum-stimulated and estradiol-inhibited proliferation of human coronary artery smooth muscle cells." *Menopause.* 2001; 8 (1): 5–9.

Slowinska-Srzednicka, J., et al. "Decreased plasma dehydroepiandrosterone sulfate and dihydrotestosterone concentrations in young men after myocardial infarction." *Z Atherosclerosis.* 1989; 79 (2–3): 197–203.

Stampfer, M. J., et al. "Postmenopausal estrogen therapy and cardiovascular disease. Ten-year follow-up from the Nurses' Health study." *New Engl J Med.* 1991; 325: 756–62.

Tomanek, R. J., et al. "Initiation of cardiac hypertrophy in response to thyroxine is not limited by age." *Am J Physiol.* 1993; 264 (4 Pt 2): H1041–47.

Tseng, K. H., et al. "Concurrent aortic and mitral valve echocardiography permits measurements of systolic time intervals as an index of peripheral tissue thyroid functional status." *J Clin Endoc Metab.* 1989; 69 (3): 633–38.

Winearls, C. G., et al. "Effect of human erythropoietin derived from recombinant DNA on the anaemia of patients maintained by chronic haemodialysis." *Lancet.* 1986; 2: 1175–78.

Wu, S. Z., et al. "Antianginal and lipid lowering effects of oral androgenic preparation (Andriol) on elderly male patients with coronary heart disease." *Chung Hua Nei Ko Tsa Chih.* 1993; 32 (4): 235–38.

Yang, R., et al. "Growth hormone improves cardiac performances in experimental heart failure." *Circulation.* 1995; 92 (2): 262–67.

Yokoyama, Y., et al. "Facilitated recovery of cardiac performance by triiodothyronine following a transient ischemic insult." *Cardiology.* 1992; 81 (1): 34–45.

Cerebrovascular Accidents

Bednarek-Tupikowska, G., et al. "Influence of dehydroepiandrosterone on platelet aggregation, superoxide dismutase activity and serum lipid peroxide concentrations in rabbits with induced hypercholesterolemia." *Med Sci Monit.* 2000; 6 (1): 40–45.

Beer, N. A., et al. "Dehydroepiandrosterone reduces plasma plasminogen activator inhibitor type 1 and tissue plasminogen activator antigen in men." *Am J Med Sci.* 1996; 311 (5): 205–10.

Bennet, A., et al. *"Ulcères de jambe post-phlébitiques et caryotype XYY: tests de fibrinolyse et fonction androgénique."* Ann Dermatol Venereol. 1987; 114: 1097–101.

Bregani, E. R., et al. "Prevention of interleukin-2-induced thrombocytopenia during the immuno-therapy of cancer by a concomitant administration of the pineal hormone melatonin." *Recent Prog Med.* 1995; 86 (6): 231–33.

Cagnacci, A., et al. "Different circulatory response to melatonin in postmenopausal women without and with hormone replacement therapy." *J Pineal Res.* 2000; 29 (3): 152–58.

Frohlich, M., et al. "Effects of hormone replacement therapies on fibrinogen and plasma viscosity in postmenopausal women." *Br J Haematol.* 1998; 100 (3): 577–81.

Gordon, G. B. "Reduction of atherosclerosis by administration of DHEA." *J Clin. Invest.* 1988; 82: 712–20.

Graettinger, J. S., et al. "A correlation of clinical and hemodynamic studies in patients with hypothyroidism." *J Clin. Invest.* 1958; 37: 502.

Hu, R. "Changes in serum thyroid hormones in acute cerebrovascular apoplexy and their clinical significance." *Chung Hua Shen Ching Ching Shen Ko Tsa Chih.* 1990; 23 (2): 87–89, 126.

Hum, P. D., et al. "Postischemic cerebral blood flow recovery in the female: effect of 17 beta-estradiol." *J Cereb Blood Flow Metab.* 1995; 15 (4): 666–72.

Kapitola, J. "Hemodynamic effects of dehydroepiandrosterone in rats." *Agressologie.* 1972; 13 (4): 247–51.

Kluft, C., et al. "Stanozolol-induced changes in fibrinolysis and coagulation in healthy adults." *Thromb Haemost.* 1984; 51: 157–64.

Lissoni, P., et al. "A biological study on the efficacy of low-dose subcutaneous interleukin-2 plus melatonin in the treatment of cancer-related thrombocytopenia." *Oncology.* 1995; 52 (5): 360–62.

Mohan, P. F., et al. "Inhibition of macrophage superoxide generation by DHEA." *Am J of Medical Sciences.* 1993; 306 (1): 10–15.

Preston, F. E., et al. "The fibrinolytic response to stanozolol in normal subjects." *Thrombos Res.* 1981; 22: 543–57.

Reinhardt, R. R., et al. "Insulin-like growth factors cross the blood-brain barrier." *Endocrinology.* 1994; 135 (5): 1753–61.

Sanmarti, A., et al. "Observational study in adult hypopituitary patients with untreated growth hormone deficiency (ODA study)." Socio-economic impact and health status. Collaborative ODA (Observational GH Deficiency in Adults) Group. *Eur J Endocrinol.* 1999; 141 (5): 481–89.

Scarabin, P. Y., et al. "Effects of oral and transdermal estrogen/progesterone regimens on blood coagulation and fibrinolysis in postmenopausal women." A randomized controlled trial. *Arterioscler Thromb Vasc Biol.* 1997; 17 (11): 3071–78.

Walker, I. D., et al. "Effect of anabolic steroids on plasma antithrombin III." *Thrombos Diathes Haemorrh (Stuttg).* 1975; 34: 106.

Wang, B. C., et al. "Vasopressin and renin responses to hemorrhage in conscious, cardiac-derervated dogs." *Am J Physiol.* 1983; 245: H399–H405.

Wuster, C., et al. "Increased prevalence of osteoporosis and arteriosclerosis in conventionally substituted anterior pituitary insufficiency: need for additional growth hormone substitution?" *Klin Wochenschr.* 1991; 18, 69 (16): 769–73.

Zumoff, B., et al. "Sex differences in twenty-four-hour mean plasma concentrations of DHEA and DHEAS and the DHEA to DHEAs ratio in normal adults." *J Clin Endocrinol Metab.* 1980; 51 (2): 330–33.

CHAPTER 10. YOUR IMMUNE SYSTEM
Immunity

Ahima, R., et al. "Type I corticosteroid receptor-like immunoreactivity in the rat CNS: distribution and regulation by corticosteroids." *J Comp Neurol.* 1991; 313 (3): 522–38.

Akbulut, K. G., et al. "The effects of melatonin on humoral immune responses of young and aged rats." *Immunol Invest.* 2001; 30 (1): 17–20.

"Annotations: Corticosteroids for tuberculous pleural effusions." *Lancet.* 1959; 1135.

Barnes, B. O. "Etiology and treatment of lowered resistance to upper respiratory infections." *Fed Proc.* 1953; 12 (1): 24.

Barnes, B. O. "Role of the thyroid in infectious diseases." *Am Med Ass An Meetng.* 1965 June 24; New York.

Barnes, O. A. "Furonculosis: etiology and treatment." *J Clin Endocrinol.* 1943; 3 (4): 243–44.

Beisel, W. R., et al. "Interrelations between adrenocortical functions and infectious illness." *N Engl Med.* 1969; 280: 541–46.

Bender, C. E. "The value of corticosteroids in the treatment of infectious mononucleosis." *JAMA.* 1967; 199: 539–31.

Block, G. "Epidemiologic evidence regarding vitamin C and cancer." *Am J Clin Nutr.* 1991; 54: 13105–45.

Boing, H., et al. "Regional nutritional pattern and cancer mortality in the Federal Republic of Germany." *Nutr Cancer.* 1985; 7 (3): 121–36.

Buiatti, F., et al. "A case-control of gastric cancer and diet in Italy: association with nutrients." *Int J Cancer.* 1990; 45: 899–901.

Carroll, K. K. "Dietary fats and cancer." *Am J Clin Nutr.* 1991; 53: 1064S-67S.

Chappel, M. R. "Infectious mononucleosis." *Southwest Med.* 1962; 43: 253–55.

Currier, N. L., "Echinacea purpurea and melatonin augment natural-killer cells in leukemic mice and prolong life span."

Degelau, J., et al. "The effect of DHEAs on influenza vaccination in aging adults." *J Am Geriatr Soc.* 1997; 45 (6): 747–51.

Diallo, K., et al. "Inhibition of human immunodeficiency virus type-1 (HIV-1) replication by immunor (IM28), a new analog of dehydroepiandrosterone." *Nucleosides Nucleotides Nucleic Acids.* 2000; 19 (10–12): 2019–24.

Dougherty, T. F., et al. "Pituitary-adrenal cortical control of antibody release from lymphocytes. An explanation of the anamnestic response." *Proc Soc Exper Biol Med.* 1945; 58: 135–40.

Ferrando, S. J., et al. "Dehydroepiandrosterone sulfate (DHEAs) and testosterone: relation to HIV illness stage and progression over one year." *J Acquir Immune Defic Syndr.* 1999; 22 (2): 146–54.

Freudenheim, J. L., et al. "Premenopausal breast cancer risk and intake of vegetables, fruits and related nutrients." *J Natl Cancer Inst.* 1996; 88: 340–48.

Fuyns, A. "Alcohol and cancer." *Proc Nutr Soc.* 1990; 49: 145–51.

Garro, A., et al. "Alcohol and Cancer." *Ann Rev Pharmacol Toxicol.* 1990; 30: 219–49.

Golditz, G. A., et al. "Increased green and yellow vegetable intake and lowered cancer deaths in an elderly population." *Am J Clin Nutr.* 1985; 41 (1): 326.

Grinspoon, S., et al. "Body composition and endocrine function in women with acquired immunodeficiency syndrome wasting." *J Clin Endocrinol Metab.* 1997; 82 (5): 1332–37.

Grunfeld, C., et al. "Indices of thyroid function and weight loss in human immunodeficiency virus infection and the acquired immunodeficiency syndrome." *Metabolism.* 1993; 42 (10): 1270–76.

Hashimoto, H., et al. "The relationship between serum levels of interleukin-6 and thyroid hormone in children with acute respiratory infection." *J Clin Endocrinol Metab.* 1994; 78 (2): 288–91.

Hurter, T., et al. "Fibrosing alveolitis responsive to corticosteroids following legionnaires' disease pneumonia." *Chest.* 1992; 101 (1): 281–83.

Inagaki, N., et al. "Drugs for the treatment of allergic diseases." *Jpn J Pharmacol.* 2001; 86 (3): 275–80. Review.

Johnson, B. E., et al. "Effect of triiodothyronine on the expression of T cell markers and immune function in thyroidectomized White Leghorn chickens." *Proc Soc Exp Biol Med.* 1992; 199 (1): 104–13.

Kai, O., et al. "Effects of hypothyroidism with treatment of an anti-thyroid drug, propylthiouracil, on immune responses in chickens." *Vet Immunol Immunopathol.* 1993; 36 (2): 123–35.

Kass, E. H., et al. "Corticosteroids and infections." *Afr Intern Med.* 1958; 9: 45–80.

Kass, E. H., et al. "Effects of adrenocorticotropic hormone in pneumonia: clinical, bacteriological and serological studies." *Ann Intern Med.* 1950; 33: 1081–98.

Khorram, O., et al. "Activation of immune function by dehydroepiandrosterone (DHEA) in age-advanced men." *J Gerontol A Biol Sci Med Sci.* 1997; 52 (1): M1–7.

Knoferl, M. W., et al. "17 beta-estradiol normalizes immuno responses in ovariectomized females after trauma-hemorrhage." *J Physiol Cell Physiol.* 2000; 279 (6): 2004–10.

Kossoy, G., et al. "Melatonin and colon carcinogenesis. IV. Effect of melatonin on proliferative activity and expression of apoptosis-related proteins in the spleen of rats exposed to 1,2-dimethylhydrazine." *Oncol Rep.* 2000; 7 (6): 1401–5.

Krause, D., et al. "Immune function did not decline with aging in apparently healthy, well-nourished women." *Mech Ageing Dev.* 1999; 112 (1): 43–57.

Lockwood, K., et al. "Partial and complete regression of breast cancer in patients in relation to dosage of coenzyme Q_{10}." *Biochem Biophys Res Commun.* 1994; 199 (3): 1504–8.

Lockwood, K., et al. "Progress on therapy of breast cancer with vitamin Q_{10} and the regression of metastases." *Biochem Biophys Res Commun.* 1995; 212 (1): 172.

Lomo, P. O., et al. "Respiratory activity of isolated liver Mitochondria following Trypanosoma congolense infection in rabbits: the role of thyroxine." *Com Biochem Physiol B.* 1993; 104 (1): 187–91.

Lu, W., et al. "Glucocorticoids rescue CD4+ T lymphocytes from activation-induced apoptosis triggered by HIV-1: implications for pathogenesis and therapy." *AIDS.* 1995; 9 (1): 35–42.

Lurie, M. B., et al. "On the role of the thyroid in native resistance to tuberculosis I. Effect of hyperthyroidism. Il. Effect of hypothyroidism. The mode of action of thyroid hormones." *Am Rev Tuberc.* 1959; 79: 152–203.

Maestroni, G. J. "The immunotherapeutic potential of melatonin." *Expert Opin Investig Drugs.* 2001; 10 (3): 467–76.

Maestroni, G. J. "Therapeutic potential of melatonin in immunodeficiency states, viral diseases, and cancer." *Adv Exp Med Biol.* 1999; 467: 217–26.

Mateiko, G. B., et al. "The efficacy of the hormonal substitute therapy of adolescents with viral hepatitis A combined with thyroid hypofunction." *Vrach Delo.* 1990; (8): 101–2.

Merle, M., et al. "Value of corticosteroids in bacterial meningitis." *Presse Med.* 1992; 21 (25): 1160–64.

Messina, M., et al. "The role of soy products in reducing the risk of cancer." *J Natl Cancer Inst.* 1991; 83: 541–46.

Norton, S. D., et al. "Administration of dehydroepiandrosterone sulfate retards onset but not progression of autoimmune disease in NZB/W mice." *Autoimmunity.* 1997; 26 (3): 161–71.

Offiah, V. N., et al. "Effects of Ehrlichia phagocytophila infection on serum thyroid hormone concentrations and on antipyrine clearance and metabolite formation in dwarf goats." *Am J Vet Res.* 1992; 53 (8): 1357–60.

Ogwu, D., et al. "Adrenal and thyroid dysfunctions in experimental Trypanosoma congolense infection in cattle." *Vet Parasitol.* 1992; 42 (1–2): 15–26.

Olivieri, A., et al. "Thyroid hypo-function related with the progression of human immunodeficiency virus infection." *J Endocrinol Invest.* 1993; 16 (6): 407–13.

Panfilov, I. A., et al. "Disorders in the hypophysis-adrenal and hypophysis-thyroid systems of patients with acute pneumonia and the ways for their therapeutic correction." *Ter Arkh.* 1990; 62 (3): 19–22.

Plaza de los Reyes, M., et al. "Influenzal pneumonia treated with cortisone and antibiotics." *Lancet.* ii, 1957; 845, 1122.

Porter, V. R., et al. "Immune effects of hormone replacement therapy in post-menopausal women." *Exp Gerontol.* 2001; 36 (2): 311–26.

Reiter, R. J., et al. *Ann NY Acad Sci.* 2000; 917: 376–86.

Rotem, C. E. "Influenzal pneumonia treated with cortisone and antibiotics." *Lancet.* ii, 1957; 948.

Rupp, M. E., et al. "Measles pneumonia. Treatment of a near-fatal case with corticosteroids and vitamin A." *Chest.* 1993; 103 (5): 1625–26.

Smadel, J. E., et al. "Treatment of typhoid fever; combined therapy with cortisone and chloramphenicol." *Ann Intern Med.* 1951; 34: 1–9.

Smith, Y. R., et al. "Long-term estrogen replacement is associated with improved nonverbal memory and attentional measures in postmenopausal women." *Fertil Steril.* 2001; 76 (6): 1101–7.

Thorn, G. W., et al. "Pharmacologic aspects of adrenocortical steroids and ACTH in man." *N Engl J Med.* 1953; 248: 232–45, 284–94, 323–37, 369–78, 414–23, 588–601, 632–46.

Tomer, Y., et al. "Infection, thyroid disease, and autoimmunity." *Endocr Rev.* 1993; 14 (1): 107–20.

Utiger, R. D. "Decreased extrathyroidal triiodothyronine production in non-thyroidal illness: benefit or harm?" *Am J Med.* 1980; 69: 807–10.

Veldhuis, J. D. "Fasting decreased mean 24h serum TSH in men." *J Clin Endocrinol Metab.* 1993; 76 (3): 587–93.

Venarucci, D., et al. "Evaluation of certain immunity parameters in rheumatoid arthritis treated with cortisone." *Panminerva Med.* 1994; 36 (4): 188–91.

Wallgren, P., et al. "Influence of experimentally induced endogenous production of cortisol on the immune capacity in swine." *Vet Immunol Immunopathol.* 1994; 42 (3–4): 301–16.

Weitzman, S., et al. "Clinical trial design in studies of corticosteroids in bacterial infections." *Ann Intern Med.* 1974; 81: 36–42.

Woodward, T. E., et al. "Treatment of typhoid fever: control of clinical manifestations with cortisone." *Ann Intern Med.* 1951; 34: 10–19.

Wu, C. Y., et al. "Glucocorticoids increase the synthesis of immunoglobulin E by interleukin 4 stimulated human lymphocytes." *J Clin Invest.* 1991; 87 (3): 870–77.

Zhang, Z., et al. "Prevention of immune dysfunction and vitamin E loss by dehydroepiandrosterone and melatonin supplementation during murine retrovirus infection." *Immunology.* 1999; 96 (2): 291–97.

Cancer

Adami, H. O., et al. "The effect of female sex hormones on cancer survival." *JAMA.* 1990; 263 (16): 2189–93.

Adami, H. O., et al. "Survival and age at diagnosis in breast cancer." *N Engl J Med.* 1987; 316: 752.

Adunsky, A., et al. "Corticosteroids in terminal cancer." *Harefuah.* 1995; 128 (5): 278–80, 335.

Akumabor, P. N. "Is pre-treatment testosterone a prognostic factor in prostate cancer?" *Cent Afr J Med.* 1993; 39 (8): 170–72.

Alberg, A. J., et al. "Serum dehydroepiandrosterone and dehydroepiandrosterone sulfate and the subsequent risk of developing colon cancer." *Cancer Epidemiol Biomarkers Prev.* 2000; 9 (5): 517–21.

Alexander, D. B., et al. "Glucocorticoids coordinately disrupt a transforming growth factor alpha autocrine loop and suppress the growth of 13762NF-derived Con8 rat mammary adenocarcinoma cells." *Cancer Res.* 1993; 53 (8): 1808–15.

Ambali, A. G., et al. "The effects of oestrogen and progesterone on re-excretion of infectious bronchitis virus strain in SPF chickens." *J Hyg Epidemiol Microbiol Immunol.* 1991; 35 (4): 429–39.

Badwe, R. A., et al. "Serum progesterone at the time of surgery and survival in women with premenopausal operable breast cancer." *Eur J Cancer.* 1994; 30A (4): 445–48.

Barni, S., et al. "A randomized study of low-dose subcutaneous interleukin-2 plus melatonin versus supportive care alone in metastatic colorectal cancer patients progressing under 5-fluorouracil and folates." *Oncology.* 1995; 52 (3): 243–45.

Bartsch, C., et al. "Melatonin in cancer patients and in tumor-bearing animals." *Adv Exp Med Biol.* 1999; 467: 247–64.

Bezwoda, W. R. "Treatment of stage D2 prostatic cancer refractory to or relapsed following castration plus oestrogens. Comparison of aminoglutethimide plus hydrocortisone with medroxyprogesterone acetate plus hydrocortisone." *Br J Urol.* 1990; 66 (2): 196–201.

Bogardus, G. M., et al. "Breast cancer and thyroid disease." *Surgery.* 1961; 49 (4): 461–68.

Boman, K., et al. "The influence of progesterone and androgens on the growth of endometrial carcinoma." *Cancer.* 1993; 71 (11): 3565–69.

Bonneterre, J., et al. "Aminoglutethimide (AG) and hydrocortisone (HC) in bone metastases: a retrospective study." *J Steroid Biochem Mol Biol.* 1993; 44 (4–6): 693–96.

Bourinbaiar, A. S., et al. "Pregnancy hormones, estrogen and progesterone, prevent HIV-1 synthesis in monocytes but not in lymphocytes." *Febs Lett.* 1992; 302 (3): 206–8.

Bulbrook, R. D., et al. "Abnormal excretion of urinary steroids by women with early breast cancer." *Lancet.* 1962; 1238–40.

Burton, J. L., et al. "Immune responses of growing beef steers treated with estrogen/progesterone implants or insulin injections." *Domest Anim Endocrinol.* 1993; 10 (1): 31–44.

Cameron, E. H. D., et al. "Benign and malignant breast disease in South Wales: a study of urinary steroids." *B Med J.* 1990; 768–71.

Chen, L. D., et al. "Melatonin's inhibitory effect on growth of ME-180 human cervical cancer cells is not related to intracellular glutathione concentrations." *Cancer Lett.* 1995; 91 (2): 153–59.

Comstock, G. W. "The relationship of serum dehydroepiandrosterone and its sulfate to subsequent cancer of the prostate." *Cancer Epidemiol Biomarkers Prev.* 1993; 2 (3): 219–21.

Cos, S., et al. "Influence of melatonin on invasive and metastatic properties of MCF-7 human breast cancer cells." *Cancer Res.* 1998; 58 (19): 4383–90.

Cos, S., et al. "Melatonin modulates growth factor activity in MCF-7 human breast cancer cells." *J Pineal Res.* 1994; 17 (1): 25–32.

Cowan, L. D., et al. "Breast cancer incidence in women with a history of progesterone deficiency." *Am J Epidemiol.* 1981; 114 (2): 209–17.

Davellaar, E. M., et al. "No increase in the incidence of breast carcinoma with subcutaneous administration of estradiol." *Ned Tijdsch Geneeskd.* 1991; 135 (14): 613–15.

De Peretti, E., et al. "Unconjugated dehydroepiandrosterone plasma levels in normal subjects from birth to adolescence in human: the use of a sensitive radioimmunoassay." *J Clin Endocrinol Metab.* 1976; 43 (5): 982–91.

Defares interview. *Privé magazine* (Nederland), January 1, 1995.

Ding, C. H., et al. "Effects of pineal body and melatonin on lymphocyte proliferation and dinoprostone production in rat spleen." *Chung Kuo Yao Li Hsueh Pao.* 1995; 16 (1): 54–57.

Edwards, C. K., et al. "In vivo administration of recombinant growth hormone or gamma interferon activities macrophages: enhanced resistance to experimental Salmonella typhimurium infection is correlated with generation of reactive oxygen intermediates." *Infect Immun.* 1992; 60 (6): 2514–21.

El-Atiq, F., et al. "Alterations in serum levels of insulin-like growth factors and insulin-like growth-factor-binding proteins in patients with colorectal cancer." *Int J Cancer.* 1994; 57 (4): 491–97.

Everilt, A., et al. "Aging and anti-aging effects of hormones." *J Gerontol.* 1989: B139–47.

Finkle, W. D., et al. "Endometrial cancer risk after discontinuing use of unopposed conjugated estrogens." *Cancer Causes Control.* 1995; 6 (2): 99–102.

Fleming, M. W., et al. "Consequences of dose-dependent immunosuppression by progesterone on parasitic worm burdens in lambs." *Am J Vet Res.* 1993; 54 (8): 1299–302.

Gambrell, R. D., Jr., et al. "Decreased incidence of breast cancer in postmenopausal estrogen-progestogen users." *Obstet Gynecol.* 1983; 62 (4): 435–43.

Gambrell, R. D., Jr. "Hormones in the etiology and prevention of breast and endometrial cancer." *South Med J.* 1984; 77 (12): 1509–15.

Gordon, G. B. "Relationship of serum levels of DHEA and DHEAs to the risk of developing postmenopausal breast cancer." *Cancer Res.* 1990; 50: 3859–62.

Hanna, N., et al. "Enhancement of tumor metastases and suppression of natural killer cell activity by beta-estradiol treatment." *J Immunol.* 1983; 130: 974–80.

Herrinton, L. J., et al. "Postmenopausal unopposed estrogens. Characteristics of use in relation to the risk of endometrial carcinoma." *Ann Epidemiol.* 1993; 3 (3): 308–18.

Hrushesky, W. J. M., et al. "Natural killer cell activity: age, estrous- and circadian-stage dependence and inverse correlation with metastatic potential." *JNCI.* 1988; 80: 1232–37.

Huang, K. F., et al. "Insulin-like growth factor 1 (IGF-1) reduces gut atrophy and bacterial trans-location after severe burn injury." *Arch Surg.* 1993; 128 (1): 47–53; discussion 53–54.

Iversen, P., et al. "Serum testosterone as a prognostic factor in patients with advanced prostatic carcinoma." *Scand J Urol Nephrol Suppl.* 1994; 157: 41–47.

Jardieu, P., et al. "In vivo administration of insulin-like growth factor-I stimulates primary B lymphopoiesis and enhances lymphocyte recovery after bone marrow transplantation." *J Immunol.* 1994; 152 (9): 4320–27.

Jick, S. S., et al. "Estrogens, progesterone, and endometrial cancer." *Epidemiology.* 1993; 4 (1): 20–24.

Karasek, M., et al. "Pineal gland, melatonin and cancer." *Neuroendocrinol Lett.* 1999; 20 (3–4): 139–44.

Karasek, M., et al. "Serial transplants of 7,12-dimethylbens(a)antraceneinduced mammary tumor in Fischer rats as model system for human breast cancer. 3. Quantitative ultrastructural studies of the pinealocytes and plasma melatonin concentration in rats bearing an advanced passage of the tumor." *Biol Signals.* 1994; 3 (6): 302–6.

Knyszynski, A., et al. "Effects of growth hormone on thymocyte development from progenitor cells in the bone marrow." *Brain Behav Immun.* 1992; 6 (4): 327–40.

Korth-Schutz, S. "Evidence for the adrenal source of androgens in precocious adrenarche." *Acta Endocrinol (Copenh).* 1976; 82: 342–52.

Kossoy, G., et al. "Melatonin and colon carcinogenesis. IV. Effect of melatonin on proliferative activity and expression of apoptosis-related proteins in the spleen of rats exposed to 1,2-dimethylhydrazine." *Oncol Rep.* 2000; 7 (6): 1401–5.

Krentz, A. J., et al. "Anthropometric, metabolic, and immunological effects of recombinant human growth hormone in AIDS and AIDS-related complex." *J Acquir Immune Defic Syndr.* 1993; 6 (3): 245–51.

Kudsk, K. A., et al. "Effect of recombinant human insulin-like growth factor I and early total parenteral nutrition on immune depression following severe head injury." *Arch Surg.* 1994; 129 (1): 66–70; discussion 70–71.

Kumar, C. A., et al. "Effect of melatonin on two-stage skin carcinogenesis in Swiss mice." *Med Sci Monit.* 2000; 6 (3): 471–75.

Laffargue, F., et al. "Estrogens, progestins and cancer of the endometrium." *Rev Prat.* 1993; 43 (20): 2603–9.

Lauritzen, C., et al. "Risks of endometrial and mammary cancer morbidity and mortality in long-term estrogen treatment." In van Herendael, H., et al. *The Climacteric—An Update.* Lancaster, England: MTP Press Ltd, 1984; 207.

Li, S., et al. "Inhibitory effects of medroxyprogesterone acetate (MPA) and the pure antiestrogen EM-219 on estrone EJ-stimulated growth of dimethylbenz(a) anthracece (DMBA)-induced mammary carcinoma in the rat." *Breast Cancer Res Treat.* 1995; 34 (2): 147–59.

Liechty, R. D., et al. "Cancer and thyroid function." *JAMA.* 1963; 183 (1): 116–18.

Lissoni, P., et al. "Amplification of eosinophilia by melatonin during the immunotherapy of cancer with interleukin-2." *J Biol Regul Homeost Agents.* 1993; 7 (1): 34–36.

Lissoni, P., et al. "Dehydroepiandrosterone sulfate (DHEAs) secretion in early and advanced solid neoplasms: selective deficiency in metastatic disease." *Int J Biol Markers.* 1998; 13 (3): 154–57.

Lissoni, P., et al. "Immunoendocrine therapy with low-dose subcutaneous interleukin-2 plus melatonin of locally advanced or metastatic endocrine tumors." *Oncology.* 1995; 52 (2): 163–66.

Lissoni, P., et al. "Oncostatic activity of pineal neuroendocrine treatment with the pineal indoles melatonin and 5-methoxytryptamine in untreatable metastatic cancer patients progressing on melatonin alone." *Neuroendocrinol Lett.* 2000; 21 (4): 319–23.

Lissoni, P., et al. "A randomized study of chemotherapy with cisplatin plus etoposide versus chemoendocrine therapy with cisplatin, etoposide and the pineal hormone melatonin as a first-line treatment of advanced non-small-cell lung cancer patients in a poor clinical state." *J Pineal Res.* 1997; 23 (1): 15–19.

Lissoni, P., et al. "A randomized study of immunotherapy with low-dose subcutaneous interleukin-2 plus melatonin vs. chemotherapy with cisplatin and etoposide as first-line therapy for advanced non-small-cell lung cancer." *Tumori.* 1994; 80 (6): 464–67.

Lundgren, S., et al. "Influence of progestins on serum hormone levels in postmenopausal women with advanced breast cancer -II. A differential effect of megestrol acetate and medroxyprogesterone acetate on serum estrone sulfate and sex hormone binding globulin." *J Steroid Biochem.* 1990; 36 (1–2): 105–9.

Luo, S., et al. "Combined effects of dehydroepiandrosterone and EM-800 on bone mass, serum lipids, and the development of dimethylbenz(A)anthracene-induced mammary carcinoma in the rat." *Endocrinology.* 1997; 138 (10): 4435–44.

Ly, L. P., et al. "A double-blind, placebo-controlled, randomized clinical trial of transdermal dihydrotestosterone gel on muscular strength, mobility, and quality of life in older men with partial androgen deficiency." *J Clin Endocrinol Metab.* 2001; 86 (9): 4078–88.

M cikova-Kalicka, K., et al. "Preventive effect of indomethacin and melatonin on 7,12-dimethybenz/a/anthracene-induced mammary carcinogenesis in female Sprague-Dawley rats." A preliminary report. *Folia Biol (Praha).* 2001; 47 (2): 75–79.

Maestroni, G. J. "T-helper-2 lymphocytes as a peripheral target of melatonin." *J Pineal Res.* 1995; 18 (2): 84–89.

Maestroni, G. J. "Therapeutic potential of melatonin in immunodeficiency states, viral diseases, and cancer." *Adv Exp Med Biol.* 1999; 467: 217–26.

Maestroni, G. J., et al. "Hematopoietic rescue via T-cell-dependent, endogenous granulocyte-macrophage colony-stimulating factor induced by the pineal neurohormone melatonin in tumor-bearing mice." *Cancer Res.* 1994; 54 (9): 2429–32.

Mantes, L. F., et al. "Chronic mucocutaneous candidiasis. Influence of thyroid status." *JAMA.* 1972; 221 (2): 156–59.

Marsh, J. A., et al. "Effect of thyroxine and chicken growth hormone on immune function in autoimmune thyroiditis (obese) strain chicks." *Proc Soc Exp Biol Med.* 1992; 199 (1): 114–22.

McCormick, D. L., et al. "Exceptional chemopreventive activity of low-dose dehydroepiandrosterone in the rat mammary gland." *Cancer Res.* 1996; 56 (8): 1724–26.

McCormick, D. L., et al. "Chemoprevention of hormone-dependent prostate cancer in the Wistar-Unilever rat." *Eur Urol.* 1999; 35 (5–6): 464–67.

Mellemgaard, A., et al. "Cancer risk in individuals with benign thyroid disorders." *Thyroid.* 1998; 8 (9): 751–54.

Melvin, W. S., et al. "Dehydroepiandrosterone-sulfate inhibits pancreatic carcinoma cell proliferation in vitro and in vivo." *Surgery.* 1997; 121 (4): 392–97.

Mendenhall, C. L., et al. "Anabolic steroid effects on immune function: differences between analogues." *J Steroid Biochem Mol Biol.* 1990; 37 (1): 71–76.

Mocchegiani, E., et al. "The immuno-reconstituting effect of melatonin or pineal grafting and its relation to zinc pool in aging mice." *J Neuroimmunol.* 1994; 53 (2): 189–201.

Moore, M. A. "Modifying influence of DHEA on the development of dihydroxy-di-n-propyl-nitrosamine-initiated lesions in the thyroid, lung and liver of F344 rats." *Carcinogenesis.* 1986; 7: 311.

Morabia, A., et al. "Thyroid hormones and duration of ovulatory activity in the etiology of breast cancer." *Cancer Epidemiol Biomakers Prev.* 1992; 1 (5): 389–93.

Morales, A., et al. "Androgen therapy in advanced carcinoma of the prostate." *CMA Journal.* 1971; 105: 71–72.

Nachtigall, L. E., et al. "Estrogen replacement II: A prospective study in the relationship to carcinoma and cardiovascular and metabolic problems." *Obstet Gynecol.* 1979; 54: 74.

Ng, E. H., et al. "Insulin-like growth factor I preserves host lean tissue mass in cancer cachexia." *Am J Physiol.* 1992; 262 (3 Pt 2): R426–31.

Nyce, J. W., et al. "Inhibition of 1,2-dimethylhydrazine-induced colon tumorigenesis in Balb/c mice by dehydroepiandrosterone." *Carcinogenesis.* 1984; 5 (1): 57–62.

Orner, G. A., et al. "Modulation of aflatoxin-B1 hepatocarcinogenesis in trout by dehydroepiandrosterone: initiation/post-initiation and latency effects." *Carcinogenesis.* 1998; 19 (1): 161–67.

Otesile, E. B., et al. "The effect of Trypanosoma brucei infection on serum biochemical parameters in boars on different planes of dietary energy." *Vet Parasitol.* 1991; 40 (3–4): 207–16.

Pedersen-Bjergaard, K., et al. "Sex hormone analyses. II. The excretion of sexual hormones by normal males, impotent males, polyarthritics, and prostatics." *Acta Med Scand.* 1948; 213: 284–97.

Peters, G. N., et al. "Estrogen replacement therapy after breast cancer: a 12-year follow-up." *Ann Surg Oncol.* 2001; 8 (10): 828–32.

Pierpaoli, W. "Pineal grafting and melatonin induce immuno-competence in nude (athymic) mice." *Int J Neurosci.* 1993; 68 (1–2): 123–31.

Rao, K. V., et al. "Chemoprevention of rat prostate carcinogenesis by early and delayed administration of dehydroepiandrosterone." *Cancer Res.* 1999; 59 (13): 3084–89.

Rao, M. S., et al. "Inhibition of spontaneous testicular Leydig cell tumor development in F-344 rats by dehydroepiandrosterone." *Cancer Lett.* 1992; 65 (2): 123–26.

Rasmussen, K. R., et al. "Dehydroepiandrosterone-induced reduction of Cryptosporidium parvum infections in aged Syrian golden hamsters." *J Parasitol.* 1992; 78 (3): 554–57.

Reiter, R. J., et al. "Melatonin and its relation to the immune system and inflammation." *Ann NY Acad Sci.* 2000; 917: 376–86.

Requintina, P. J., et al. "Synergistic sedative effect of selective MAO-A, but not MAO-B, inhibitors and melatonin in frogs." *J Neural Transm Suppl.* 1994; 41: 141–44.

Reynard, J. M., et al. "Prostate-specific antigen and prognosis in patients with metastatic prostate cancer—a multivariable analysis of prostate cancer mortality. *Br J Urol.* 1995; 75 (4): 507–15.

Rosenfeld, R. S., et al. "Metabolism and interconversion of dehydroisoandrosterone and dehydroisoandrosterone sulfate." *J Clin Endocrinol Metab.* 1972; 35 (2): 187–93.

Rutanen, E. M., et al. "Relationship between carbohydrate metabolism and serum insulin-like growth factor system in postmenopausal women: comparison of endometrial cancer patients with healthy controls." *J Clin Endocrinol Metab.* 1993; 77 (1): 199–204.

Schatzl, G., et al. "Endocrine patterns in patients with benign and malignant prostatic diseases." *Prostate.* 2000; 44 (3): 219–24.

Schatzl, G., et al. "Endocrine status in elderly men with lower urinary tract symptoms: correlation of age, hormonal status, and lower urinary tract function. The Prostate Study Group of the Austrian Society of Urology." *Urology.* 2000; 55 (3): 397–402.

Schwartz, A. G., et al. "Protective effect of DHEA against aflatoxin B1- and 7,12-dimethylbenzaantracene-induced cytotoxicity and transformation in cultured cells." *Cancer Res.* 1975; 35: 2482–87.

Schwartz, S. B. S. "The relationship of thyroid deficiency to cancer: a 50-year retrospective study." *J IAPM* 1977; VI (1): 9–21.

Screpanti, I., et al. "Estrogen and antiestrogen modulation of the levels of mouse natural killer activity and large granula lymphocytes." *Cell Immunol.* 1987; 106: 191–202.

Shao, Z. M., et al. "Thyroid hormone enhancement of estradiol stimulation of breast carcinoma proliferation." *Exp Cell Res.* 1995; 218 (1): 1–8.

Shelton, B. K. "Hypothyroidism in cancer patients." *Nurse Pract Forum.* 1998; 9 (3): 185–91.

Slotman, B. J., et al. "Survival of patients with ovarian cancer. Apart from stage and grade, tumor progesterone receptor content is a prognostic indicator." *Cancer.* 1990; 66 (4): 740–44.

Spencer, J. G. "Influence of thyroid deficient disease in malignancy." *Br J Cancer.* 1954; 8: 393.

Suzuki, H., et al. "Inhibition of growth and increase of acid phosphatase by testosterone on androgen-independent murine prostatic cancer cells transfected with androgen receptor cDNA." *Prostate.* 1994; 25 (6): 310–19.

Thomas, J. L., et al. "Behaviour of thyroid tissue from patients with Graves' disease in nude mice." *J Clin Endocrinol Metab.* 1984; 59 (1): 175–77.

Twycross, R. "The risks and benefits of corticosteroids in advanced cancer." *Drug Saf.* 1994; 11 (3): 163–78.

Tymchuk, C. N., et al. "Evidence of an inhibitory effect of diet and exercise on prostate cancer cell growth." *J Urol.* 2001; 166 (3): 1185–89.

Van Weerden, W. M., et al. "Effect of adrenal androgens on the transplantable human prostate tumor." *Endocrinology.* 1992; 131 (6): 2909–13.

Verges, B., et al. "Endocrine abnormalities in HIV infections." *Presse Med.* 1990; 19 (27): 1267–70.

Vijayalaxmi, et al. "Melatonin protects human blood lymphocytes from radiation-induced chromosome damage." *Mutat Res.* 1995; 346 (1): 23–31.

Villette, J. M., et al. "Circadian variations in plasma levels of hypophyseal, adrenocortical and testicular hormones in men infected with human immunodeficiency virus." *J Clin Endocrinol Metab.* 1990; 70 (3): 572–77.

White, A. "Influence of endocrine secretions on the structure and function of lymphoid tissue." *Harvey Lectures Ser.* Springfield, Illinois: Thomas, 1947–48; 43: 43–70.

Wingo, P. A., et al. "The risk of breast cancer in postmenopausal women who have used estrogen replacement therapy." (Published erratum appears in *JAMA.* 1987; 257 [18]: 2438.) *JAMA.* 1987; 257 (2): 209–15.

Wise, T., et al. "Effects of neonatal sexual differentiation, growth hormone and testosterone on thymic weights and thymosin-beta 4 in hypophysectomized rats." *J Reprod Immunol.* 1991; 19 (1): 43–54.

Wolf, D. A., et al. "Synthetic androgens suppress the transformed phenotype in human prostate carcinoma cell line LNCaP." *Br J Cancer.* 1991; 64 (1): 47–53.

Wolf, R. F., et al. "Growth hormone and insulin reverse net whole body and skeletal muscle protein catabolism in cancer patients." *Ann Surg.* 1992; 216 (3): 280–88; discussion 288–90.

Ying, S. W., et al. "Human malignant melanoma cells express high-affinity receptors for melatonin: antiproliferative effects of melatonin and 6-chloromelatonin." *Eur J Pharmacol.* 1993; 246 (2): 89–96.

Yonei, Y., et al. "Primary hepatocellular carcinoma with severe hypoglycemia: involvement of insulin-like growth factors." *Liver.* 1992; 12 (2): 90–93.

CHAPTER 11. SUPER SEX (NO VIAGRA NECESSARY)

Alexander, G. M., et al. "Androgen-behavior correlations in hypogonadal men and eugonadal men. I. Mood and response to auditory sexual stimuli." *Horm Behav.* 1997; 31 (2): 110–19.

Arvers, S., et al. "Improvement of sexual function in testosterone deficient men treated for 1 year with a permeation enhanced testosterone transdermal system." *J Urol.* 1996; 155 (5): 1604–8.

Blache, D., et al. "Inhibition of sexual behaviour and the luteinizing hormone surge by intracerebral progesterone implants in the female sheep." *Brain Res.* 1996; 741 (1–2): 117–22.

Casson, P. R., et al. "Dehydroepiandrosterone supplementation augments ovarian stimulation in poor responders: a case series." *Hum Reprod.* 2000; 15 (10): 2129–32.

Dabbs, J. M. Jr. "Testosterone and pupillary response to auditory sexual stimuli." *Physiol Behav.* 1997; 62 (4): 909–12.

Davis, S. R. "The clinical use of androgens in female sexual disorders." *J Sex Marital Ther.* 1998; 24 (3): 153–63.

Dudley, R. E., et al. "Comparative pharmacokinetics of three doses of per-cutaneous dihydrotestosterone gel in healthy elderly men—a clinical research center study." *J Clin Endocrinol Metab.* 1998; 83 (8): 2749–57.

Guay, A. T. "Decreased testosterone in regularly menstruating women with decreased libido: a clinical observation." *J Sex Marital Ther.* 2001; 27 (5): 513–19.

Halpern, C. T., et al. "Monthly measures of salivary testosterone predict sexual activity in adolescent males." *Arch Sex Behav.* 1998; 27 (5): 445–65.

Kapicioglu, S., et al. "Inhibition of penile erection in rats by a long-acting somatostatin analogue, octreotide (SMS 201–995)." *Br J Urol.* 1998; 81 (1): 142–45.

Karabelyos, C., et al. "Effect of neonatal triiodothyronine (T_3) treatment (hormonal imprinting) on the sexual behavior of adult rats." *Acta Physiol Hung.* 1997–98; 85 (1): 11–15.

Keast, Jr., et al. "Testosterone has potent, selective effects on the morphology of pelvic autonomic neurons which control the bladder, lower bowel and internal reproductive organs of the male rat." *Neuroscience.* 1998; 85 (2): 543–56.

Mani, S. K., et al. "Dopamine requires the unoccupied progesterone receptor to induce sexual behavior in mice" (Published erratum appears in *Mol Endocrinol.* 1997; 11 (4): 423). *Mol Endocrinol.* 1996; 10 (12): 1728–37.

Meston, C. M., et al. "The neurobiology of sexual function." *Arch Gen Psychiatry.* 2000; 57 (11): 1012–30.

Mills, T. M., et al. "Androgenic maintenance of inflow and veno-occlusion during erection in the rat." *Biol Reprod.* 1998; 59 (6): 1413–18.

Mills, T. M., et al. "Androgens and penile erection: a review." *J Androl.* 1996; 17 (6): 633–38.

Nishihara, M., et al. "Different female reproductive phenotypes determined by human growth hormone (hGH) levels in hGH-transgenetic rats." *Biol Reprod.* 1997; 56 (4): 847–51.

Penson, D. F., et al. "Androgen and pituitary control of penile nitric oxide synthase and erectile function in the rat." *Biol Reprod.* 1996; 55 (3): 567–74.

Rakic, Z., et al. "Testosterone treatment in men with erectile disorder and low levels of total testosterone in serum." *Arch Sex Behav.* 1997; 26 (5): 495–504.

Reilly, C. M., et al. "Androgenic regulation of NO availability in rat penile erection." *J Androl.* 1997; 18 (2): 110–15.

Reiter, W. J., et al. "Dehydroepiandrosterone in the treatment of erectile dysfunction: a prospective, double-blind, randomized, placebo-controlled study." *Urology.* 1999; 53 (3): 590–94; discussion 594–95.

Reiter, W. J., et al. "Placebo-controlled dihydroepiandrosterone substitution in elderly men." *Gynakol Geburtshilfliche Rundsch.* 1999; 39 (4): 208–9.

Reiter, W. J., et al. "Serum dehydroepiandrosterone sulfate concentrations in men with erectile dysfunction." *Urology.* 2000; 55 (5): 755–58.

Riters, L. V., et al. "Effects of brain testosterone implants on appetitive and consummatory components of male sexual behavior in Japanese quail." *Brain Res Bull.* 1998; 47 (1): 69–79.

Roberts, R. L., et al. "Sexual differentiation in prairie voles: the effects of corticosterone and testosterone." *Physiol Behav.* 1997; 62 (6): 1379–83.

Sarrel, P., et al. "Estrogen and estrogen-androgen replacement in post-menopausal women dissatisfied with estrogen-only therapy. Sexual behavior and neuroendocrine responses." *J Reprod Med.* 1998; 43 (10): 847–56.

Sarrel, P. M. "Ovarian hormones and vaginal blood flow: using laser Doppler velocimetry to measure effects in a clinical trial of post-menopausal women." *Int J Impot Res.* 1998; 10 (Suppl 2): S91–93; discussion S98–101.

Sarrel, P. M. "Psychosexual effects of menopause: role of androgens." *Am J Obstet Gynecol.* 1999; 180 (3 Pt 2): S319–24.

Sato, Y., et al. "Restoration of sexual behavior and dopaminergic neurotransmission by long-term exogenous testosterone replacement in aged male rats." *J Urol.* 1998; 160 (4): 1572–75.

Shabsigh, R. "The effects of testosterone on the cavernous tissue and erectile function." *World J Urol.* 1997; 15 (1): 21–26.

Szczypka, M. S., et al. "Dopamine-stimulated sexual behavior is testosterone dependent in mice." *Behav Neurosci.* 1998; 112 (5): 1229–35.

Tutten, A., et al. "Discrepancies between genital responses and subjective sexual function during testosterone substitution in women with hypothalamic amenorrhea." *Psychosom Med.* 1996; 58 (3): 234–41.

Van Goozen, Z. H., et al. "Psychoendocrinological assessment of the menstrual cycle: the relationship between hormones, sexuality, and mood." *Arch Sex Behav.* 1997; 26 (4): 359–82.

Velasquez-Urzola, A. "Hypoplasia of the penis: etiologic diagnosis and results of treatment with delayed-action testosterone." *Arch Pediatr.* 1998; 5 (8): 844–50.

Wang, C., et al. "Transdermal testosterone gel improves sexual function, mood, muscle strength, and body composition parameters in hypogonadal men." *J Clin Endocrinol Metab.* 2000; 85 (8): 2839–53.

Wu, S. C., et al. "Influence of erythropoietin treatment on gonadotropic hormone levels and sexual function in male uremic patients." *Scand J Urol Nephrol.* 2001; 35 (2): 136–40.

Yang, S., et al. "Sexual dimorphism in secretion of hypothalamic gonadotropin-releasing hormone and norepinephrine after coitus in rabbits." *Endocrinology.* 1996; 137 (7): 2683–93.

Zumpe, D., et al. "Effects of progesterone on the sexual behavior of castrated, testosterone-treated male cynomolgus monkeys *(Macaca fascicularis)*." *Physiol Behav.* 1997; 62 (1): 61–67.

CHAPTER 12. SLEEPING BEAUTIFULLY

Antonijevic, I. A., et al. "Modulation of the sleep electroencephalogram by estrogen replacement in postmenopausal women." *Am J Obstet Gynecol.* 2000; 182 (2): 277–82.

Astrom, C., et al. "Growth hormone-deficient young adults have decreased deep sleep." *Neuroendocrinology.* 1990; 51 (1): 82–84.

Astrom, C., et al. "The influence of growth hormone on sleep in adults with growth hormone deficiency." *Clin Endocrinol (Oxf).* 1990; 33 (4): 495–500.

Bäckström, T., et al. "Ovarian steroid hormones." *Acta Obstet Gynecol Scand Suppl.* 1985; 130: 19.

Cagnaccid, A., et al. "Hypothermic effect of melatonin and nocturnal core body temperature decline are reduced in aged women." *J Appl Physiol.* 1995; 78 (1): 314–17.

Chiba, S., et al. "The influence of sleep breathing disorder on growth hormone secretion in children with tonsil hypertrophy." *Nippon Jibiinkoka Gakkai Kaiho.* 1998; 101 (7): 873–78.

Claustrat, B., et al. "Melatonin and jet lag: confirmatory result using a simplified protocol." *Biol Psychiatry.* 1992; 15; 32 (8): 705–11.

Freeman, E. W., et al. "Anxiolytic metabolites of progesterone: correlation with mood and performance measures following oral progesterone administration to healthy female volunteers." *Neuroendocrinology.* 1993; 58 (4): 478–84.

Friedman, T. C., et al. "Decreased delta-sleep and plasma delta-sleep-inducing peptide in patients with Cushing syndrome." *Neuroendocrinology.* 1994; 60 (6): 626–34.

Friess, E., et al. "DHEA administration increases rapid eye movement sleep and EEG power in the sigma frequency range." *Am Physiological Society.* 1995; E107–13.

Garfinkel, D., et al. "Improvement of sleep quality in elderly people by controlled-release melatonin." *Lancet.* 1995; 346 (8974): 541–44.

Greenbaum, A. L. "Changes in body composition and respiratory quotient of adult female rats treated with purified growth hormone." *Biochem J.* 1953; 54: 400.

Holland, M., et al. "Serum testosterone: a possible marker for colorectal cancer." *Medicine B Aires.* 1993; 53 (2): 117–23.

Hollander, L. E., et al. "Sleep quality, estradiol levels, and behavioral factors in late reproductive age women." *Obstet Gynecol.* 2001; 98 (3): 391–97.

Hughes, J. T. "Electromagnetic fields and brain tumours: a commentary." *Teratog Carcinog Mutagen.* 1994; 14 (5): 213–17.

Kayumov, L., et al. "A randomized, double-blind, placebo-controlled crossover study of the effect of exogenous melatonin on delayed sleep phase syndrome." *Psychosom Med.* 2001; 63 (1): 40–48.

Keefe, D. L., et al. "Hormone replacement therapy may alleviate sleep apnea in menopausal women: a pilot study." *Menopause.* 1999; 6 (3): 196–200.

Langer, M., et al. "Androgen receptors, serum androgen levels and survival of breast cancer patients." *Arch Gynecol Obstet.* 1990; 247 (4): 203–9.

Mathur, P. P., et al. "Effect of sleep deprivation on the physiological status of rat testis." *Andrologia.* 1991; 23 (1): 49–51.

Monti, J. M., et al. "A critical assessment of the melatonin effect on sleep in humans." *Biol Signals Recept.* 2000; 9 (6): 328–39.

Montplaisir, J., et al. "Sleep in menopause: differential effects of two forms of hormone replacement therapy." *Menopause*. 2001; 8 (1): 10–16.

Nave, R., et al. "Melatonin improves evening napping." *Eur J Pharmacol*. 1995; 275 (2): 213–16.

Obal, F., Jr., et al. "Growth hormone-releasing hormone antibodies suppress sleep and prevent enhancement of sleep after sleep deprivation." *Am J Physiol*. 1992; 263 (5 Pt 2): R1078–85.

Opstad, P. K. "Androgenic hormones during prolonged physical stress, sleep, and energy deficiency." *J Clin Endocrinol Metab*. 1992; 74 (5): 1176–83.

Paul, M. A., et al. "Melatonin and zopiclone as pharmacologic aids to facilitate crew rest." *Aviat Space Environ Med*. 2001; 72 (11): 974–84.

Picazo, O., et al. "Anti-anxiety effects of progesterone and some of its reduced metabolites: an evaluation using the burying behavior test." *Brain Res*. 1995; 680 (1–2): 135–41.

Poland, R. E., et al. "Effects of low-dose dexamethasone on sleep EEG patterns, plasma cortisol and the TSH response to TRH in major depression." *Pharmacopsychiatry*. 1993; 26 (3): 79–83.

Schiavi, R. C., et al. "Pituitary-gonadal function during sleep in healthy aging men." *Psychoneuroendocrinology*. 1992; 17 (6): 599–609.

Werner, A. A. "The male climacteric." *JAMA*. 1946; 132 (4): 188–94.

Wieland, S., et al. "Anxiolytic activity of the progesterone metabolite 5 alpha-pregnan-3 alpha-ol-20-one." *Brain Res*. 1991; 565 (2): 263–68.

CHAPTER 13. REMEMBERING NOT TO FORGET

Alexander, G. M., et al. "Androgen-behavior correlations in hypogonadal men and eugonadal men. II. Cognitive abilities." *Horm Behav*. 1998; 33 (2): 85–94.

Applezwig, M. H., et al. "The pituitary-adrenocortical system in avoidance learning." *Psychol Rep*. 1955; 1: 417–20.

Asthana, S., et al. "High-dose estradiol improves cognition for women with AD: results of a randomized study." *Neurology*. 2001; 57 (4): 605–12.

Bastianetto, S., et al. "Dehydroepiandrosterone (DHEA) protects hippocampal cells from oxidative stress-induced damage." *Brain Res Mol Brain Res*. 1999; 66 (1–2): 35–41.

Bennet, A., et al. "Ulcères de jambe post-phlébitiques et caryotype XYY: tests de fibrinolyse et fonction androgénique." *Ann Dermatol Venereol*. 1987; 114: 1097–101.

Bohus, B., et al. "Effects of adrenocorticotropic hormone on avoidance behaviour in intact and adrenalectomized rats." *Int J Neuropharmacol*. 1968; 7: 307–14.

Bonnet, K. A., et al. "Cognitive effects of DHEA replacement therapy." In *The Biological Role of DHEA*, eds. W. Regelson and M. Kalimi. Berlin: Walter de Gruyter & Co., 1990; 65–79.

Cherrier, M. M., et al. "Testosterone supplementation improves spatial and verbal memory in healthy older men." *Neurology*. 2001; 57 (1): 80–88.

Christiansen, K. "Sex hormone-related variations of cognitive performance in Kung San hunter-gatherers of Namibia." *Neuropsychobiology.* 1993; 27 (2): 97–107.

Constant, E. L., et al. "Cerebral blood flow and glucose metabolism in hypothyroidism: a positron emission tomography study." *J Clin Endocrinol Metab.* 2001; 86 (8): 3864–70.

Corpechot, C., et al. "Pregnenolone and its sulfate ester in the rat brain." *Brain Res.* 1983; 270 (1): 119–25.

Darnaudery, M., et al. "The promnesic neurosteroid pregnenolone sulfate increases paradoxical sleep in rats." *Brain Res.* 1999; 818 (2): 492–98.

Deijen, J. B., et al. "Cognitive changes during growth hormone replacement in adult men." *Psychoneuroendocrinology.* 1998; 23 (1): 45–55.

De Wied, D. "Influence of anterior pituitary on avoidance learning and escape behavior." *Am J Physiol.* 1964; 207: 255–59.

Delwaide, P. J., et al. "Acute effect of drugs upon memory of patients with senile dementia." *Acta Psychiatr Belg.* 1980; 80: 748–54.

Dinu, M., et al. "The effects of vitamin D_2 on the lipid profile and on the platelet and cardiovascular activities in castrated or testosterone-treated male rats." *Rev Med Chir Soc Med Nat Lasi.* 1990; 94 (1): 123–27.

Erkkola, R. "Female menopause, hormone replacement therapy and cognitive processes." *Maturitas.* 1996; 23 suppl: 527–30.

Fekete, M., et al. "The ACTH-(4-9) analog ORG 2766 and desglycinamide[9]—(Arginine[8])—vasopressin reverse the retrograde amnesia induced by disrupting circadian rhythms in rats." *Peptides.* 1986; 7: 563–68.

Flood, J. F., et al. "Age-related decrease of plasma testosterone in SAMP8 mice: replacement improves age-related impairment of learning and memory." *Physiol Behav.* 1995; 57 (4): 669–73.

Flood, J. F., et al. "Dehydroepiandrosterone and its sulfate enhance memory retention in mice." *Brain Res.* 1988; 447 (2): 269–78.

Flood, J. F., et al. "Dehydroepiandrosterone sulfate improves memory in aging mice." *Brain Res.* 1988; 448 (1): 178–81.

Flood, J. F., et al. "Memory-enhancing effects in male mice of pregnenolone and steroids metabolically derived from it." *Proc Natl Acad Sci USA.* 1992; 89: 1567–71.

Freedman, D. S., et al. "Relation of serum testosterone levels to high density lipoprotein cholesterol and other characteristics in men." *Arterioscler Thromb.* 1991; (2): 307–15.

Gauchie, C., et al. "The relationship between testosterone levels and cognition ability patterns." *Psychoneuroendocrinology.* 1991; 16 (4): 323–34.

Gutai, J., et al. "Plasma testosterone, high density lipoprotein cholesterol and other lipoprotein factions." *Am J Cardiol.* 1981; 48: 897–902.

Hoff, A. L., et al. "Association of estrogen levels with neuropsychological performance in women with schizophrenia." *Am J Psychiatry.* 2001; 158 (7): 1134–39.

Hughes, G. S., et al. "Fish oil produces an atherogenic lipid profile in hypertensive men." *Atherosclerosis.* 1990; 84 (2–3): 229–37.

Jandhi, C., et al. "Corticosterone facilitates long-term memory formation via enhanced glycoprotein synthesis." *Neuroscience.* 1995; 69 (4): 1087–93.

Jean-Louis, G., et al. "Melatonin effects on sleep, mood, and cognition in elderly with mild cognitive impairment." *J Pineal Res.* 1998; 25 (3): 177–83.

Kampen, D. L., et al. "Estradiol is related to visual memory in healthy young men." *Behav Neurosci.* 1996; 110 (3): 613–17.

Kopp, C. B., et al. "Relationship between sex hormones and haemostatic factors in healthy middle-aged men." *Atherosclerosis.* 1988; 71: 71–76.

Koppeschaar, H. P., "Growth hormone, insulin-like growth factor I and cognitive function in adults." *Growth Horm IGF Res.* 2000; 10 Suppl B: S69–73.

Laczi, F., et al. "Differential effect of desglycinamide 9-(Arg 8)-vasopressin, vasopressin on cognitive functions of diabetes insipidus and alcoholic patients." *Acta Endocrinol (Copenh).* 1987; 115: 393–98.

Lanthier, A., et al. "Sex steroids and 5-en-3 beta-hydroxysteroids in specific regions of the human brain and cranial nerves." *J Steroid Biochem.* 1986; 25: 445–49.

Legros, J. J., et al. "Influence of vasopressin on learning and memory." *Lancet.* 1978; 1 (8054): 41–42.

Legros, J. J., et al. "Vasopressin and memory in the human." In Gotto, A. M., Jr., et al., eds. *Brain peptides: a new endocrinology.* Amsterdam: Elsevier/North-Holland. 1979; 347–64.

Linzmayer, L., et al. "Double-blind, placebo-controlled psychometric studies on the effects of a combined estrogen-progestin regimen versus estrogen alone on performance, mood and personality of menopausal syndrome patients." *Arzneimittelforschung.* 2001; 51 (3): 238–45.

Lotmar, R. "Histopathologische Befunde in Gehirnen von kongenitale Myxoëdem (thyreoplasie), un Kachexia thyreopriva." *Monatschr Neurol Psychiatry.* 1929; 119: 491.

Marinesco, G. M. "Contribution à l'étude des lésions du myxoedème congénital." *Encéphale.* 1924; 19: 265.

Mayo, W., et al. "Pregnenolone sulfate and aging of cognitive functions: behavioral, neurochemical, and morphological investigations." *Horm Behav.* 2001; 40 (2): 215–17.

Miller, L. H., et al. "A neuroheptapeptide influence on cognitive functioning in the elderly." *Peptides.* 1980; 55–57.

Molsa, P. K., et al. "Epidemiology of dementia in a Finnish population." *Acta Neurol Scand.* 1982; 654: S41–S52.

Nebes, R. D., et al. "The effect of vasopressin on memory in the healthy elderly." *Psychiatr Res.* 1984; 11: 49–59.

Peeters, B. W. M. M., et al. "Involvement of corticosteroids in the processing of stressful life-events." *J Steroid Biochem Mol Biol.* 1994; 49 (4–6): 417–27.

Pharoah, P. O., et al. "Relationship between maternal thyroxine levels during pregnancy and memory function in childhood." *Early Hum Dev.* 1991; 25 (1): 43–51.

Rasika, S., et al. "Testosterone increases the recruitment and/or survival of new high vocal center neurons in adult female canaries." *Proc Natl Acad Sci USA.* 1994; 91 (17): 7854–58.

Reiter, R. J., et al. "A review of the evidence supporting melatonin's role as an antioxydant." *J Pineal Res.* 1995; 18 (1): 1–11.

Robel, P., et al. "Neuro-steroids: 3 beta-hydroxy-delta 5-derivatives in rat and monkey brain." *J Steroid Biochem.* 1987; 27: 649–55.

Roberts, E. "Dehydroepiandrosterone (DHEA) and its sulfate (DHEAs) as neural facilitators: effects on brain tissue in culture and on memory in young and old mice. A cyclic GMP hypothesis of action of DHEA and DHEAs in nervous system and other tissues." In *The Biological Role of DHEA,* eds. W. Regelson and M. Kalimi. Berlin: Walter de Gruyter & Co., 1990; 13–42.

Rollero, A., et al. "Relationship between cognitive function, growth hormone and insulin-like growth factor I plasma levels in aged subjects." *Neuropsychobiology.* 1998; 38 (2): 73–79.

Roozendaal, B., et al. "Amygdaloid nuclei lesions differentially affect glucocorticoid-induced memory enhancement in an inhibitory avoidance task." *Neurobiol Learn Mem.* 1996; 65 (1): 1–8.

Ruiz, Marcos, et al. "Thyroxine treatment and the recovery of the cerebral cortex from changes induced by juvenile-onset hypothyroidism." *J Neurobiological.* 1994; 25 (7): 808–18.

Sandstrom, N. J., et al. "Memory retention is modulated by acute estradiol and progesterone replacement."

Sandyk, R. "Estrogen's impact on cognitive functions in multiple sclerosis." *Int J Neurosci.* 1996; 86 (1–2): 23–31.

Schreiber, P., et al. "Correlative observations of cerebral metabolism and cardiac output in myxedema." *J Clin Invest.* 1950; 29: 1139.

Sekiguchi, R., et al. "Analysis of the influence of vasopressin neuropeptides on social memory of rats." *Eur Neuropsychopharmacol.* 1991; 2: 123–26.

Sharma, M., et al. "Effect of chronic treatment of melatonin on learning, memory and oxidative deficiencies induced by intracerebroventricular streptozotocin in rats." *Pharmacol Biochem Behav.* 2001; 70 (2–3): 325–31.

Sherwin, B. B. "Can estrogen keep you smart? Evidence from clinical studies." *J Psychiatry Neurosci.* 1999; 24 (4): 315–21.

Sherwin, B. B. "Estrogen and/or androgen replacement therapy and cognitive functioning in surgically menopausal women." *Psychoneuroendocrinology.* 1988; 13 (4): 345–57.

Smith, Y. R., et al. "Long-term estrogen replacement is associated with improved nonverbal memory and attentional measures in postmenopausal women." *Fertil Steril.* 2001; 76 (6): 1101–7.

Stein, D. G. "Brain damage, sex hormones and recovery: a new role for progesterone and estrogen?" *Trends Neurosci.* 2001; 24 (7): 386–91.

Sternberg, S. "High-speed scanning in human memory." *Science.* 1966; 153: 652–54.

Stocker, S., et al. "Exogenous testosterone differentially affects myelination and neurone soma sizes in the brain of canaries." *Neuroreport.* 1994; 5 (12): 1449–52.

Tan, R. S. "Memory loss as a reported symptom of andropause." *Arch Androl.* 2001; 47 (3): 185–89.

Tan, R. S., et al. "The andropause and memory loss: is there a link between androgen decline and dementia in the aging male?"

Vallee, M., et al. "Role of pregnenolone, dehydroepiandrosterone and their sulfate esters on learning and memory in cognitive aging." *Brain Res Rev.* 2001; 37 (1–3): 301–12.

van Dam, P. S., et al. "Effects of dehydroepiandrosterone replacement in elderly men on event-related potentials, memory, and well-being." *J Gerontol A Biol Sci Med Sci.* 1998; 53 (5): M385–90.

Van Goozen, S. H., et al. "Activating effects of androgens on cognitive performance: causal evidence in a group of female-to-male transsexuals." *Neuropsychologia.* 1994; 32 (10): 1153–57.

Van Ree, J. M. "Memory and Neuropeptides." In Morley, J. E., et al., eds. *Endocrinology and metabolism in the elderly.* Oxford: Blackwell Science, 1992; 500–24.

Van Ree, J. M., et al. "Neurohypophyseal principles and memory processes." *Biochem Pharmacol.* 1978; 27: 1793–1800.

Wolter, R., et al. "Neuropsychological study in treated thyroid dysgenesis." *Acta Paediatr Scand Suppl.* 1979; 227: 41–46.

Yamada, K., et al. "Long-term deprivation of oestrogens by ovariectomy potentiates beta-amyloid-induced working memory deficits in rats." *Br J Pharmacol.* 1999; 128 (2): 419–27.

CHAPTER 14. IN THE RIGHT MOOD
Anxiety

Abelson, J. L., et al. "Blunted growth hormone response to clonidine in patients with generalized anxiety disorder." *Arch Gen Psychiatry.* 1991; 48 (2): 157–62.

Arlt, W., et al. "DHEA replacement in women with adrenal insufficiency—pharmacokinetics, bioconversion and clinical effects on well-being, sexuality and cognition." *Endocr Res.* 2000; 26 (4): 505–11.

Arlt, W., et al. "Dehydroepiandrosterone replacement in women with adrenal insufficiency." *N Engl J Med.* 1999; 341 (14): 1013–20. Comment in *N Engl J Med.* 1999; 341 (14): 1073–74.

Bauer, M., et al. "Psychological and endocrine abnormalities in refugees from East Germany: Part I. Prolonged stress, psychopathology, and hypothalamic-pituitary-thyroid axis activity." *Psychiatry Res.* 1994; 51 (1): 61–73.

Bitran, D., et al. "Anxiolytic effect of progesterone is mediated by the neurosteroid allopregnenolone at brain GABA receptors." *J Neuroendocrinol.* 1995; 7 (3): 171-77.

Diamond, P., et al. "Trait anxiety, submaximal physical exercise and blood androgens." *Eur J Appl Physiol Occup Physiol.* 1989; 58 (7): 699–704.

Flood, J. F. "DHEA and its sulfate enhance memory retention mice." *Brain Research.* 1988; 447: 269–78.

Freeman, E. W., et al. "Anxiolytic metabolites of progesterone: correlation with mood and performance measures following oral progesterone administration to healthy female volunteers." *Neuroendocrinology.* 1993; 58 (4): 478–84.

Gallo, M. A., et al. "Progesterone withdrawal decreases latency to and increases duration of electrified prod burial: a possible rat model of PMS anxiety." *Pharmacol Biochem Behav.* 1993; 46 (4): 897–904.

Golombek, D. A., et al. "Melatonin as an anxiolytic in rats: time dependence and interaction with the central GABAergic system." *Eur J Pharmacol.* 1993; 237 (2–3): 231–36.

Hammond, C. B., et al. "Current status of estrogen therapy for the menopause." *Fertil Steril.* 1982; 37: 5–25.

Hughes, G. "Management of thyrotoxic crisis with a beta-adrenergic blocking agent (pronethalol)." *Br J Clin Pract.* 1966; 20: 579.

Kleemann, D. O., et al. "Exogenous progesterone and embryo survival in Booroolacross ewes." *Reprod Fertil Dev.* 1991; 3 (1): 71–77.

Lissoni, P., et al. "Modulation of cancer endocrine therapy by melatonin: a phase II study of tamoxifen plus melatonin in metastatic breast cancer patients progressing under tamoxifen alone." *Br J Cancer.* 1995; 71 (4): 854–56.

McCaul, K. D., et al. "Winning, losing, mood, and testosterone." *Horm Behav.* 1992; 26 (4): 486–504.

Melchior, C. L., et al. "Dehydroepiandrosterone is an anxiolytic in mice on the plus maze." *Pharmacol Biochem Behav.* 1994; 47 (3): 437–41.

Montgomery, B. M., et al. "Effect of oestrogen and testosterone implants on psychological disorders in the climacteric." *Lancet.* 1987; 1 (8528): 297–99.

Nava, F., et al. "Melatonin reduces anxiety induced by lipopolysaccharide in the rat." *Neurosci Lett.* 2001; 307 (1): 57–60.

Obal, F., Jr., et al. "Inhibition of growth hormone-releasing factor suppresses both sleep and growth hormone secretion in the rat." *Brain Res.* 1991; 557 (1–2): 9–53.

Petitti, D. B., et al. "Noncontraceptive estrogens and mortality: long-term follow-up of women in the Walnut Creek Study." *Obstet Gynecol.* 1987; 70 (3 Pt 1): 289–93.

Picazo, O., et al. "Anti-anxiety effects of progesterone and some of its reduced metabolites: an evaluation using the burying behavior test." *Brain Res.* 1995; 680 (1–2): 135–41.

Stabler, B. "Impact of growth hormone (GH) therapy on quality of life along the lifespan of GH-treated patients." *Horm Res.* 2001; 56 Suppl 1: 55–58.

Tancer, M. E., et al. "Growth hormone response to intravenous clonidine in social phobia: comparison patients with panic disorder and healthy volunteers." *Biol Psychiatry*. 1993; 34 (9): 591–95.

Wallymahmed, M. E., et al. "The quality of life of adults with growth hormone deficiency: comparison with diabetic patients and control subjects." *Clin Endocrinol (Oxf)*. 1999; 51 (3): 333–38.

Wieland, S., et al. "Anxiolytic activity of the progesterone metabolite 5-alpha-pregnan-3 alpha-o1-20-one." *Brain Res*. 1991; 565 (2): 263–68.

Wiren, L., et al. "A prospective investigation of quality of life and psychological well-being after the discontinuation of GH treatment in adolescent patients who had GH deficiency during childhood." *J Clin Endocrinol Metab*. 2001; 86 (8): 3494–98.

Zhdanova, I. V., et al. "Sleep-inducing effects of low doses of melatonin ingested in the evening." *Clin Pharmacol. Ther*. 1995; 57 (5): 552–58.

Depression

Arlt, W., et al. "Dehydroepiandrosterone replacement in women with adrenal insufficiency." *N Engl J Med*. 1999; 341 (14): 1013–20.

Barrett-Connor, E., et al. "Endogenous levels of dehydroepiandrosterone sulfate, but not other sex hormones, are associated with depressed mood in older women: the Rancho Bernardo Study." *J Am Geriatr Soc*. 1999; 47 (6): 685–91.

Barry, S., et al. "Neuroendocrine challenge tests in depression: a study of growth hormone, TRH and cortisol release." *J Affect Disord*. 1990; 18 (4): 229–34.

Bloch, M., et al. "Dehydroepiandrosterone treatment of midlife dysthymia." *Biol Psychiatry*. 1999; 45 (12): 1533–41.

Bouwer, C., et al. "Prednisone augmentation in treatment-resistant depression with fatigue and hypocortisolaemia: a case series." *Depress Anxiety*. 2000; 12 (1): 44–50.

Cleghorn, R. A. "Adrenal cortisol insufficiency: psychological and neurological observations." *Canad Med Ass J*. 1951; 65: 449.

Cleghorn, R. A., et al. "Psychologic changes in 3 cases of Addison's disease during treatment with cortisone." *J Clin Endocrinol Metab*. 1954; 14: 344–52.

Dahl, R. E., et al. "Regulation of sleep and growth hormone in adolescent depression." *J Am Acad Child Adolesc Psychiatry*. 1992; 31 (4): 615–21.

Degerblad, M., et al. "Physical and psychological capabilities during substitution therapy with recombinant growth hormone in adults with growth hormone deficiency." *Acta Endocrinol (Copenh)*. 1990; 123: 185–93.

de Lignières, B. "Conséquences cliniques de la ménopause." *La Revue du Praticien*. 1984; 34 (25): 1323–37.

de Lignières, B., et al. "Differential effects of exogenous oestradiol and progesterone on mood in postmenopausal women: individual dose/effect relationship." *Maturitas*. 1982; 4: 67–72.

Dinan, T. G., et al. "Responses of growth hormone to desipramine in endogenous and non-endogenous depression." *Br J Psychiatry*. 1990; 156: 680–84.

Dow, M. G., et al. "Hormonal treatments of sexual unresponsiveness in postmenopausal women: a comparative study." *Br J Obstet Gynaecol.* 1983; 90: 361–66.

Fava, M., et al. "Psychological behavioral and biochemical factors for coronary artery disease among American and Italian male corporate managers." *Am J Cardiol.* 1992; 70: 1412–16.

Flood, J. F. "Memory-enhancing effects in male mice of pregnenolone and steroids metabolically derived from it." *Proc Natl Acad Sci USA.* 1992; 89: 1567–71.

Fountoulakis, K. N., et al. "Morning and evening plasma melatonin and dexamethasone suppression test in patients with nonseasonal major depressive disorder from northern Greece (latitude 40–41.5 degrees)." *Neuropsychobiology.* 2001; 44 (3): 113–17.

Hannan, C. J., Jr., et al. "Psychological and serum homovanillic acid changes in men administered androgenic steroids." *Psychoneuroendocrinology.* 1991; 16 (4): 335–43.

Harro, J., et al. "Association of depressiveness with blunted growth hormone response to maximal physical exercise in young healthy men." *Psychoneuroendocrinology.* 1999; 24 (5): 505–17.

Jarrett, D. B., et al. "Recurrent depression is associated with a persistent reduction in sleep-related growth hormone secretion." *Arch Gen Psychiatry.* 1990; 47 (2): 113–18.

Jarett, D. B., et al. "Sleep-related growth hormone secretion is persistently suppressed in women with recurrent depression: a preliminary longitudinal analysis." *J Psychiatr Res.* 1994; 28 (3): 211–23.

Lesch, K. P., et al. "A receptor responsivity in unipolar depression. Evaluation of ipsapirone-induced ACTH and cortisol secretion in patients and controls." *Biol. Psychiatry.* 1990; 28 (7): 620–28.

Linkowski, P., et al. "24-hour profiles of adrenocorticotropin, cortisol, and growth hormone in major depressive illness: effect of antidepressant treatment." *J Clin Endocrinol Metab.* 1987; 65 (1): 141–52.

McCaul, K. D., et al. "Winning, losing, mood, and testosterone." *Horm Behav.* 1992; 26 (4): 486–504.

McGauley, G. A., et al. "Psychological well-being before and after growth hormone treatment in adults with growth hormone deficiency." *Horm Res.* 1990; 33 (suppl 4): 52–54.

Morales, A., et al. "Effects of replacement dose of DHEA in men and women of advancing age." *J Clin Endocrinol Metab.* 1994; 78: 1360–67.

Nagata, C., et al. "Serum concentrations of estradiol and dehydroepiandrosterone sulfate and soy product intake in relation to psychologic well-being in peri- and postmenopausal Japanese women." *Metabolism.* 2000; 49 (12): 1561–64.

Nakamura, T., et al. "Comparison of thyroid function between responders and nonresponders to thyroid hormone supplementation in depression." *Jpn J Psychiatry Neurol.* 1992; 46 (4): 905–9.

Raghavendra, V., et al. "Anti-depressant action of melatonin in chronic forced swimming-induced behavioral despair in mice, role of peripheral benzodiazepine receptor modulation." *Eur Neuropsychopharmacol.* 2000; 10 (6): 473–81.

Rubin, R. T., et al. "Neuroendocrine aspects of primary endogenous depression. X: Serum growth hormone measures in patients and matched control subjects." *Biol Psychiatry.* 1990; 27 (10): 1065–82.

Souche, A., et al. "Treatment of depression by a combination of clomipramine and triiodothyronine." *Encephale.* 1991; 17 (1): 37–42.

Steiger, A., et al. "The sleep EEG and nocturnal hormonal secretion studies on changes during the course of depression and on effects of CNS-active drugs." *Prog Neuropsychopharmacol Biol Psychiatry.* 1993; 17 (1): 125–37.

Steiger, A., et al. "Sleep EEG and nocturnal secretion of testosterone and cortisol in patients with major endogenous depression during acute phase and after remission." *J Psychiatr Res.* 1991; 25 (4): 169–77.

Steiger, A., et al. "Studies of nocturnal penile tumescence and sleep electroencephalogram in patients with major depression and in normal controls." *Acta Psychiatr Scand.* 1993; 87 (5): 358–63.

Voderholzer, U., et al. "Profiles of spontaneous 24-hour and stimulated growth hormone secretion in male patients with endogenous depression." *Psychiatry Res.* 1993; 47 (3): 215–27.

Werner, A. A. "The male climacteric." *JAMA.* 1946; 132 (4): 188–94.

Wolf, O. T., et al. "Effects of a two-week physiological dehydroepiandrosterone substitution on cognitive performance and well-being in healthy elderly women and men." *J Clin Endocrinol Metab.* 1997; 82 (7): 2363–67.

Wolkowitz, U. M., et al. "Antidepressant and cognition-enhancing effects of DHEA in major depression." *Ann NY Acad Sci.* 1995; 774: 337–39.

Yaffe, K., et al. "Neuropsychiatric function and dehydroepiandrosterone sulfate in elderly women: a prospective study." *Biol Psychiatry.* 1998; 43 (9): 694–700.

CHAPTER 15. STRESSING HEALTH

Alexander, S. L., et al. "Effect of isolation stress on concentrations of arginine, vasopressin, alpha-melanocyte-stimulating hormone and ACTH in the pituitary venous effluent of the normal horse." *J Endocrinol.* 1988; 116: 325–34.

Armario, A., et al. "Dissociation between corticosterone and growth hormone adaptation to chronic stress in the rat." *Horm Metab Res.* 1984; (16): 142–45.

Armario, A., et al. "Influence of intensity and duration of exposure to various stressors on serum TSH and GH levels in adult male rats." *Life Sciences.* 1989; 44 (3): 215–27.

Briski, K. P., et al. "Comparative effects of various stressors on immunoreactive versus bioreactive protection release in old and young male rats." *Neuroendocrinology.* 1990; 51: 625–31.

Briski, K. P., et al. "Endogenous opiate involvement in acute and chronic stress-induced change in plasma LH concentrations in the male rat." *Life Sciences.* 1984; 34 (25): 2485–93.

Cameron, O. G., et al. "Venous plasma epinepherine levels and the symptoms of stress." *Psychosom Med.* 1990; 52 (4): 411–24.

Caroff, S., et al. "Diurnal variation of growth hormone secretion following thyrotropin-releasing hormone infusion in normal men." *Psychosom Med.* 1989; 46 (1): 59.

Collu, R., et al. "Role of catecholamines in the inhibitory effect of immobilisation stress on testosterone secretion in rats." *Biol. Reprod.* 1984; 30: 416–22.

Culebras, A., et al. "Differential response of growth hormone, cortisol, and prolactin to seizures and stress." *Epilepsie.* 1987; 28: 564–70.

Du Ruisseau, P., et al. "Pattern of adenohypophyseal hormone changes various stressors in female and male rats." *Neuroendocrinology.* 1978; 27: 257–71.

Fredrikson, M., et al. "Cortisol excretion during the defence reaction in humans." *Psychosom Med.* 1985; 47 (4): 313–19.

Gaillard, R. C., et al. "Stress and pituitary adrenal axis." *Bailliere's Clin End Metab.* 1987; 1 (2): 319–54.

Goncharov, N. P., et al. "Levels of adrenal and gonodal hormones in rhesus monkeys during chronic hypokinesia." *Endocrinology.* 1984; 115: 129–35.

Heim, C., et al. "The potential role of hypocortisolism in the pathophysiology of stress-related bodily disorders." *Psychoneuroendocrinology.* 2000; 25 (1): 1–35.

Jacobs, S., et al. "Psychological distress, depression and prolactin responses in stressed persons." *J Hum Stress.* 1986; 113–18.

Jacobs, S. C. "Bereavement and catecholamines." *Psychosomatic Res.* 1986; 30 (4): 489–96.

Johansson, G., et al. "Examination stress affects plasma levels of TSH and thyroid hormone differently in females and males." *Psychosom Med.* 1987; 49: 390–96.

Langer, P., et al. "Immediate increase of thyroid hormone release during acute stress in rats: effect of biogenic amines rather than that of TSH." *Acta Endocrinol (Copenh).* 1983; 104: 443–49.

Leedy, M. G., et al. "Testosterone and cortisol levels in crewmen of U. S. air force fighter and cargo planes." *Psychosom Med.* 1985; 47 (4): 333–38.

Meyerhoff, J. L., et al. "Psychologic stress increases plasma levels of prolactin, cortisol and POMC-derived peptides in man." *Psychosom Med.* 1988; 50: 28–29.

Reichlin, S., et al. "The role of stress in female reproductive dysfunction." *J Human Stress.* 1979; 5 (2): 38–45.

Rivier, C., et al. "Diminished responsiveness of the hypothalamic-pituitary-adrenaline axis of the rat during exposure to prolonged stress: a pituitary medicated mechanism." *Endocrinology.* 1987; 121: 1320–28.

Rivier, C., et al. "Involvement of corticotropin-releasing factor and somatostatin in stress-induced inhibition of growth hormone secretion in the rat." *Endocrinology.* 1985; 117: 2478–82.

Schaeffer, M. A., et al. "Adrenal cortisol response to stress at Three Mile Island." *Psychosom Med.* 1984; 46 (3): 227.

Selye, H. "The general adaptation syndrome and the diseases of adaptation." *J Clin Endocrinol.* 1946; 6: 117–230.

Semple, C. G., et al. "Endocrine effects of examination stress." *Clinical Science.* 1988; 74: 255–59.

Taché, Y., et al. "Pattern of adenohypophyseal hormone changes in male rats following chronic stress." *Neuroendocrinology.* 1978; 26: 208–19.

Wheeler, G. D., et al. "Endurance training decreases serum testosterone levels in men without change in LH pulsatile release." *J Clin Endocrinol Metab.* 1991; 72: 422–29.

White, A. J., et al. "Thyroid diseases and mental illnesses: a study of thyroid disease in psychiatric admissions." *J Psychosom Res.* 1988; 32 (1): 99–106.

CHAPTER 16. A MORE ENERGETIC YOU

Abbasi, A., et al. "Association of dehydroepiandrosterone sulfate, body composition, and physical fitness in independent community-dwelling older men and women." *J Am Geriatr Soc.* 1998; 46 (3): 263–73.

Arlt, W., et al. "DHEA replacement in women with adrenal insufficiency—pharmacokinetics, bioconversion and clinical effects on well-being, sexuality and cognition." *Endocr Res.* 2000; 26 (4): 505–11.

Arver, S., et al. "Long-term efficacy and safety of a permeation-enhanced testosterone transdermal system in hypogonadal men." *Clin Endocrinol (Oxf).* 1997; 47 (6): 727–37.

Bäckström. T., et al. "Ovarian steroid hormones." *Acta Obstet Gynecol Scand Suppl.* 1985; 130: 19.

Bahrke, M. S., et al. "Psychological moods and subjectively perceived behavioral and somatic changes accompanying anabolic-androgenic steroid use." *Am J Sports Med.* 1992; 20 (6): 717–24.

Barrett-Connor, E. "A prospective study of DHEAs, mortality and cardiovascular disease." *N Engl J Med.* 1986; 315 (24): 1519–24.

Bixo, M., et al. "Progesterone distribution in the brain of the PMSG treated female rat." *Acta Physiol Scand.* 1984; 122: 355.

Boone, J. B., Jr., et al. "Resistance exercise effects on plasma cortisol, testosterone and creatine kinase activity in anabolic-androgenic steroid users." *Int J Sports Med.* 1990; 11 (4): 293–97.

Cleare, A. J., et al. "Hypothalamo-pituitary-adrenal axis dysfunction in chronic fatigue syndrome, and the effects of low-dose hydrocortisone therapy." *J Clin Endocrinol Metab.* 2001; 86 (8): 3545–54.

Cleare, A. J., et al. "Urinary free cortisol in chronic fatigue syndrome." *Am J Psychiatry.* 2001; 158 (4): 641–43.

Cuneo, R. C., et al. "Growth hormone treatment in growth hormone-deficient adults. I. Effects on muscle mass and strength." *J Appl Physiol.* 1991; 70 (2): 688–94.

Cuneo, R. C., et al. "Growth hormone treatment in growth hormone-deficient adults. II. Effects on exercise performance." *J Appl Physiol.* 1991; 70 (2): 695–700.

Cuneo, R. C., et al. "Skeletal muscle performance in adults with growth hormone deficiency." *Horm Res.* 1990; 33 (Suppl 4): 55–60.

Demitrack, M. A., et al. "Evidence for impaired activation of the hypothalamic-pituitary-adrenal axis in patients with chronic fatigue syndrome." *J Clin Endocrinol Metab.* 1991; 73 (6): 1224–34.

Flood, J. F. "DHEA and its sulfate enhance memory retention in mice." *Brain Research.* 1988; 447: 269–78.

Friedl, K. E., et al. "Comparison of the effects of high dose testosterone and 19-nortestosterone to a replacement dose of testosterone on strength and body composition in normal men." *J Steroid Biochem Mol Biol.* 1991; 40 (4–6): 607–12.

Granner, D. K. "The role of glucocorticoid hormones as biologic amplifiers." In *Glucocorticoid Hormone Action,* Baxter, J. D., et al., eds. New York: Springer-Verlag, 1979; 593–611.

Hadley, O., et al. "Adrenal androgens and cortisol in major depression." *Am J Psychiatry.* 1993; 150 (5): 806–9.

Herrington, D. M. "Plasma DHEA and DHEAs in patients undergoing diagnostic coronary angiography." *J Am Coll Cardiology.* 1990; 16 (4): 862–70.

Hunt, P. J., et al. "Improvement in mood and fatigue after dehydroepiandrosterone replacement in Addison's disease in a randomized, double-blind trial." *J Clin Endocrinol Metab.* 2000; 85 (12): 4650–56.

Ingle, D. J., et al. *Physiological and therapeutic effects of corticotropin (ACTH) and cortisone.* Springfield, Illinois: Thomas, 1953; 40.

Jefferies, W. *Safe Uses of Cortisone.* Springfield, Illinois: Thomas, 1981; 9.

John, T. M., et al. "Influence of chronic melatonin implantation on circulating levels of catecholamines, growth hormone, thyroid hormones, glucose and free fatty acids in the pigeon." *Gen Comp Endocrinol.* 1990; 79 (2): 226–32.

Kudsk, K. A., et al. "Effect of recombinant human insulin-like growth factor I and early total parenteral nutrition on immune depression following severe head injury." *Arch Surg.* 1994; 129 (1): 66–70; discussion 70–71.

Levin, M. E., et al. "Fatal coma due to myxoedema." *Am J Med.* 1955; 18: 1017.

Li Voon Chong, J. S., et al. "Elderly people with hypothalamic-pituitary disease and growth hormone deficiency: lipid profiles, body composition and quality of life compared with control subjects." *Clin Endocrinol (Oxf).* 2000; 53 (5): 551–59.

McGauley, G. A., et al. "Psychological well-being before and after growth hormone treatment in adults with growth hormone deficiency." *Horm Res.* 1990; 33 (Suppl 4): 52–54.

Moorkens, G., et al. "Characterization of pituitary function with emphasis on GH secretion in the chronic fatigue syndrome." *Clin Endocrinol (Oxf).* 2000; 53 (1): 99–106.

Nicolson, N. A., et al. "Salivary cortisol patterns in vital exhaustion." *J Psychosom Res.* 2000; 49 (5): 335–42.

O'Brien, I. A. D., et al. "Abnormal circadian rhythm of melatonin in diabetic autonomic neuropathy." *Clinical Endocrinology.* 1986; 24: 359–64.

Paul, M. A., et al. *Aviat Space Environ Med.* 2001; 72 (11): 974–84.

Rabkin, J. G., et al. "A double-blind, placebo-controlled trial of testosterone therapy for HIV-positive men with hypogonadal symptoms." *Arch Gen Psychiatry.* 2000; 57 (2): 141–47; discussion 155–56.

"Report International Health Foundation": ref 10 A 32 b.

Sandyk, R., et al. "Pineal calcification and its relationship to the fatigue of multiple sclerosis." *Int J Neurosci.* 1994; 74 (1–4): 95–103.

Schinberg, P., et al. "Correlative observations of cerebral metabolism and cardiac output in myxedema." *J Clin Invest.* 1950; 29: 1139.

Scott, L. V., et al. "Small adrenal glands in chronic fatigue syndrome: a preliminary computer tomography study." *Psychoneuroendocrinology.* 1999; 24 (7): 759–68.

van der Pompe, G., et al. "An exploratory study into the effect of exhausting bicycle exercise on endocrine and immune responses in post-menopausal women: relationships between vigour and plasma cortisol concentrations and lymphocyte proliferation following exercise." *Int J Sports Med.* 2001; 22 (6): 447–53.

Wendlova, J. "Effect of Kliogest on bone metabolism, bone mineral density and quality of life in postmenopausal patients." *Vnitr Lek.* 1998; 44 (8): 464–68.

Werner, A. A. "The male climacteric." *JAMA.* 1946; 132 (4): 188–94.

Whitcomb, J. E., et al. "Randomized trial of oral hydrocortisone and its effect on emergency physicians during night duty." *WMJ.* 2000; 99 (7): 37–41, 46.

Whybrow, P. C. "Behavioral and psychiatric aspects." In Ingbar, S., et al., eds. *Werner's The Thyroid.* Philadelphia: Lippincott Company, 1986; 1205.

Wing, S. S., et al. "Glucocorticoids activate the ATP-ubiquitin-dependent proteolytic system in skeletal muscle during fasting." *Am J Physiol.* 1993; 264 (4 Pt 1): E668–76.

Wuster, C., et al. "Increased prevalence of osteoporosis and arteriosclerosis in conventionally substituted anterior pituitary insufficiency: need for additional growth hormone substitution?" *Klin Wochenschr.* 1991; 69 (16): 769–73.

CHAPTER 17. THE HORMONE SOLUTION DIET
Food

Arts, C. J., et al. "Effect of wheat bran on excretion of radioactively labeled estradiol-17 beta and estrone-glucoronide injected intravenously in male rats." *J Steroid Biochem Mol Biol.* 1992; 42 (1): 103–11.

Berrino, F., et al. "Reducing bioavailable sex hormones through a comprehensive change in diet: the diet and androgens (DIANA) randomized trial." *Cancer Epidemiol Biomarkers Prev.* 2001; 10 (1): 25–33.

Boukhliq, R., et al. "Role of glucose, fatty acids and protein in regulation of testicular growth and secretion of gonadotropin, prolactin, somatotropin and insulin in the mature ram." *Reprod Fertil Dev.* 1997; 9 (5): 515–24.

Bubenik, G. A. "The effect of food deprivation on brain and gastrointestinal lisine levels of tryptophan, serotonin, 5-hydrocyindo-leacetic acid, and melatonin." *J Pineal Res.* 1992; 12 (1): 7–16.

Cai, X., et al. "High-fat diet increases the weight of rat ventral prostate." *Prostate.* 2001; 49 (1): 1–8.

Cai, X., et al. "Pilot study of dietary fat restriction and flaxseed supplementation in men with prostate cancer before surgery: exploring the effects on hormonal levels, prostate-specific antigen, and histopathologic features." *Urology.* 2001; 58 (1): 47–52.

Clarke, I. J., et al. "Effect of high-protein feed supplements on concentrations of GH, insulin-like growth factor-I (IGF-1) and IGF-binding protein-3 in plasma and on the amounts of GH and messenger RNA for GH in the pituitary glands of adult rams." *J Endocrinol.* 1993; 138 (3): 421–27.

Crave, J. C., et al. "Effects of diet and metformin administration on sex hormone-binding globulin, androgens, and insulin in hirsute and obese women." *J Clin Endocrinol Metab.* 1995; 80 (7): 2057–62.

Dorgan, J. F., et al. "Effects of dietary fat and fiber on plasma and urine androgens and estrogens in men: a controlled feeding study." *Am J Clin Nutr.* 1996; 64 (6): 850–55.

Dorgan, J. F., et al. "Relation of energy, fat, and fiber intakes to plasma concentrations of estrogens and androgens in premenopausal women." *Am J Clin Nutr.* 1996; 64 (1): 25–31.

Fraser, W. M., et al. "Effect of L-tryptophan on growth hormone and prolactin release in normal volunteers and patients with secretory pituitary tumors." *Horm Metab Res.* 1979; 11 (2): 149–55.

Friedrich, M. "Effects of diet enrichment with glucose and casein on blood cortisol concentration of calves in early postnatal period." *Arch Vet Pol.* 1995; 35 (1–2): 117–25.

Ginsburg, E. "Effects of alcohol ingestion on estrogens in postmenopausal women." *JAMA.* 1996; 276 (21): 1747–51.

Hill, P. B., et al. "Effect of a vegetarian diet and dexamethasone on plasma prolactin, testosterone and dehydroepiandrosterone in men and women." *Cancer Lett.* 1979; 7 (5): 273–82.

Inglett, G. E., et al. "Dietary fiber and personality factors as determinants of stool output." *Gastroenterology.* 1981; 81 (5): 879–83.

Ingram, D. M., et al. "Effect of low-fat diet on female sex hormone levels." *J Natl Cancer Inst.* 1987; 79 (6): 1225–29.

Jakubowicz, D. J. "Disparate effects of weight reduction by diet on serum dehydroepiandrosterone-sulfate levels in obese men and women." *J Clin Endocrinol Metab.* 1995; 80 (11): 3373–76.

Kalk, W. J., et al. "Thyroid hormone and carrier protein interrelationships in children recovering from kwashiorkor." *Am J Clin Nutr.* 1986; 43 (3): 406–13.

Keagy, E. M., et al. "Thyroid function, energy balance, body composition and organ growth in protein-deficient chicks." *J Nutr.* 1987; 117 (9): 1532–40.

Laessle, R. E., et al. "Gonadotropin secretion in bulimia nervosa." *J Clin Endoc Metab.* 1992; 74 (5): 112–17.

Lammoglia, M. A., et al. "Effects of dietary fat on follicular development and circulating concentrations of lipids, insulin, progesterone, estradiol-17 beta,

13, 14-dihydro-15-keto-prostaglandin F(2 alpha), and GH in estrous cyclic Brahman cows." *J Anim Sci.* 1997; 75 (6): 1591–600.

Lu, L. J. et al. "Decreased ovarian hormones during a soya diet: implications for breast cancer prevention." *Cancer Res.* 2000; 60 (15): 4112–21.

Maghnié, M., et al. "Diagnosing GH deficiency: the value of short-term hypocaloric diet." *J Clin Endocrinol Metab.* 1983; 77 (5): 1372–78.

Nagata, C., et al. "Relationships between types of fat consumed and serum estrogen and androgen concentrations in Japanese men." *Nutr Cancer.* 2000; 38 (2): 163–67.

Ohtsoka, A., et al. "Reduction of corticosterone-induced muscle proteolysis and growth retardation by a combined treatment with insulin, testosterone and high-protein-high-fat diet in rats." *Nutr Sci Vitaminol. Tokyo.* 1992; 38 (1): 83–92.

Oliva, A., et al. "Contribution of environmental factors to the risk of male infertility." *Hum Reprod.* 2001; 16 (8): 1768–76.

Petridou, E., et al. "Pregnancy estrogens in relation to coffee and alcohol intake." *Ann Epidemiol.* 1992; 2 (3): 241–47.

Remer, T., et al. "Short-term impact of a lactovegetarian diet on adrenocortical activity and adrenal androgens." *J Clin Endocrinol Metab.* 1998, 83 (6): 2132–37.

Remer, T., et al. "The short-term effect of dietary pectin on plasma levels and renal excretion of dehydroepiandrosterone sulfate." *Z Ernahrungswiss.* 1996; 35 (1): 32–33.

Rojdmark, S., et al. "Effect of short-term fasting on nocturnal melatonin secretion in obesity." *Metabolism.* 1992; 41 (10): 1106–9.

Santolaria, F., et al. "Effects of alcohol and liver cirrhosis on the GH-IGF-1 axis." *Alcohol Alcohol.* 1995; 30 (6): 703–8.

Schmitz, M. M. "Disrupted melatonin-secretion during alcohol withdrawal." *Prog Neuropsychopharmacol Biol Psychiatry.* 1996; 20 (6): 983–95.

Sudi, K. M., et al. "Effects of weight loss on leptin, sex hormones, and measures of adiposity in obese children." *Endocrine.* 2001; 14 (3): 429–35.

Takeuchi, T., et al. "Oral glucose challenge effects on growth and sex steroid hormones in normal women and women with hypothalamic amenorrhea." *Int J Gynaecol Obstet.* 1998; 61 (2): 171–78.

Van Niekerk, F. E., et al. "The effect of dietary protein on reproduction in the mare. IV. Serum progestagen, FSH, LH and melatonin concentrations during the anovulatory, transitional and ovulatory periods in the non-pregnant mare." *J S Afr Vet Assoc.* 1997; 68 (4): 114–20.

Volek, J. S., et al. "Effects of a high-fat diet on postabsorptive and postprandial testosterone responses to a fat-rich meal." *Metabolism.* 2001; 50 (11): 1351–55.

Volek, J. S., et al. "Testosterone and cortisol in relationship to dietary nutrients and resistance exercise." *J Appl Physiol.* 1997; 82 (1): 49–54.

Wade, C. E. "Upon-admission adrenal steroidogenesis is adapted to the degree of illness in intensive care unit patients." *J Clin Endocrinol Metab.* 1988; 67 (2): 223–27.

Winlamowska, A. "Food restriction enhances melatonin effects on the pituitary-gonadal axis in female rats." *J Pineal Res.* 1992; 13 (9): 1–5; 1993; 64 (5): 221–25.

Zaouali-Ajina, M., et al. "Dietary docosahexaenoic acid-enriched phospholipids normalize urinary melatonin excretion in adult (n-3) polyunsaturated fatty acid-deficient rats." *J Nutr.* 1999; 129 (11): 2074–80.

Zgliczynksi, W., et al. "Alcohol decreases the alfa subunit, LH and testosterone secretion in response to LH-RH." *Endocrinol Pol.* 1992; 43 (3): 257–62.

Vitamins and Trace Elements

Bricq, B. "La logique des oligoéléments." *Laboratoire Boiron.* 1993; 257.

Burch, G. E., et al. "The importance of magnesium deficiency in cardiovascular disease." *Am Heart J.* 1987; 94: 649–57.

Coppen, A., et al. "Tryptophan and depressive illness." *Psychological Med.* 1978; 59–57.

Gordon, T., et al. "Drinking and coronary heart disease: the Albary study." *Am Heart J.* 1985; 110: 331–34.

Hercberq, S. "Les vitamines." *Dossiers du Praticien, Impact Médecin.* 1993; 178: 24.

Joborn, C., et al. "Psychiatric symptomatology in patients with primary lympaperparathyroitom." *Ups J Med Sci.* 1986. 91 (1): 77–87.

Kleppin, J., et al. *Receuil de données sur la composition des aliments.* Paris: CFIV, Produits Roche, 1989; 252.

Le Grusse, J., et al. "Les vitamines. Données biochimiques nutritionnelles et cliniques." Produits Roche. 1973; 30: 277–83.

Lieberman, J. A., et al. "Acute antidepressant effect of lithium in unipolar depression." *Psychosomatics.* 1984; 25 (12): 932–33.

Menkes, M. S., et al. "Serum betacarotene, vitamins A and E, selenium and the risk of lung cancer." *New Engl J Med.* 1986; 15: 1250.

Schultz, B. M., et al. "Iron deficiency in the elderly." *Baillieres Clin. Haenatole.* 1987; 291–313.

Stampfer, M. J., et al. "Effect of vitamin E on lipids." *Am J Clin Path.* 1983; 79 (6): 71–78.

Vaufraechein, J. R. D., et al. "Coenzyme 9_{10} and physical performance," in *Bio Med Clinique. Aspects of Coenzyme 9_{10}.* Folhers, K., et al., eds. 1981; 3: 235–41.

Vodoevitch, V. P., et al. "Effect of B group vitamin complex on the blood content of saturated and unsaturated fatty acids in patients with ischemic heart disease and hypotension." *Vopr Pitan.* 1986; 2: 9–11.

Vollestad, N. K., et al. "Biochemical correlates with fatigue." *Eur J Appl Physiol.* 1988; 57: 336–47.

CHAPTER 18. THE HORMONE SOLUTION TREATMENT PLANS

Kim, M. K., et al. "The steady-state permeation rates of testosterone in the ethanol/water systems increased exponentially as the volume fraction of ethanol increased, reaching the maximum value (2.69+/-0.69 microg cm(-2)h(-1)) at 70% (v/v) ethanol in water, and then decreasing with further increases in the ethanol volume fraction. Skin permeation of testosterone and its ester derivatives in rats." *J Pharm Pharmacol.* 2000; 52 (4): 369–75.

Simon, J. A., et al. "Safety profile: transdermal testosterone treatment of women after oophorectomy." *Obstet Gynecol.* 2001; 97 (4 Suppl 1): S10–S11.

Wang, C., et al. "Comparative pharmacokinetics of three doses of percutaneous dihydrotestosterone gel in healthy elderly men—a clinical research center study." *J Clin Endocrinol Metab.* 1998; 83 (8): 2749–57.

INDEX

casein, 232
catalase, and skin, 103, 105
catecholamines, 182
cellulite, 91–92
cerebral hemorrhage, 154
cheeks, 95, 104–5
chin, double, 104
cholesterol:
   HDL and LDL, 94, 141, 143
   and heart, 142–44
   and unsaturated fat, 141, 144
   and water, 140
Chris (erectile dysfunction), 186–87
chromium:
   and cholesterol, 94
   for heart, 141, 142
   and insulin, 94
   for weight loss, 93, 94
chronic fatigue syndrome, 123–24,
   225–26
circulation, 138
   activity and, 122
   and memory, 201
   protection of, 149–50
   self-test on, 45–48
   and thyroid hormones, 118, 234
claudication, 152
clitoris, 185
coffee and tea, 248
colds, catching, 176
cold sores, 103
collagen, 119
colon cancer, 166, 167
concentration, 202, 204, 206
confusion, 204–5, 217, 226
copper:
   for anxiety and depression, 210, 211
   and hair color, 104, 110
   for heart, 141, 142
   for joint pain, 117
   and skin care, 103, 105, 107
CoQ10 (coenzyme Q10):
   for energy, 233
   for immune system, 173, 174
   for weight loss, 93, 94
cortical bone, 134
corticosteroids, 146
cortisol, 57–58
   for anxiety and depression, 214,
    217–18, 220
   and appetite, 95
   and blood pressure, 147, 156
   and blood sugar, 147, 226

   and bone loss, 135, 137
   and buffalo hump, 88
   and cancer, 165–66
   catabolic effects of, 120
   and cerebral arteries, 154
   and confusion, 204–5, 206
   and DHEA, 120, 135, 137
   diagnostic tests of, 77
   and digestive problems, 226
   effects of aging on, 7
   and face swelling, 87–88
   and hair problems, 108, 109, 111
   and heart, 152, 156
   in Hormone Solution Diet, 251
   and immune system, 163, 177
   and infections, 170
   and insulin, 90
   and joint pain, 119–20, 121, 126
   and lupus, 125
   overuse of, 120
   self-test on, 26–27
   and sex, 182, 185, 188
   and skin problems, 106
   and sleep, 193, 195
   and stress, 214, 217–18, 226, 228,
    234–35, 239
   and thyroid hormones, 87
   too much, 218
   treatment plan, 262–63
   water and salt retention, 147,
   and weight problems, 96
crow's feet, 104
cryptococcidiosis, 171
cysteine, 104, 105, 110

dairy products:
   appetite for, 90
   and bone loss, 130
   and energy, 231, 232
   in Hormone Solution Diet, 247, 250
   and weight control, 92
   and yeast infections, 89
dandruff, 104, 108
defeat, feelings of, 217
delta brain waves, 191
dendrites, 199
depression, 133–34, 209
   decoding your deficiencies, 215–19
   and nutrition, 209–11
   summary, 220
DHEA (dehydroepiandrosterone), 58–59
   as anabolic hormone, 120
   for anxiety, 212–13, 220

ABOUT THE AUTHORS

THIERRY HERTOGHE, M.D., is a member of the International Advisory Board of the American Academy of Anti-Aging Medicine. He lectures regularly to medical professionals and laypeople in the United States and abroad on the subject of hormone deficiencies.

JULES-JACQUES NABET, M.D., practices general medicine in Paris and London, specializing in longevity. He is a member of the European Academy of Quality of Life and Longevity Medicine (EAQUALL) and the American Academy of Anti-Aging Medicine.

COURSES ▪ SEMINARS ▪ CONFERENCES

Conferences and seminars in practical medical therapies oriented toward improvement of quality of life and longevity are organized regularly in the United States and Europe by the European Academy of Quality of Life and Longevity (EAQUALL), the European association of anti-aging medicine. Most focus on hormone therapy in aging adults and are intended for physicians and other health professionals, although some are suitable for the general public. If you are interested, please send your name, profession, address, e-mail address, and phone and fax numbers to the following address to receive information about upcoming events:

EAQUALL
95 avenue Albert Giraud
B-1030 Brussels
Belgium
Fax: 00-32-2-732-57-43
www.Eaquall.net